Elsevier's Integrated
Genetics

Elsevier's Integrated
Genetics

Linda R. Adkison PhD

Professor of Genetics
and
Professor of Obstetrics and Gynecology
Mercer University School of Medicine
Macon, Georgia

Michael D. Brown PhD

Associate Professor of Genetics
Mercer University School of Medicine
Macon, Georgia

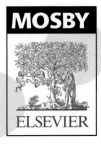

MOSBY

ELSEVIER

MOSBY
ELSEVIER

1600 John F. Kennedy Blvd
Suite 1800
Philadelphia, PA 19103-2899

ELSEVIER'S INTEGRATED GENETICS   ISBN-13: 978-0-323-04329-8

Notice

Knowledge and best practice in this field are constantly changing. As new research and experience broaden our knowledge, changes in practice, treatment and drug therapy may become necessary or appropriate. Readers are advised to check the most current information provided (i) on procedures featured or (ii) by the manufacturer of each product to be administered, to verify the recommended dose or formula, the method and duration of administration, and contraindications. It is the responsibility of the practitioner, relying on their own experience and knowledge of the patient, to make diagnoses, to determine dosages and the best treatment for each individual patient, and to take all appropriate safety precautions. To the fullest extent of the law, neither the Publisher nor the Authors assume any liability for any injury and/or damage to persons or property arising out or related to any use of the material contained in this book.

The Publisher

Library of Congress Cataloging-in-Publication Data

Adkison, Linda R.
  Elsevier's integrated genetics / Linda R. Adkison, Michael D. Brown.
    p. ; cm. — (Elsevier's integrated series)
  Includes index.
  ISBN-13: 978-0-323-04329-8
  ISBN-10: 0-323-04329-1
  1. Medical genetics. I. Brown, Michael D. (Michael Dean), 1963–
II. Title III. Series.
  [DNLM: 1. Genetics, Medical. QZ 50 A236e 2007]
  RB155A2565 2007
  616'.042—dc22

                                    2007000523

Acquisitions Editor: Alex Stibbe
Developmental Editor: Andrew Hall

Printed in China

Last digit is the print number: 9 8 7 6 5 4 3 2 1

This textbook is dedicated to the memory of E. Peter Volpe, PhD (1927–2004), whose 50 years as an academician and mentor of many faculty laid the foundation for this book, and to our students who constantly challenge the boundaries of our knowledge and allow learning to remain fun. Finally, without the support and understanding of our families, this project could not have been completed.

Preface

Though the youngest of all the medical specialties, genetics embodies the essence of all normal and abnormal development and all normal and disease states. Perhaps because of its recent recognition as a discipline and perhaps because of its derivation from research in several areas, it is easy for genetics to be an "integrated" discipline. Approaching genetics as "a particular gene located on a specific chromosome and inherited in a specific manner" loses the appreciation of spatial and temporal dimensions of expression and the many, many factors affecting every single aspect of development, survival, and even death.

Every medical discipline is connected to human well-being through the mechanisms of gene expression, environmental influences, and inheritance. Genetics underscores the many biochemical pathways, physiologic processes, and pathologic mechanisms presented in other volumes of this series. It explains better the morphologic variation observed in embry-ologic development and anatomic presentation. It provides better insight into susceptibility to infection and disease. It offers insight into neurologic and behavorial abnormalities. It is providing a glimpse into possibilities of gene therapy and pharmacogenomics. For these reasons, it has been exciting to put this book together.

This text focuses on well-known and better described diseases and disorders that students and practitioners are likely to read about in other references. Many of these do not occur at a high frequency in populations, but they underscore major mechanisms and major concepts associated with many other medical situations. It is our hope that this text will be as stimulating to read as it was to write.

Linda R. Adkison, PhD
Michael D. Brown, PhD

Editorial Review Board

Contents

Series Preface

How to Use This Book

The idea for Elsevier's Integrated Series came about at a seminar on the USMLE Step 1 exam at an American Medical Student Association (AMSA) meeting. We noticed that the discussion between faculty and students focused on how the exams were becoming increasingly integrated—with case scenarios and questions often combining two or three science disciplines. The students were clearly concerned about how they could best integrate their basic science knowledge.

One faculty member gave some interesting advice: "read through your textbook in, say, biochemistry, and every time you come across a section that mentions a concept or piece of information relating to another basic science—for example, immunology—highlight that section in the book. Then go to your immunology textbook and look up this information, and make sure you have a good understanding of it. When you have, go back to your biochemistry textbook and carry on reading."

This was a great suggestion—if only students had the time, and all of the books necessary at hand, to do it! At Elsevier we thought long and hard about a way of simplifying this process, and eventually the idea for Elsevier's Integrated Series was born.

The series centers on the concept of the *integration box*. These boxes occur throughout the text whenever a link to another basic science is relevant. They're easy to spot in the text—with their color-coded headings and logos. Each box contains a title for the integration topic and then a brief summary of the topic. The information is complete in itself—you probably won't have to go to any other sources—and you have the basic knowledge to use as a foundation if you want to expand your knowledge of the topic.

You can use this book in two ways. First, as a review book . . .
When you are using the book for review, the integration boxes will jog your memory on topics you have already covered. You'll be able to reassure yourself that you can identify the link, and you can quickly compare your knowledge of the topic with the summary in the box. The integration boxes might highlight gaps in your knowledge, and then you can use them to determine what topics you need to cover in more detail.

Second, the book can be used as a short text to have at hand while you are taking your course . . .
You may come across an integration box that deals with a topic you haven't covered yet, and this will ensure that you're one step ahead in identifying the links to other subjects (especially useful if you're working on a PBL exercise). On a simpler level, the links in the boxes to other sciences and to clinical medicine will help you see clearly the relevance of the basic science topic you are studying. You may already be confident in the subject matter of many of the integration boxes, so they will serve as helpful reminders.

At the back of the book we have included case study questions relating to each chapter so that you can test yourself as you work your way through the book.

Online Version

An online version of the book is available on our Student Consult site. Use of this site is free to anyone who has bought the printed book. Please see the inside front cover for full details on the Student Consult and how to access the electronic version of this book.

In addition to containing USMLE test questions, fully searchable text, and an image bank, the Student Consult site offers additional integration links, both to the other books in Elsevier's Integrated Series and to other key Elsevier textbooks.

Books in Elsevier's Integrated Series

The nine books in the series cover all of the basic sciences. The more books you buy in the series, the more links that are made accessible across the series, both in print and online.

 Anatomy and Embryology

 Histology

 Neuroscience

 Biochemistry

 Physiology

 Pathology

 Immunology and Microbiology

 Pharmacology

 Genetics

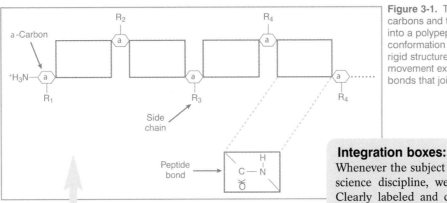

Figure 3-1. The peptide bond linking α-carbons and their side chains together into a polypeptide. The *trans* conformation is favored, producing a rigid structure that restricts freedom of movement except for rotation around bonds that join to the α-carbons.

Artwork:
The books are packed with 4-color illustrations and photographs. When a concept can be better explained with a picture, we've drawn one. Where possible, the pictures tell a dynamic story that will help you remember the information far more effectively than a paragraph of text.

Integration boxes:
Whenever the subject matter can be related to another science discipline, we've put in an Integration Box. Clearly labeled and color-coded, these boxes include nuggets of information on topics that require an integrated knowledge of the sciences to be fully understood. The material in these boxes is complete in itself, and you can use them as a way of reminding yourself of information you already know and reinforcing key links between the sciences. Or the boxes may contain information you have not come across before, in which case you can use them a springboard for further research or simply to appreciate the relevance of the subject matter of the book to the study of medicine.

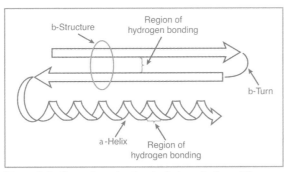

Figure 3-3. Secondary structure includes α-helix and β-pleated sheet (β-sheet).

MICROBIOLOGY

Prion Diseases

Prions (PrP^{Sc}) are formed from otherwise normal neurologic proteins (PrP) and are responsible for encephalopathies in humans (Creutzfeldt-Jakob disease, kuru), scrapie in sheep, and bovine spongiform encephalopathy. Contact between the normal PrP and PrP^{Sc} results in conversion of the secondary structure of PrP from predominantly α-helical to predominantly β-pleated sheet. The altered structure of the protein forms long, filamentous aggregates that gradually damage neuronal tissue. The harmful PrP^{Sc} form is highly resistant to heat, UV irradiation, and protease enzymes.

Since proline has no free hydrogen to contribute to helix stability, it is referred to as a "helix breaker." The α-helix is found in most globular proteins and in some fibrous proteins (e.g., α-keratin).

Text:
Succinct, clearly written text, focusing on the core information you need to know and no more. It's the same level as a carefully prepared course syllabus or lecture notes.

-structure) consists of

tabilized by hydrogen f adjacent sequences.

(parallel) or opposite (antiparallel) direction. β-Structures are found in 80% of all globular proteins and in silk fibroin.

Supersecondary Structure and Domains

Supersecondary structures, or *motifs*, are characteristic combinations of secondary structure 10–40 residues in length that recur in different proteins. They bridge the gap between the less specific regularity of secondary structure and the highly specific folding of tertiary structure. The same motif can perform similar functions in different proteins.

- The four-helix bundle motif provides a cavity for enzymes to bind prosthetic groups or cofactors.
- The β-barrel motif can bind hydrophobic molecules such as retinol in the interior of the barrel.
- Motifs may also be mixtures of both α and β conformations.

Basic Mechanisms

1

The essence of genetics is an understanding of the hereditary material within a cell and the influence it has on survival of the cell through every function and response the cell and its organelles undertake. Without these fundamental concepts, no aspect of human development and well-being can be adequately explained.

●●● CHROMATIN

One of the finest triumphs of modern science has been the elucidation of the chemical nature of chromatin and its role in the transfer of information from nucleic acids into proteins, known as the central dogma. James Watson built on his earlier work, which outlined the fundamental unit and chemical composition of the complex molecule composing chromatin deoxyribonucleic acid (DNA). Briefly stated, the central dogma "oversimplifies" the mechanism whereby the chemical message held in DNA is transferred to RNA through transcription and this RNA blueprint is translated into protein: DNA → RNA → Protein. Other proteins associated with DNA contribute to its structure and may play roles in regulating functions. In its simplest form, chromatin is composed of DNA and histone proteins.

Histones are small, highly conserved, positively charged proteins that bind to DNA and to other histones. The five major histones are H1, H2A, H2B, H3, and H4. The presence of 20% to 30% lysine and arginine account for the positive charge of histones and distinguish these from most other proteins. All histones except H1 are highly conserved among eukaryotes.

DNA is packaged into the nucleus by winding of the double helix twice around an octamer of histones; this DNA-histone structure is called a nucleosome (Fig. 1-1). Each nucleosome is composed of two of each histone except H1

and approximately 150 nucleotide pairs wrapped around the histone core. H1 histone anchors the DNA around the core. This structure leads to a superhelix of turns upon turns upon turns called a solenoid structure. In the solenoid structure, each helical turn contains six nucleosomes and approximately 1200 nucleotide pairs. Additional turns form minibands that when tightly stacked upon each other give the structure recognized as a chromatid. In each nucleus, chromatin is organized into 46 chromosomes. In a fully relaxed configuration, DNA is approximately 2 nm in diameter; chromatids are approximately 840 nm in diameter. Twisting and knotting are extremely effective at compacting DNA within the nucleus (Fig. 1-2).

A DNA molecule comprises two long chains of nucleotides arranged in the form of a double helix. Its shape may be compared to a twisted ladder in which the two parallel supports of the ladder are made up of alternating deoxyribose sugars and phosphate molecules. Each rung of the ladder is composed of one pair of nitrogenous bases, held together by specific hydrogen bonds. Hydrogen bonds are weak bonds; however, the total number of hydrogen bonds between the two strands assures that the two strands of the double helix are firmly associated with each other under conditions commonly found in living cells.

The molar concentration of adenine equals thymine and of guanine equals cytosine. This information is best accommodated in a stable structure if the double-ring purines (adenine or guanine) lay opposite the smaller, single-ring pyrimidines (thymine or cytosine). The combination of one purine and

BIOCHEMISTRY

DNA Confirmation

There are three basic three-dimensional configurations of DNA. The most common is the B-form in which DNA is wound in a right-handed direction with 10 bp per turn. Within the turned structure are a major groove and a minor groove, where proteins can bind. The A-form also has a right-handed turn and is composed of 11 bp per turn. This form is seen in dehydrated DNA such as in oligonucleotide fibers or crystals. The third form, Z-form DNA, was named for its zigzag appearance and has a left-handed turn composed of 12 bp per turn. This form occurs in regions of DNA with alternating pyrimidine-purines: CGCGCG.

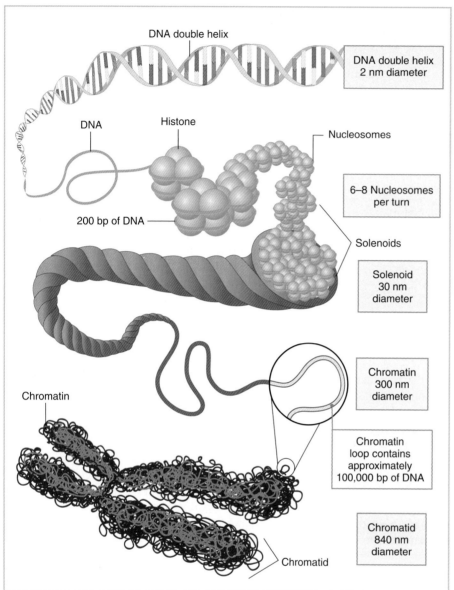

Figure 1-1. Chromosome organization. The shortening, or condensation, of chromatin results in a diminished volume of each chromosome and a reduction in the exposed chromosome surface. This is a dynamic process beginning with the least condensed form, the DNA double helix, and proceeding to chromatin visible in interphase and prophase. The level of greatest condensation occurs at metaphase.

Labels in figure:
- DNA double helix
- DNA double helix 2 nm diameter
- DNA
- Histone
- Nucleosomes
- 200 bp of DNA
- 6–8 Nucleosomes per turn
- Solenoids
- Solenoid 30 nm diameter
- Chromatin
- Chromatin 300 nm diameter
- Chromatin loop contains approximately 100,000 bp of DNA
- Chromatid 840 nm diameter
- Chromatid

one pyrimidine to make up each cross-connection is conveniently called a *base pair* (bp). In a DNA base pair, adenine (A) forms two hydrogen bonds with thymine (T), and guanine (G) and cytosine (C) share three hydrogen bonds. The sequence of one strand of DNA automatically implies the sequence of the opposite strand because of the precise pairing rule A = T and C = G.

Because of the configuration of the phosphodiester bonds between the 3′ and 5′ positions of adjacent deoxyribose molecules, every linear polynucleotide can have a free, unbounded 3′ hydroxyl group at one pole of the polynucleotide (*3′ end*) and a free 5′ hydroxyl at the other pole (*5′ end*). There are theoretically two possible ways for the two polynucleotides to be oriented in a double helix. They could have the same polarity—i.e., be parallel, with both strands having 3′ ends at one pole and 5′ ends at the other pole. Or, by rotating one strand 180 degrees with respect to the other, they could have opposite polarity—i.e., be *antiparallel*—with

a 3′ and a 5′ end at one pole of the double helix and a 5′ and a 3′ end at the other pole of the double helix. Only the antiparallel orientation actually occurs. The antiparallel nature of the double helix dictates that a new DNA chain being replicated must be copied in the opposite direction from the template (Fig. 1-3).

BIOCHEMISTRY

Nitrogenous Bases

Purines are adenosine (A) and guanine (G). Pyrimidines are cytosine (C) and thymine (T). In the double helix structure, A binds to T with two hydrogen bonds; C binds to G with three hydrogen bonds.

Uracil (U) is found in RNA in place of T in DNA. The structure of U is T without the methyl group at carbon 5. Hypoxanthine is found in certain tRNAs.

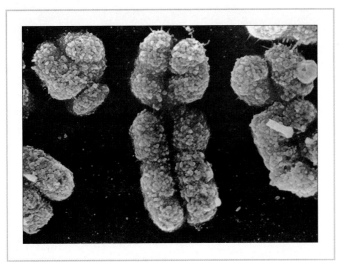

Figure 1-2. Generally, chromosomes are shown as in this photograph—in a highly condensed stage known as metaphase. This structure, however, represents one chromosome that has been replicated and is composed of two identical sister chromatids. At a later stage, the sister chromatids will separate at the centromere, and two chromosomes will exist. Note: when in doubt about the number of chromosomes present, count the number of centromeres present!

●●● CHROMOSOME ORGANIZATION

DNA of eukaryotes is repetitive—i.e., there are many DNA sequences of various lengths and compositions that do *not* represent functional genes. Three subdivisions of DNA are recognized: *unique* DNA, *middle repetitive* DNA, and *highly repetitive* DNA. Unique DNA is present as a single copy or as only a few copies. The proportion of the genome taken up by repetitive sequences varies widely among taxa. In mammals, up to 60% of the DNA is repetitive. The highly repetitive fraction is made up of short sequences, from a few to hundreds of nucleotides long, which are repeated on the average of 500,000 times. The middle repetitive fraction consists of hundreds or thousands of base pairs on the average, which appear in the genome up to hundreds of times.

Most unique-sequence genes code for proteins and are essentially "structural" genes. Analysis of data from completion of the Human Genome Project in April 2003 suggests that human DNA encodes 20,000 to 25,000 different gene products. The sequence of more than 10,000 of these genes is known, but the number of variations that occur within these is harder to predict; however, a phenotype, or an observable feature of specific gene expression, is associated with a smaller proportion of these. (See the *Online Mendelian Inheritance of Man,*

BIOCHEMISTRY

Phosphodiester Bonds and Deoxyribose Molecules

A phosphodiester bond occurs between carbon 5 on one deoxyribose and carbon 3 on an adjacent deoxyribose. The sugar in DNA is deoxyribose: H replaces OH at carbon 2. The energy to form this bond is derived from the cleavage of two phosphates from the ribonucleotide triphosphate.

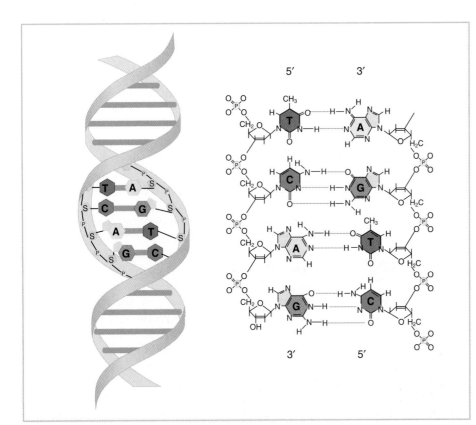

Figure 1-3. DNA is organized in an antiparallel configuration: one strand is 5′ to 3′ in one direction and the other strand is 5′ to 3′ in the opposite direction. A purine is bound to a pyrimidine by hydrogen bonds: A:T and G:C. The helix occurs naturally because of the bonds in the phosphate backbone.

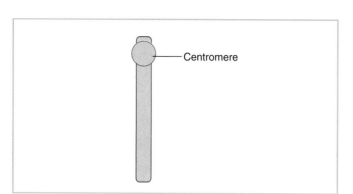

Figure 1-4. Acrocentric chromosome—a chromosome whose centromere is near the end.

available at: http://www3.ncbi.nlm.nih.gov/omim.) Much of the time, variations in genes are discussed relative to abnormal gene expression and disease; however, many mutations may have either no effect on gene expression or little effect on the function of the protein in the individual. For example, a protein may have less than 100% activity with little or no effect until the activity drops below a certain level.

Middle repetitive sequences represent redundant, tandemly arrayed copies of a given gene and may be transcribed just as unique-sequence genes. Specifically, these sequences refer to genes coding for transfer RNA and ribosomal RNA. Because these RNAs are required in such large quantities for the translation process, several hundred copies of RNA-specifying genes are expected. As a striking example, the 18S and 28S fractions of ribosomal RNA are coded by about 200 copies of DNA sequences, localized in the tip regions of five acrocentric chromosomes in the human genome (Fig. 1-4). It is estimated that human DNA is about 20% middle repetitive DNA.

Highly repetitive DNA is usually not transcribed, apparently lacking promoter sites on which RNA polymerase can initiate RNA chains. These highly repeated sequences may be clustered together in the vicinity of centromeres, or may be more evenly distributed throughout the genome. Presumably, the clustered sequences are involved in binding particular proteins essential for centromere function. The most common class of dispersed sequences in mammals is the *Alu* elements. The name derives from the fact that many of these repetitious sequences in humans contain recognition sites for the restriction enzyme *Alu*I. The entire group has been referred to as the *Alu* family. The *Alu* sequences are 200 to 300 bp in length, of which there are an estimated million copies in the human genome. They constitute between 5% and 10% of the human genome. Various

debatable roles have been ascribed to the *Alu* elements, from "molecular parasites" to initiation sites of DNA synthesis.

GENE ORGANIZATION

Each cell has 23 pairs of chromosomes, or 46 separate DNA double helices, with one chromosome from each pair inherited maternally and the other paternally. Twenty-two pairs are called *autosomes* and one pair is called the *sex chromosomes*. Each pair of autosomes is identical in size and organization of genes. The genes on these *homologous chromosomes* are organized to produce the same proteins. However, slight variations may occur, which changes the organization of the base pairs and can lead to a change in a protein. These changes can be called polymorphisms (from Greek "having many forms") and result from mechanisms creating changes, or mutations, within the DNA. Another name for variation in the same gene on homologous chromosomes is allele. Stated another way, an allele is an alternative form of a gene. It is possible for a gene to have identical alleles; i.e., two alleles that are present in an individual at the same place on two homologous chromosomes may be exactly the same or they may be different. The presence of few alleles indicates the gene has been highly conserved over the years, whereas genes with hundreds of alleles have been less stringently conserved. An example of the latter is the gene responsible for cystic fibrosis, which may have one or more of over 1000 reported changes, or mutations. Different alleles, or combinations of alleles, may cause different presentations of a disease within an individual, although some alleles may not lead to any appreciable change in the clinical presentation.

As noted above, the central dogma states that DNA is transcribed into RNA, which is then translated into protein. It is now known that a gene may express RNA that is not translated into a protein; these genes represent less than 5% of the genome. More commonly, a gene is a coding sequence that ultimately results in the expression of a protein. The sequence of bases in unique DNA provides a code for the sequence of the amino acids composing polypeptides. This DNA code is found in triplets—i.e., three bases taken together code for one amino acid. Only one of the two strands of the DNA molecule (called the transcribed, or template, strand) serves as the genetic code. More precisely, one strand is

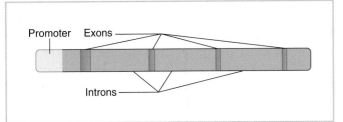

Figure 1-5. Organization of a gene showing the upstream promoter region, exons, and introns. Introns are removed by splicing during the formation of mRNA.

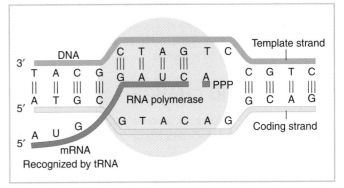

Figure 1-6. RNA is transcribed from the template strand and has a complementary sequence to the coding strand. Therefore, the coding strand sequence more accurately reflects the genetic code.

consistent for a given gene, but the strand varies from one gene to another.

The eukaryotic gene contains unexpressed sequences that interrupt the continuity of genetic information. The coding sequences are termed *exons*, whereas the noncoding intervening sequences are called *introns* (Fig. 1-5). The coding region of the gene begins downstream from the promoter at the initiation codon (ATG). It ends at a termination codon (UAG, UAA or UGA). Sequences before the first exon and after the last exon are generally transcribed but not translated in protein.

The 5′ region of the gene contains specific sites important for the transcription of the gene. This region, called the *promoter*, has two types of binding sites. The core promoter, also referred to as the TATA box because its seven-base-pair sequence is TATAAAA, is part of all protein-coding genes. More than 50 proteins bind to this sequence or to the transcription factors binding to this site. Other binding sites within the promoter may vary from gene to gene. As imagined, this is an extremely complex region. Many genes in different cells may share the same promoter-binding proteins. It is the unique combination of different proteins binding that regulates differential expression of the gene in different cells and tissues.

Some gene expression may be facilitated by transcription factors binding to special sequences known as *enhancers*. Enhancers may be found hundreds to thousands of base pairs away from the promoter, upstream or downstream of the gene or even within the gene. Binding of these sites increases

the rate of transcription. It is suggested that the factor binding to the enhancer may cause DNA to loop back onto the promoter region and interact with the proteins binding in this region to increase initiation.

The entire gene is transcribed as a long RNA precursor, commonly referred to as the primary RNA transcript, or premessenger RNA; this is sometimes called heterogenous nuclear RNA (hnRNA). Through *RNA processing*, the introns of the primary RNA transcript are excised and the exons spliced together to yield the shortened, intact coding sequence in the mature mRNA. Specific enzymes that recognize precise signals at intron-exon junctions in the primary transcript assure accurate "cutting and pasting." There is no rule that governs the number of introns. The gene for the β-chain of human hemoglobin contains two introns, whereas the variant gene that causes Duchenne type muscular dystrophy has more than 60 introns. Nearly all bacteria and viruses have streamlined their structural genes to contain no introns.

The concept, mentioned above, of only one strand being transcribed for a gene can be confusing when trying to understand how the DNA code is transferred to RNA, which is, in turn, the message used to translate the code into a precise amino acid sequence of a protein. As noted, the two DNA strands of the double helix are antiparallel, with a 5′ and 3′ end at each end of the molecule. Transcription occurs in a 5′ to 3′ direction from the transcribed, or template, strand (Fig. 1-6). The sequence of this hnRNA, and subsequently the mRNA, is complementary to the antiparallel strand that is the

BIOCHEMISTRY

DNA Orientation: Basic Concepts

DNA is arranged in a 5′ to 3′ orientation. By convention, the 5′ end is to the left and the 3′ end is to the right. Similarly, sequences to the left of a point are upstream and those to the right are downstream. For example, the promoter is upstream of the initiation site. Therefore, although these sequences are not transcribed, they are important for binding proteins to allow proper binding of polymerase and initiation of transcription. Similarly, sequences at the end of the gene are important for termination, and signaling sites are important for the addition of polyadenosine (polyA) that is not specified in the DNA template.

BIOCHEMISTRY

Transcription and RNA Processing

Transcription is the synthesis of RNA from a DNA template, requiring RNA polymerase II. RNA is single stranded with an untranslated 5′ cap and 3′ polyA tail.

Small nuclear ribonucleoproteins (snRNPs) stabilize intron loops, in a complex called a spliceosome, for removal of introns. snRNPs are rich in uracil and are identified as U and a number: U1, U2, U3, etc.

opposite the template strand. The antiparallel strand is also referred to as the coding strand. The anticodons of tRNA find the appropriate three-base-pair complementary mRNA codon to attach the amino acid specified.

●●● GENETIC CHANGE

Variability in genetic information occurs naturally through fertilization when two gametes containing 23 chromosomes join to make a unique individual. No two individuals except identical twins have identical DNA patterns. DNA changes are more likely to occur within highly repetitive sequences than within genes transcribing nontranslated RNAs and functional genes in which change could lead to a failure to function and potentially threaten the existence of the cell and ultimately the individual. Changes within the repetitive regions usually have little consequence on the cell because of the apparent lack of function. Repetitive sequences are similar but not identical among individuals and represent a great reservoir for mutational changes. These sequences represent the DNA "fingerprint" of an individual because these regions demonstrate the same heritability observed with expressed regions of the chromosomes.

Aside from fertilization, which brings together chromosomes that have undergone recombination during gamete formation and chromosomes that have assorted randomly into gametes, changes in genetic material are generally observed as numerical or structural. These changes are called mutations. Numerical changes generally occur as a result of nondisjunction. This error in the separation of chromosomes may occur in the division of somatic cells, called *mitosis*, or in the formation of gametes, called *meiosis*. In meiosis, nondisjunction may occur in either the first or second stages of meiosis, called meiosis I or meiosis II. The greatest consequences of nondisjunction are those observed in meiosis because the resulting embryo has too many or too few chromosomes. Humans do not tolerate either excess or insufficient DNA well. Except for a few situations, the absence of an entire chromosome (monosomy) or the addition of an entire chromosome (trisomy) is incompatible with life for more than a few weeks to perhaps as long as a few months (see Chapter 2).

Changes in genetic material, less dramatic than in an entire chromosome, are generally tolerated inversely to the size of the change: the smaller the change, the better the cell may tolerate the change. Changes may occur at a single nucleotide, a *point mutation*, or involve a large portion of a chromosome. At the nucleotide level, a purine may be replaced by another purine, or a pyrimidine by another pyrimidine. This substitution process is known as a *transition*. If, however, a purine replaces a pyrimidine, or vice versa, a *transversion* occurs. Any consequences of these changes depend on where the change occurs. Obviously, there is a greater opportunity for an effect within a gene rather than within highly repetitive, noncoding sequences. Even within a gene, the location of the change is important. If the change results in the creation of a stop codon, known as a *nonsense* mutation, the resulting protein may be truncated and hence either nonfunc-

tional or with reduced function. If the change results in a different codon being presented for translation, the change may cause a different amino acid at a certain position (*missense* mutation) within the protein and the consequences would depend on the importance of that particular amino acid. Other changes may alter a splice site recognition sequence or sites of posttranscriptional or posttranslational modification. It is also possible that a change in a nucleotide may have no consequence, owing to the redundancy of the genetic code or the importance of the amino acid in the protein, and thus it is a silent mutation.

More observable changes can occur when regions of a chromosome are deleted or duplicated. Loss of genetic material may occur from within a chromosome or at the termini and results in what may be called partial monosomy. Just as with base changes, a single nucleotide may be added or deleted from a sequence, the consequences depending on its location. These changes, called *frameshift* mutations, within a coding sequence can alter the reading frame of the mRNA during translation. These may create a stop codon, or incorrect amino acids will be inserted into the protein, resulting in suboptimal function.

Many deletions of larger regions of chromosomes have been described in which partial monosomies result in specific syndromes. As might be expected, a deletion that involves more than one gene may have a worse effect than a mutation in a single gene. Many of the described disorders involve deletions of millions of base pairs and numerous genes. Most of these are de novo mutations and have such significant presentations that the individuals do not pass the deletion on to another generation (Box 1-1). Duplication of genetic material results from errors in replication. These may occur when a segment of DNA is copied more than once or when unequal exchange of DNA occurs between homologous chromosome pairs. The results may be a direct, or tandem, repeat or an inverted repeat of the DNA. Unequal exchange, or recombination, occurs in meiosis when homologous chromosomes do not align properly. The recombination results in a deletion for one chromosome and a duplication for the other. In either case, DNA that has been gained or lost can result in unbalanced gene expression.

Genetic material may also be moved from one location to another without the loss of any material. Such movements may occur within a chromosome or between chromosomes. Within a chromosome, movements are usually seen as inversions. Inversions either include the centromere (pericentric

BOX 1-1. EXAMPLES OF DELETION SYNDROMES

Cri du chat syndrome (5p15)
Prader-Willi syndrome (15q11-13)
Angelman syndrome (15q11-13)
DiGeorge syndrome (22q11.2)
Smith-Magenis syndrome (17p11.2)
Wolf-Hirschhorn syndrome (4p16.3)

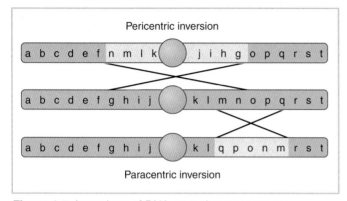

Pericentric inversion

a b c d e f n m l k   j i h g o p q r s t

a b c d e f g h i j   k l m n o p q r s t

a b c d e f g h i j   k l q p o n m r s t

Paracentric inversion

Figure 1-7. Inversions of DNA on a chromosome are distinguished by the involvement of the centromere. Pericentric inversions include the centromere. Paracentric inversions occur in either the p or q arm.

inversion) or are in one arm of the chromosome (paracentric inversion) (Fig. 1-7). These changes provide significant challenges to the chromosome during meiosis. Proper alignment of homologous chromosomes is impossible. If recombination is attempted, distribution of genetic material to gametes becomes unbalanced; some gametes may receive duplicate copies of DNA segments while others lack these DNA segments.

The movement of genetic material between chromosomes is called a *translocation*. Translocations that exchange material between two chromosomes are called reciprocal translocations. These translocations generally have little consequence for the individual in whom they arise. However, translocations become important during the formation of gametes and segregation of the chromosomes. Some gametes will receive extra copies of genetic material while others will be missing genetic material (see Chapter 2).

A common rearrangement is the fusion of two long arms of acrocentric chromosomes leading to the formation of two new chromosomes. When this fusion occurs at the centromere, it is called a Robertsonian translocation. There are five acrocentric chromosomes among the 23 pairs (chromosomes 13, 14, 15, 21, and 22), and all are commonly seen in translocations. Robertsonian translocations are the most common chromosomal rearrangement. In a balanced arrangement, no problems are evident in the individual. However, the unbalanced form presents the same concerns as partial monosomy or partial trisomy.

As noted, a mutation is a heritable change in genetic material. It may be spontaneous, as with some nondisjunction insertions or deletions, or induced by an external factor. This external factor, a *mutagen*, is any physical or chemical agent that increases the rate of mutation above the spontaneous rate; the spontaneous rate of mutation for any gene is 1×10^{-6} per generation. Therefore, determining whether a mutation results from a spontaneous event within the cell or from a mutagen requires evaluation and comparison of the rates of mutation.

Mutagens are generally chemicals and irradiation (Box 1-2). Chemical mutagens can be classified as (1) base analogs that mimic purines and pyrimidines; (2) intercalating agents that alter the structure of DNA, resulting in nucleotide insertions and frameshifts; (3) agents that alter bases, resulting in different base properties; and (4) agents that alter the structure of DNA, resulting in noncoding regions, cross-linking of strands, or strand breaks.

Ionizing radiation damages cells through the production of free radicals of water. The free radicals interact with DNA and protein, leading to cell damage and death. Obviously, those cells most vulnerable to damage are rapidly dividing cells. The extent of the damage is dose dependent. Cells that are not killed have damage—mutations—to the DNA at sublethal doses. Such damage is demonstrated by base mutations, DNA cross-linking, and breaks in DNA. Breaks in the DNA of chromosomes may result in deletions, rearrangements, or even loss.

Ultraviolet (UV) radiation is non-ionizing because it produces less energy. UV-A (≥320 nm) is sometimes called "near-UV" because it is closer to visible light wavelength. UV-B (290–320 nm) and UV-C (190–290 nm) cause the greatest damage. The most damaging lesion is the formation of pyrimidine dimers from covalent bonds formed between adjacent pyrimidines. These dimers block transcription and replication.

BIOCHEMISTRY

Genetic Code

Three nucleotides code for one amino acid. A change in the third nucleotide may have no effect on the code for a particular amino acid; this is the "wobble effect." For example, arginine is coded for by CGU, CGC, CGA, and CGG. A change in the first or second nucleotide will change the amino acid inserted into the protein. The third position has no effect and is referred to as the wobble effect. There is one codon for methionine and tryptophan. Other amino acids may be specified by two to six codons (none are specified by five). There are three stop, or "nonsense," codons.

1st position (5′ end)	2nd position (middle)				3rd position (3′ end)
	U	C	A	G	
U	Phe F	Ser S	Tyr Y	Cys C	U
	Phe F	Ser S	Tyr Y	Cys C	C
	Leu L	Ser S	STOP	STOP	A
	Leu L	Ser S	STOP	Trp W	G
C	Leu L	Pro P	His H	Arg R	U
	Leu L	Pro P	His H	Arg R	C
	Leu L	Pro P	Gln Q	Arg R	A
	Leu L	Pro P	Gln Q	Arg R	G
A	Ile I	Thr T	Asn N	Ser S	U
	Ile I	Thr T	Asn N	Ser S	C
	Ile I	Thr T	Lys K	Arg R	A
	Met M	Thr T	Lys K	Arg R	G
G	Val V	Ala A	Asp D	Gly G	U
	Val V	Ala A	Asp D	Gly G	C
	Val V	Ala A	Glu E	Gly G	A
	Val V	Ala A	Glu E	Gly G	G

●●● ERRORS IN DNA AND DNA REPAIR

DNA mutations can be significant if the expression of a gene, or its alleles, and its allelic products are altered and the alteration cannot be repaired. Cells obviously have mechanisms to repair DNA damage, since each individual encounters many spontaneous mutations that do not progress to a disease state. Daily exposure to UV radiation results in pyrimidine dimers, even from UV-A. These dimers are split by photolyases in a process known as photoreactivation in many organisms. The enzyme monomerizes the dimers, but the precise mechanism of binding the substrate and utilizing light energy to effect repair is unclear. The enzyme, or protein, responsible for this process is not known in humans, and presumably photoreactivation does not occur in humans. Three general steps are involved in DNA repair: (1) mutated DNA is recognized and excised, (2) the original DNA sequence is restored with DNA polymerase, and (3) the ends of the replaced DNA are ligated to the existing strand. The mechanisms employed by cells to accomplish these steps include base excision, nucleotide excision, and mismatch repair.

Individual bases need replacing because of oxidative damage, alkylation, deamination, or a structural error in which no base is attached to phosphate-sugar backbone. Unlike other types of mutations, these examples cause little

distortion of the DNA and are repaired by *base excision* (Fig. 1-8). DNA glycosylases release the base by cleaving the glycosidic bonds between the deoxyribose and the base. DNA polymerase I replaces the base to restore the appropriate pairing (A:T or G:C) followed by ligation to repair the ends. *Glycosylases are specific for the base being removed,* and if there is a deficiency of a particular glycosylase, repair is compromised.

More extensive damage to DNA than single base pairs may distort the DNA structure. Damage of this type requires the removal of several nucleotides to accomplish repair. *Nucleotide excision repair* (Fig. 1-9) differs from base excision repair, which requires specific enzyme recognition of the base needing repair and of the size of the repair. The general mechanism of nucleotide excision repair is recognition of a bulky distortion, cleavage of the bonds on either side of the distortion with an endonuclease, removal of the bases, replacement of the fragment with DNA polymerase I, and ligation of the ends to the DNA strand.

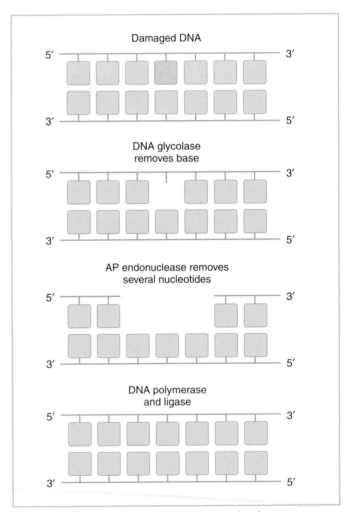

Figure 1-8. Base excision repair is the mechanism most commonly employed for incorrect or damaged bases. Specificity of repair is conferred by specific DNA *N*-glycosylases such as uracil DNA *N*-glycosylase. These glycosylases hydrolyze the *N*-glycosidic bond between the base and the deoxyribose. AP, apurinic/apyrimidinic.

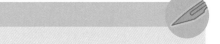

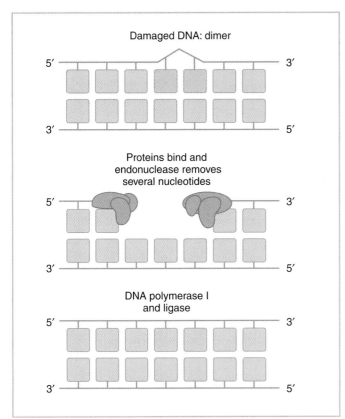

Figure 1-9. Nucleotide excision repair. Damaged DNA is recognized on the basis of its abnormal structure or abnormal chemistry. A multiprotein complex binds to the site to initiate excision and repair by a DNA polymerase and ligase.

Nucleotide excision repair requires a complex system of proteins to stabilize the bulky region of the DNA being removed and then to resynthesize the correct segment matching the template. More than 30 proteins are involved. Any of these proteins can be mutated and affect the repair process. This is exactly what is seen in the inherited disease named xeroderma pigmentosum. Mutations in many genes yield the same general clinical presentation (Table 1-1). Patients have flaking skin with abnormal pigmentation and numerous skin cancers, such as basal and squamous cell

PATHOLOGY

Skin Tumors

Basal cell carcinoma is a slow-growing tumor that rarely metastasizes. It presents as pearly papules with subepidermal telangiectasias and basaloid cells in the dermis. Squamous cell carcinoma is the most common tumor resulting from sun exposure. The in situ form does not invade the basement membrane but has atypical cellular and nuclear morphology. Invasive forms occur when the basement membrane is invaded.

Melanoma of the skin demonstrates a variation in pigmentation with irregular borders. Some malignant melanomas may develop from dysplastic nevi, but the association of multiple dysplastic nevi with malignant melanoma is strongest for familial forms of melanoma.

carcinomas as well as melanomas. Combinations of different mutated genes result in variations in the severity and spectrum of disease presentation. For example, Cockayne's syndrome, another DNA repair disorder, shares several clinical features with xeroderma pigmentosum, such as sensitivity to sunlight. Two primary genes have been identified as causing Cockayne's syndrome: *csa* and *csb*. However, abnormal proteins involved in the DNA repair process have not only been identified in Cockayne's syndrome but some are also responsible for xeroderma pigmentosum. Clinical features of these two distinct syndromes become less distinct when similar mutations are shared.

The mechanism of *mismatch repair* (Fig. 1-10) does not recognize *damage* to DNA; it recognizes bases that do not match those of the template strand. Proteins of the mismatch repair system recognize a mispairing and bind to the DNA. Other proteins bind to the site, and several nucleotides are excised by an exonuclease and replaced by DNA polymerase III and ligase. The DNA template strand and the newly synthesized strand can be distinguished early in the replication process by methylation present on specific nucleotides of the template strand, allowing the repair machinery to

TABLE 1-1. Specific Genes Associated with Xeroderma Pigmentosum*

Locus Name	Gene Symbol	Chromosome Locus	Protein
XPA	XPA	9q22.3	DNA repair protein complementing XP-A cells
XPB	ERCC3	2q21	TFIIH basal transcription factor complex helicase XPB subunit
XPC	XPC	3p25	DNA repair protein complementing XP-C cells
	ERCC2	19q13.2-q13.3	TFIIH basal transcription factor complex helicase subunit
XPD	DDB2	11p12-p11	DNA damage binding protein 2
XPE	ERCC4	16p13.3-p13.13	DNA repair protein complementing XP-F cells
XPF	ERCC5	13q33	DNA repair protein complementing XP-G cells
XP variant	POLH	6p21.1-p12	Error-prone DNA photoproduct polymerase

*Mutations in these genes, as well as in others, may cause clinical features of the disease. These represent locus heterogeneity, or a condition in which more than one gene can cause the same presentation.

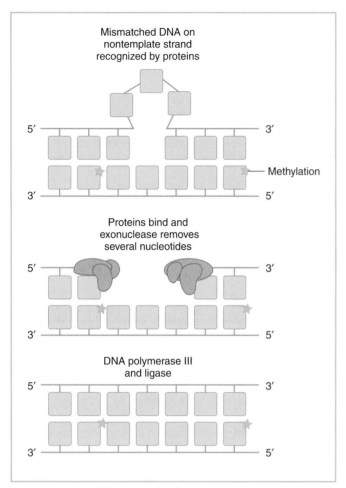

Mismatched DNA on
nontemplate strand
recognized by proteins

5'   3'

Methylation

3'   5'

Proteins bind and
exonuclease removes
several nucleotides

5'   3'

3'   5'

DNA polymerase III
and ligase

5'   3'

3'   5'

Figure 1-10. Mismatch repair. Mismatches most commonly occur during replication; however, they may occur from other mechanisms such as deamination of 5-methylcytosine to produce thymidine improperly paired to G. This mechanism is best understood in *Escherichia coli,* but many of these proteins have homologs in humans and the human mechanism has many similarities to *E. coli.* Mismatch repair mutations are characteristic in hereditary nonpolyposis colon cancer (HNPCC).

differentiate between correct and incorrect nucleotides at the mismatch site.

Hereditary nonpolyposis colon cancer (HNPCC) is one of the most common of all hereditary cancers. Mutations in proteins of the mismatch repair system have been identified in almost all cases of HNPCC. Because repair is defective,

mutations accumulate in cells, leading to normal to abnormal cancer cell progression (see Chapter 5).

Overall, the combination of DNA polymerase 3'→5' proof-reading and the above three postreplication DNA repair mechanisms reduce the error rate of DNA replication to 10^{-9} to 10^{-12}.

Chromosomes in the Cell 2

CONTENTS

The replication and segregation of chromosomes from progenitor cells to daughter cells is a fundamental requirement for the viability of a multicellular organism. Defects in the replication and distribution of this chromosomal material during cell division give rise to numerical (aneuploidy) or structural (translocations, deletions, duplications, or inversions) chromosomal defects. Down syndrome is a well-known example of a disorder that can be caused by either a numerical error or a structural error and is discussed several times in this chapter; other disorders are highlighted to a lesser extent. These and many other abnormalities have *pleiotropic* consequences, or multiple effects from a single event, and can result in severe clinical presentations that are readily recognizable. The field of cytogenetics, the study of chromosome abnormalities, has been enabled by visualization techniques that allow for rapid and inexpensive determination of an individual's chromosomal complement.

●●● CHROMOSOME STRUCTURE AND NOMENCLATURE

Genetic information in DNA is organized on chromosomes as genes. As noted in Chapter 1, each cell has 22 autosomal pairs and one pair of sex chromosomes. The autosome pairs are numbered 1 to 22, in descending order of length, and further classified into seven groups, designated by capital letters A through G. Each pair of autosomes is identical in size, organization of genes, and position of the centromere (Fig. 2-1). The genes on these *homologous chromosomes* are organized to produce the same protein. In addition, there are two *sex chromosomes*, which are unnumbered and of different sizes. The male has one X chromosome and one Y chromosome. The female has two X chromosomes of equal size and no Y chromosome. Thus, the complement of 46 human chromosomes comprises 22 pairs of autosomes plus the sex chromosome pair—XX in normal females and XY in normal males—and the female is described as 46,XX and the male as 46,XY.

Cytogenetic analysis and preparation of a karyotype provide physical identification of metaphase chromosomes. At this stage of visualization, each chromosome is longitudinally doubled, and the two strands (or chromatids) are held together at a primary constriction, known as the centromere. A chromosome with a medially located centromere is technically called *metacentric*. When the centromere is located away from the midline, one arm of the chromosome appears longer than the other. Such a chromosome is termed *submetacentric*. In *acrocentric* chromosomes, the centromere is nearly terminal in position (Fig. 2-2). Cytogeneticists betrayed their sense of humor by designating the short arm of the chromosome as *p* (for petit) and the long arm as *q* (the next letter of the alphabet!).

Identification of Chromosomes

Chromosomes are most easily identified in the metaphase stage of the cell cycle. Here, each homologous chromosome has doubled and has a sister chromatid; the sister chromatids are held together by a single centromere. Beginning with a sample of blood, phytohemagglutinin, which stimulates cell division in human white blood cells, and colchicine, which arrests cell division at the metaphase stage, can be used to provoke a large number of cells to the metaphase stage. At this point, chromosomes are ordinarily stained for visualization under the light microscope. Two of the more traditionally employed techniques are Q-banding and G-banding.

Quinacrine dye stains chromosomes and is detected with a fluorescent microscope. The banding pattern produced is called *Q-banding*. Pretreating cells with the enzyme trypsin, which partially digests the chromosomal proteins, and then staining the preparation with Giemsa dye, results in the formation of *G-bands*, which are visible under the ordinary light microscope as demonstrated in Figure 2-1. The Giemsa bands, those stained with the dye, are rich in adenine and thymine (AT-rich), whereas the light bands are rich in guanine

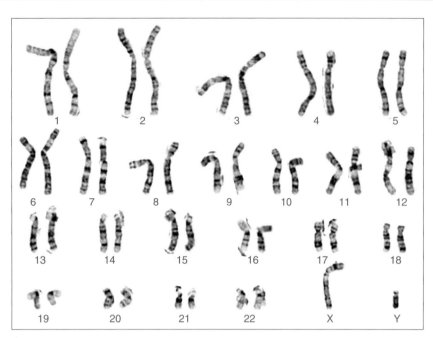

A

Figure 2-1. A, Normal karyotype. (Courtesy of Dr. Linda Pasztor, Sonora Quest Laboratories.) **B**, Characteristics of metaphase chromosomes showing groups with similar lengths and centromere positions. (Data from the International System for Chromosome Nomenclature, 2005.)

Group	Number	Diagrammatic Representation	Relative Length*
Large chromosomes			
A	1		8.4
	2		8.0
	3		6.8
B	4		6.3
	5		6.1
Medium chromosomes			
C	6		5.9
	7		5.4
	8		4.9
	9		4.8
	10		4.6
	11		4.6
	12		4.7
D	13		3.7
	14		3.6
	15		3.5
Small chromosomes			
E	16		3.4
	17		3.3
	18		2.9
F	19		2.7
	20		2.6
G	21		1.9
	22		2.0
Sex chromosomes			
	X		5.1 (group C)
	Y		2.2 (group G)

* Percentage of the total combined length of a haploid set of 22 autosomes.

B

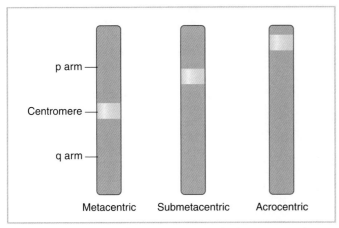

Figure 2-2. Anatomy of a chromosome. A chromosome is divided by a centromere into a long arm (q) and a short arm (p). By convention the p arm is always at the top. The centromere is designated by its location as metacentric, submetacentric, or acrocentric.

and cytosine (GC-rich). Quinacrine and Giemsa dyes produce identical banding patterns. The advantage of Giemsa over quinacrine is that it does not necessitate expensive fluorescent microscopy. These banding procedures are the cornerstones of karyotypic analysis.

The key point in karyotypic analysis is that each chromosome is visualized as consisting of a continuous series of dark and light bands. In each chromosome arm, the bands are numbered from the centromere to the terminus. In describing a particular site, the chromosome number is listed first, followed by the arm (p or q), then the region number within an arm, and finally the specific band within that region. For example, 1q32 refers to chromosome 1, long arm, region 3, and band 2. Higher-resolution techniques have permitted the portrayal of prophase chromosomes and, concomitantly, the subdivision of existing bands. To indicate a subband, a decimal point is placed after the original band designation, followed by the number assigned to the subband. In the example used, the identification of two subbands would be designated 1q32.1 and 1q32.2.

Technical advances have continued to accumulate that promise (or threaten) to render the more classical procedures obsolete. Today, researchers identify a given region or a particular gene-specific sequence on a chromosome spread with a fluorescent DNA-specific probe that hybridizes with its corresponding sequence on the chromosome. The hybridized probe is revealed by fluorescence under ultraviolet light. This nonradioactive technique is called *fluorescent in situ hybridization*, or FISH. The technique is useful in defining specific chromosome sequences in both interphase and metaphase nuclei. It has been favored in recent years for detecting many chromosomal aberrations prenatally. Each chromosome can also be labeled by chromosome-specific fluorophores, a technique known as *chromosome painting*, and readily distinguished (Fig. 2-3). This technique is particularly useful for the detection of an abnormal chromosome number or a rearrangement between chromosomes.

●●● CELL CYCLE AND MITOSIS

Cells can be described as existing within a cell cycle. The cell cycle has two essential components: *mitosis*, the period of cell division, and *interphase*, and the period between mitoses. Interphase is defined by three stages: the first gap phase (G_1), the synthesis (S) phase, and the second gap (G_2) phase. Cells in a state of quiescence are in G_0 but can be stimulated to reenter G_1. Progression through the cell cycle occurs rapidly or quite slowly, and often this is controlled by the length of time that the cell spends in the G_1 phase. The S phase is the period of DNA replication, and each G_1 chromosome that had been a single chromosome now comprises two identical (sister) chromatids. Thus, at the end of the G_2 phase, each chromosome is represented as a pair of homologous chromosomes and each member of the pair is composed of two sister chromatids. The cell is now ready for mitosis (Fig. 2-4).

During mitosis, the cell undergoes fission and each daughter cell receives a complete genetic complement that is identical to the progenitor cell. This is a highly complex phase of the cell cycle with five distinct phases. *Prophase* begins mitosis and is characterized by a condensation of the chromosomes and the initial stages of the mitotic spindle formation. A pair of organelles called centrioles form

BIOCHEMISTRY

Cell Cycle
Regulation of the cell cycle is very complex. Some important features include the following:

- Cyclin-dependent kinases (CDKs) along with cyclins are major control switches regulating transitions from G_1 to S and G_2 to M.
- CDKs and cyclins trigger progression through the cell cycle.

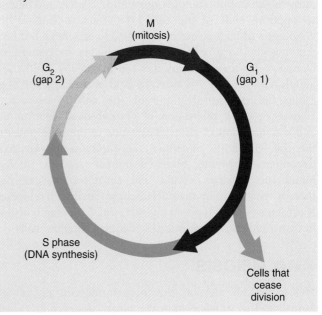

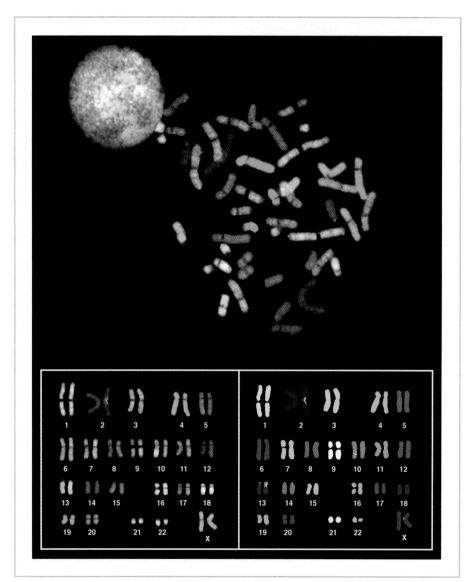

Figure 2-3. Spectral karyotyping (SKY) and multiplex fluorescence in situ hybridization (M-FISH) of human chromosomes permit simultaneous visualization of all chromosomes in different colors. Chromosome-specific probes are generated from flow-sorted chromosomes that are amplified by polymerase chain reaction and fluorescently labeled. Each human chromosome absorbs a unique combination of fluorochromes. Both spectral karyotyping and M-FISH (multiplex-FISH) use spectrally distinguishable fluorochromes, but they employ different methods of detection. (Courtesy of Evelin Schröck, Stan du Manoir, and Thomas Ried, National Institutes for Health.)

microtubule/mitotic spindle organization centers and migrate to opposite ends of the cell. *Prometaphase* features the dissolution of the nuclear membrane and attachment of each chromosome to a spindle microtubule via its centromere. During *metaphase*, chromosomes are maximally condensed, and thus most easily visualized by light microscopy, and align along the equatorial plane of the cell. *Anaphase* is characterized by replication of chromosomal centromeres and the migration of sister chromatids to opposite poles of the cell. Finally, in *telophase*, the chromosomes begin to decondense, spindle fibers disappear, and a nuclear membrane re-forms around the chromosomal material, thereby reconstituting the nucleus. Associated with telophase is cytokinesis, or cytoplasm division, which ultimately results in two complete, chromosomally identical daughter cells.

●●● MEIOSIS

Meiosis is cell division that occurs only during gamete formation. This variation from the mitosis observed in somatic cells is essential because human somatic cells—including gamete progenitor cells—are *diploid*, containing two complete copies of each chromosome. The genetic material must be reduced by 50%, to a *haploid* state, during gamete formation for a newly formed zygote to have a complete chromosomal complement. Meiosis involves two separate cell divisions that are conceptually similar to the stages of mitosis (Fig. 2-5). The first cell division, *meiosis I*, is referred to as a "reductive division"

HISTOLOGY

Centrioles

Centrioles occur as a pair of organelles in the cell, and they are arranged perpendicular to each other. They are composed of microtubules—nine sets of triplets—and organize the spindle apparatus of spindle fibers and astral rays on which chromosomes move during mitosis and meiosis. Similarly to mitochondria, centrioles replicate autonomously.

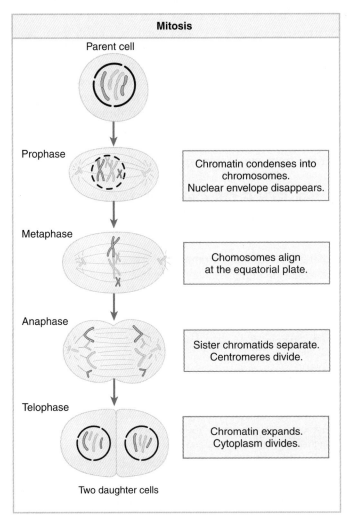

Figure 2-4. Mitosis is the process of forming identical daughter cells. There are four basic stages: prophase, metaphase, anaphase, and telophase.

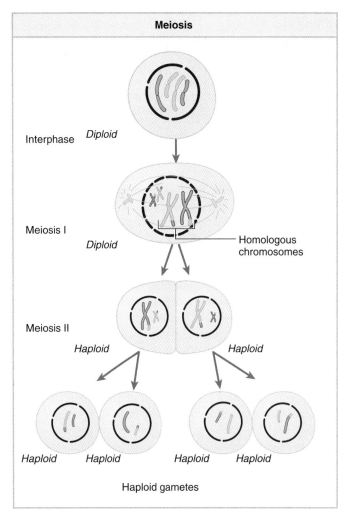

Figure 2-5. Meiosis occurs in gonads and results in the formation of gametes. In the first stage, meiosis I, homologous pairs of chromosomes are separated, thereby reducing the number of chromosomes to 23. In meiosis II, sister chromatids are separated, resulting in gametes with 23 chromosomes.

because the chromosomal number is reduced to a haploid number in the resulting daughter cells. Here, homologous chromosomes, each comprising two sister chromatids, line up along the equatorial plate during metaphase I and separate during anaphase I. *Meiosis II* directly follows meiosis I in the absence of further DNA replication. During anaphase of meiosis II, centromeres are duplicated and sister chromatids segregate to opposite poles of the cell. Each gamete formed contains a haploid genome consisting of 23 chromosomes.

Prophase of meiosis I is the signature event of the meiotic process, since it is here that *genetic recombination* takes place. This stage is complex and is subdivided into five stages. During *leptotene*, chromosomes begin to condense to the point where they are easily visible. The chromosomes are represented by pairs, each with a single centromere and two sister chromatids. In *zygotene*, homologous chromosomes associate with each other and pair, via the synaptonemal complex, along the entire length of the chromosomes. Further coiling and condensing of the chromosomes and completion of the synapsis process characterize *pachytene*. Synapsed,

paired homologous chromosomes are termed bivalent—indicating two joined or synapsed chromosomes—or tetrad—representing the four separate chromatids in the bivalent structure. Importantly, bivalent chromosomes in pachytene undergo an exchange of chromatid material in a process called recombination or crossing-over. In practice, genetic recombination is vital to the chromosomal exchange of parental genetic material during gamete formation. This process is the major source of genetic variation in humans, and it permits an extremely high degree of genetic variability among gametes produced by an individual. Homologous chromosomes begin to pull apart in *diplotene*, and chiasmata—points of attachment between paired chromosomes—are apparent. Chiasmata indicate positions where crossing-over has occurred. In the next stage, *diakinesis*, homologous chromosomes continue to separate from each other and attain a maximally condensed state.

Following diakinesis, the rest of meiosis I proceeds quite similarly to mitosis. During metaphase I, a spindle apparatus forms and the paired chromosomes align along the equatorial pole of the cell. During anaphase I, the individual bivalents completely separate from each other; then homologous chromosomes, with their cognate centromere, are separated and drawn to opposite poles of the cell. Finally, in telophase I, the haploid chromosomal complement has segregated to both poles of the cell and cytoplasmic cleavage yields two daughter cells. Two critical features can be appreciated at this point. First, *the number of chromosomes has been reduced from diploid (46 chromosomes) in one cell to haploid (23 chromosomes) in daughter cells.* Second, genetic recombination has generated a new arrangement of genetic material, which originated from parental chromosomes, in each of the daughter cells. Each chromosome in the daughter cell can be thought of as hybrid, or recombinant, representing a unique combination of the two parental chromosomes.

Meiosis II proceeds just as in mitosis except the starting cell is haploid and no DNA replication (typically an interphase event) occurs. Each of the 23 chromosomes is represented by two sister chromatids sharing a centromere. These chromosomes thicken and align along the equatorial plane of the cell. Each chromatid is then pulled to opposite poles of the cell during anaphase II. Subsequent cytoplasmic division yields two haploid (23 single chromatid chromosomes with one centromere) gametes. Overall, a single gamete progenitor cell may yield four independent gametes.

Meiosis and Gamete Formation

Meiosis is the signature event in gamete formation. However, marked sex-specific differences exist in the production of sperm and egg. By birth, females have nearly completed oogenesis as primary oocytes—derived from oogonia via roughly 30 mitotic divisions—and have initiated prophase of meiosis I. The primary oocytes are suspended at dictyotene until sexual maturity is reached and ovulation occurs. At this point, the oocyte completes meiosis I, producing a secondary oocyte that contains most of the cytoplasm from the primary oocyte. The second cell of this division forms the first polar body, which contains little cytoplasm and undergoes atresia. The secondary oocyte initiates meiosis II, but this process is completed only at fertilization of a mature ovum at which point a second polar body is formed. Hence, in females, only one mature, haploid gamete is produced during gameto-

genesis, and the process may take from 10 to 50 years. Spermatogenesis, on the other hand, is a much more rapid and dynamic process, taking roughly 60 days to complete. Here, puberty signals the mitotic maturation of diploid spermatogonia to diploid primary spermatocytes. Primary spermatocytes undergo meiosis I to form haploid secondary spermatocytes, which, in turn, proceed through meiosis II to form spermatids that differentiate further into mature sperm. In contrast to oogenesis, four mature, haploid gametes are derived from one primary spermatocyte.

●●● ROLE OF CHROMOSOMAL ABNORMALITIES IN HUMAN MEDICAL GENETICS

Having considered chromosomal structure, nomenclature, and behavior during gamete formation, it is now possible to consider the impact of chromosomal defects on human health.

Chromosomal abnormalities generally fall into two categories: numerical or structural. Each category is considered separately.

Chromosomal Numerical Abnormalities

Euploidy versus Aneuploidy

Cells with normal chromosome complements have *euploid* karyotypes (Greek eu, "good"; ploid, "set"). The euploid states in humans are the haploid (23 chromosomes) germ cells (gametes) and the diploid (46 chromosomes) somatic cells. *Aneuploid* cells have an incomplete or unbalanced chromosome complement owing to deficiency or excess of individual chromosomes. A cell lacking one chromosome of a diploid complement is called *monosomic* (46 − 1). A trisomic cell has a complete chromosome complement plus a single extra chromosome (46 + 1). Tetrasomics (46 + 2) carry a particular chromosome in quadruplicate; the remaining chromosomes are present twice as homologous pairs. *Polyploidy* describes the condition in which a complete extra chromosomal set is present, e.g., 69 or 92 chromosomes. Only aneuploidy is relevant for live births, since polyploidy is incompatible with life.

Cause and Incidence of Aneuploidy

Down syndrome, trisomy 21, illustrates the principles of aneuploidy (Fig. 2-6). The additional extra chromosome 21 in somatic cells of individuals with Down syndrome was initially thought to be the *next-to-smallest* chromosome. When improved karyotypic techniques revealed that chromosome 21 is actually smaller than chromosome 22, no reversal in numbers occurred because of the firm association of number 21 with Down syndrome. Geneticists acknowledge the prevailing inconsistency that chromosome 21 (not 22) is in reality the smallest chromosome in the human complement.

Down syndrome is the most common congenital chromosomal disorder associated with severe mental retardation. The clinical features of this syndrome are quite distinctive and readily discernible at birth. Characteristic features include a prominent forehead, a flattened nasal bridge, a habitually open mouth, a projecting lower lip, a protruding tongue, slanting eyes, and epicanthic folds. Additional features are shown in Box 2-1.

Many of these features are variably expressed and not present in all affected individuals. Even the highly unusual iris of a Down infant is not universal. White (or light yellow) cloud-like specks may circumscribe the outer layer of the iris (Fig. 2-7) and are known as Brushfield's spots. The specks are rarely associated with brown irides and have not been found in black infants with Down syndrome. The ultimate confirmation of Down syndrome must come from analysis of the chromosome complement. Individuals with Down syndrome have 47 chromosomes rather than 46.

The incidence of Down syndrome rises markedly with maternal age—from about one in 2000 live births at maternal age 20 years to one in 100 at age 40 (Fig. 2-8). Among infants born to women over age 45, one in 40 are expected to be affected with Down syndrome. It was immediately surmised

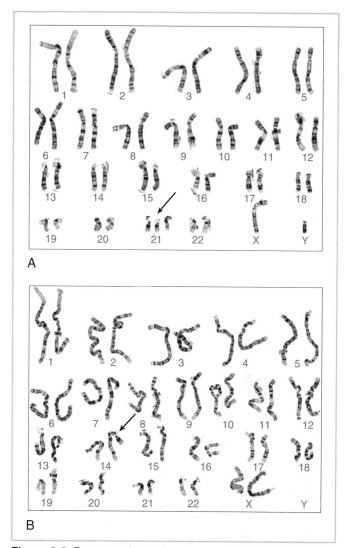

Figure 2-6. Down syndrome karyotypes. **A**, Trisomy Down syndrome: 47,XX,+21. **B**, Translocation Down syndrome: 46,XY, t(14q;21q). (Courtesy of Dr. Linda Pasztor, Sonora Quest Laboratories.)

that the extra chromosome in the affected infant is acquired during the production of the egg by the mother. As noted above, all eggs a woman produces during her reproductive life are present from the moment of birth. At birth, the ovaries contain 1 to 2 million germ cells; by puberty this number has declined to 300,000 to 400,000 germ cells through normal follicular atresia. There is a progressive decline in the number of eggs that mature perfectly as the woman ages. By age 50, the production of functional eggs is drastically diminished.

For numerous years, scientists were comfortable in the belief that the eggs of the human female are subject to the hazards of aging and that aging alone accounted for most trisomy cases. However, the simple focus on older women and aged eggs is inadequate. Since 1970, the mean maternal age for all live births has declined substantially because of the decreasing number of children born to women over 35 years

Box 2-1.   CLINICAL FEATURES ASSOCIATED WITH DOWN SYNDROME

Hypotonia	Flat, depressed nasal bridge
Mental retardation	Palpebral fissures slant upwards
Short stature	Brushfield spots
Prematurity	Single palmar crease
Lower birth weight	Posterior-rotated ears
Brachycephaly	Upturned nose
Macroglossia	Flattened occiput
Small mandible and maxilla	Short, broad hands
Excess nuchal skin	Clinodactyly of the fifth finger
Epicanthal folds	Diastasis

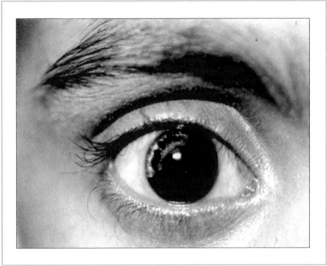

Figure 2-7. Brushfield spots. Brushfield spots are white or yellow colored spots seen on the anterior surface of the iris. The spots may be arranged concentrically to the pupils or as seen here along the pupillary periphery. They are present in 85% of blue- or hazel-eyed patients with trisomy 21. Only 17% of Down syndrome patients with a brown iris have Brushfield spots, since they can be obscured by pigment. (Courtesy of Dr. Usha Langan, New Delhi, India)

of age. *Women under age 35 are currently responsible for more than 90% of all births.* Presently, women under the age of 35 have 75% of the children affected with Down syndrome, demonstrating that some factors in its etiology are still not understood. Data show that the egg is not always at fault, as surmised earlier. In 5% to 15% of the cases of Down syndrome, the extra chromosome is of paternal origin.

Origin of Trisomy 21: Nondisjunction in Meiosis

The process of meiosis is complex and subject to error. It does not always proceed normally. Accidents occur that affect the normal functioning of the spindle fibers and impede the proper migration of one or more chromosomes. During the first meiotic division, a given pair of *homologous chromosomes* may fail to separate from each other. This failure of separation, known as *nondisjunction*, can result in a gamete containing a pair of chromosomes from one parent rather than a single chromosome homolog (Fig. 2-9). Stated another way, nondisjunction of chromosome 21 homologs during oogenesis results in an egg cell that possesses two copies of chromosome 21 rather than the usual one. Fertilization by a normal sperm gives rise to an individual that is trisomic for chromosome 21.

It should be noted in Figure 2-9 that nondisjunction of one chromosome pair in meiosis I results in two types of cells in equal proportions at the end of meiosis I; one cell contains both members of the chromosome pair and the other lacks the particular chromosome. In normal meiosis, the gametes formed at the end of meiosis II have a single homolog of each chromosome and fertilization returns the zygote to a diploid state with homologous pairs of chromosomes. If a normal sperm fertilizes an egg cell lacking the particular chromosome, the outcome is *monosomy*. Theoretically, autosomal monosomies should be equally as common as autosomal trisomies. However, *monosomy, when it occurs in the autosomes, is largely incompatible with life.* In fact, any rare viable newborn with one autosome completely missing is short-lived. Ironically, a person can survive with one missing X chromosome; 45,X is known as Turner syndrome. Indeed, of all

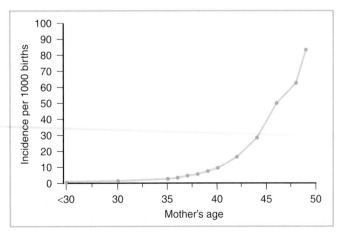

Figure 2-8. Maternal age versus Down syndrome.

PATHOLOGY

Screening and Diagnostic Tests for Down Syndrome

The triple screen is a noninvasive screening test to determine whether there is an increased risk for Down syndrome. It is only a screening test and not a diagnostic test. Increased risk is associated with the following:

- Low maternal serum α-fetoprotein (MSAFP)
- Low unconjugated estriol (uE$_3$)
- Elevated human chorionic gonadotropin (hCG)

Diagnostic tests include amniocentesis, chorionic villus sampling (CVS), and percutaneous umbilical blood sampling (PUBS).

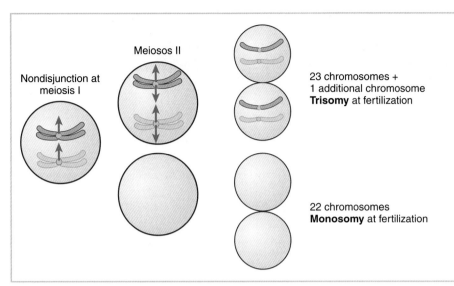

A

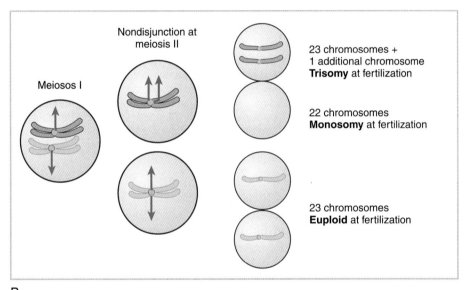

B

Figure 2-9. Nondisjunction.
A, Nondisjunction occurs in meiosis I when homologous chromosome pairs segregate to the same daughter cell.
B, Nondisjunction occurs in meiosis II when sister chromatids segregate to the same daughter cell. When nondisjunction occurs in meiosis I, all gametes are abnormal, whereas when it occurs in meiosis II, there is a 50% chance that a normal gamete will be fertilized.

disorders involving missing or additional chromosomes, those involving the sex chromosomes are the most likely to demonstrate survival beyond the early days and months of life.

Meiotic nondisjunction may occur during *either* the first *or* the second meiotic division (see Fig. 2-9). If nondisjunction occurs in a primary spermatocyte during meiosis I, then all sperm derived from the primary spermatocyte will be abnormal and all zygotes will have an aberrant chromosome complement. If nondisjunction occurs in a secondary spermatocyte undergoing meiosis II, only two of the four sperm will be abnormal and only two of the zygotes will be chromosomally abnormal; the other two will be normal euploids. There is also a difference in chromatids, and therefore in alleles present on chromatids, depending on whether nondisjunction occurs during meiosis I or meiosis II. If nondisjunction occurs during meiosis I, all three chromatids in a fertilized egg have unique parental (or really grandparental) origin. If nondis-

junction occurs during meiosis II, the result is two chromatids that originated from the replication of the same DNA strand and one unique chromatid occurring in the fertilized egg. The potential for inheriting similar alleles is more likely with nondisjunction in meiosis II than in meiosis I even if consideration is not given to the recombination that may occur. In both cases—nondisjunction in meiosis I and meiosis II—the result is aneuploidy, or an abnormal number of chromosomes. The nomenclature is somewhat burdensome, since the standard terminology differs for the gamete and the zygote. For a gamete, *nullisomic* (23 − 1) signifies the absence of one chromosome in the haploid complement and *disomic* (23 + 1) signifies the addition of one chromosome in the haploid complement. For a zygote, *monosomic* (46 − 1) specifies the absence of one chromosome in the diploid set and trisomic (46 + 1) specifies the presence of one additional chromosome in the diploid set.

Other Trisomies

Several thorough investigations have revealed that 40% to 50% of first-trimester spontaneous abortuses are trisomic for one of the autosomes. All human autosomal trisomic conditions are associated with marked developmental disorders. The frequencies of trisomies in different autosomal groups vary widely. Trisomies for chromosomes 13, 16, 18, 21, and 22 occur most often, especially chromosome 16. For reasons not well understood, chromosome 16 appears to be particularly vulnerable to nondisjunction. Trisomy 16 is the most common (one-third) autosomal trisomy found in abortuses. Interestingly, trisomy 16 in abortuses shows little association with increasing maternal age, suggesting that an unusual age-independent mechanism is responsible for this extraordinarily common trisomic condition.

Other than in Down syndrome, the trisomic condition is rare in live-born infants. Two autosomal trisomies other than trisomy 21 demonstrate survival to term and occur with significant frequency to be well-described syndromes—namely, trisomy 13 (Patau syndrome, Fig. 2-10) and trisomy 18 (Edwards syndrome, Fig. 2-11). Both disorders are associated with severe mental retardation and a broad spectrum of severe developmental anomalies (Table 2-1). Prominent features of a trisomy 13 baby are bilateral clefts of the lip and palate, a forehead that slopes backward, defective eye development, and an excess number of fingers and toes

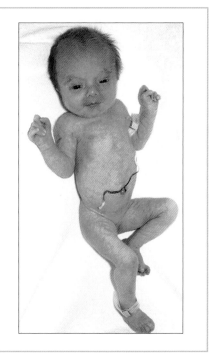

Figure 2-11. Features of trisomy 18 (Edwards syndrome). Trisomy 18 female infant with a characteristic clenched fist, short sternum, narrow pelvis, hypertelorism, short palpebral fissures, and rocker bottom feet. (From Moore KL, Persaud TVN. *The Developing Human: Clinically Oriented Embryology,* 7th ed. Philadelphia, WB Saunders, 2003, p 164.)

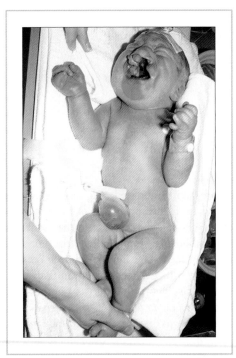

Figure 2-10. Features of trisomy 13 (Patau syndrome). Trisomy 13 female infant with cleft palate and bilateral lip, low-set malformed ears, hypotelorism, and postaxial polydactyly of the left hand. This infant also has an omphalocele. (From Moore KL, Persaud TVN. *The Developing Human: Clinically Oriented Embryology,* 7th ed. Philadelphia, WB Saunders, 2003, p 164.)

(polydactyly). Common clinical features of trisomy 18 infants are recessed chin, elongated head, small eyes, "rocker-bottom" feet, and tightly clenched hands and fingers with the second and fifth fingers overlapping the third and fourth. Estimates for trisomy 13 and trisomy 18 range widely from 1 in 4000 to 1 in 10,000 live births. Each leads to death in early infancy, invariably within a year of birth.

Mitotic Nondisjunction and Mosaicism

A small percentage (1% to 3%) of infants with Down syndrome have two populations of cell types with respect to chromosome 21. Such *mosaic* individuals, with both normal (46 chromosomes) and trisomic (47 chromosomes) cells, typically have less severe features of Down syndrome. Actually, there is appreciable phenotypic variability among mosaics, depending on the proportion of trisomic cells.

One route to mosaicism is nondisjunction during the early cleavage stages of the zygote. A mitotic nondisjunction at the first cleavage division leads to two dissimilar cell populations; one cell line will be trisomic and the other will be mono-somic. If the monosomic cell line perishes, then only trisomic cells remain. Now, if nondisjunction occurs during the second cleavage division, three different cell types arise. If the monosomic cell line perishes (as is usually the case), then the embryo will be a mosaic consisting of cells with a normal chromosome number and cells with a trisomic number of chromosomes. When several thousand normal divisions ensue before a

TABLE 2-1. Comparison of Trisomy 13 and Trisomy 18

Feature	Trisomy 13	Trisomy 18
Life span	50% die by age 1 month 75% die by age 6 months	90% die by age 1 year
Clinical presentation	Seizures Microcephaly; micrognathia Scalp defects (absent skin) Cleft lip, cleft palate Hypotelorism Coloboma defects of the iris Low-set, abnormally shaped ears Polydactyly Simian crease Hernias Cryptorchidism Hypotonia Severe mental and motor retardation	Clenched fist; second and fifth fingers overlap the third and fourth Intrauterine growth retardation (IUGR) Rocker bottom feet Micrognathia, prominent occiput, micro-ophthalmia Low-set ears Cardiac defects Generalized muscle spasticity Renal anomalies Mental retardation
Associated disorders	Congenital heart defects in 80% Dextrocardia in 20–50% (heart is on right side of chest rather than left) Omphalocele in 10% Holoprosencephaly in 66%	Congenital heart defects in 90% Joint contractures Spina bifida in 6% Eye abnormalities in 10% Hearing loss — high Radial bone aplasia in 5–10%

Problems associated with survival past 1 month of age:
  Feeding difficulties
  Gastroesophageal reflux
  Slow postnatal growth
  Apnea
  Seizures
  Hypertension
  Kidney defects
  Developmental disability
  Scoliosis

mitotic error occurs, the mosaicism may be clinically inconsequential inasmuch as the number of normal cells far exceeds the abnormal cells. Mosaics may also arise by *chromosome loss*, better designated as *anaphase lag*. In this situation, one chromatid may lag so far behind during anaphase that it fails to become incorporated in a daughter nucleus.

Sex Chromosome Numerical Abnormalities

Unlike autosome pairs that are the same size and contain homologous alleles, sex chromosomes are strikingly different in size with little similarity in the genes found on each. This discrepancy is critically important in the developing embryo because the two X chromosomes found in cells of females represent twice as many coding genes, and potentially gene products, as the one X chromosome found in cells of males.

It is now understood that most conditions of aneuploidy, with the exception of chromosome 21 and some combinations of sex chromosomes, are lethal. Therefore, the finding of two X chromosomes in females but only one in males raised several questions. Why do females survive with twice as much gene product as males? Or, why do males survive with only half as much gene product as females?

The answers to these questions became clear with a better understanding of the mechanism of compensation for this apparent gene dosage discrepancy. In the 1940s, Murray Barr and Ewart Bertram noted differences in the position of a darkly staining mass in the nuclei of interphase cells. They further noted that the darkly staining mass, which became know as a *Barr body*, was associated only with interphase cells from females. This led to the speculation that the Barr body was a tightly condensed X chromosome. Because of its correlation with the X chromosome, Barr bodies are also referred to as *sex chromatin.*

A common method to observe sex chromatin is on a buccal smear of cells scraped from the inside the cheek, spread on a glass slide, stained, and examined with a light microscope. The number of Barr bodies observed is the number of X chromosomes minus 1. In embryos, it is first observed around the sixteenth day of development. Although easy to detect, disadvantages of Barr body analysis are that structural abnormalities of the X chromosome are not detected and that mosaicism can be missed. Currently, FISH analysis followed by G-banding is preferred over buccal smears for X chromosome studies.

In 1959, the first male with *Klinefelter syndrome* and a karyotype of 47,XXY was identified. As expected, these males possess a Barr body, because of the presence of an extra X chromosome, whereas normal males do not. At about the same time, a female with gonadal dysgenesis was described with a karyotype of 45,X, and the disorder became known as *Turner syndrome.* These two events, along with research data, led scientists to recognize the importance of the Y chromosome in sexual development and underscored the importance of two normal X chromosomes for female development (see Chapter 11). An embryo develops as a male in the presence of a Y chromosome and as a female in the absence of a Y chromosome.

Lyonization and Dosage Compensation

In 1961, Mary Lyon proposed the inactive-X hypothesis to explain what happens to genes on the Barr body. She hypothesized that (1) the genes found on the condensed X chromosome are genetically inactive, (2) inactivation occurs very early in development during the blastocyst stage, and (3) inactivation occurs randomly in each blastocyst cell. The net effect of this inactivation would equalize the phenotypes in males and females through a phenomenon known as dosage compensation. The process of X chromosome inactivation is called lyonization. Contrary to Lyon's original hypothesis that X inactivation occurs randomly, it has now been demonstrated that gene inactivation may not always be random and that the inactive X chromosome has some genes that are indeed expressed. This work also highlights the need for two active X chromosomes in early development for normal female development but not normal male development (see Chapter 11).

Chromosomal Structural Abnormalities

Certain chromosomal defects do not involve numerical deficiency or excess. Rather, they feature morphologic or structural abnormalities such as translocations, deletions, duplications, or inversions.

Translocation Errors

One chromosomal aberration that does not involve nondisjunction is translocation—the transfer of a part of one chromosome to another, generally a nonhomologous chromosome. This occurs when two chromosomes break and then rejoin in another combination. The exchange of broken parts is often reciprocal and may not involve loss of chromosomal material. The first translocation observed was reported in the bone marrow cells of an infant with Down syndrome born to a mother only 21 years old. They found 46 chromosomes in the affected child instead of the expected 47. However, detailed examination of the chromosomes revealed that one of the chromosomes had an unusual configuration. It appeared to consist of two chromosomes fused together (see Fig. 2-6B). The interpretation was that the affected child had inherited an extra chromosome, but this extra chromosome had become integrally joined to another chromosome. Stated another way, one chromosome was in fact represented three times, but the third instance was concealed as part of another chromosome.

Translocations that exchange material between two chromosomes are called *reciprocal translocations* (Fig. 2-12). These translocations generally have little consequence for the individual in whom they arise. However, reciprocal translocations become an important issue during the formation of gametes and segregation of the chromosomes. Some gametes will receive extra copies of genetic material while others will be missing genetic material.

A common rearrangement is the fusion of two long arms of acrocentric chromosomes leading to the formation of a new chromosome. This fusion occurs at the centromere and is called a *Robertsonian translocation.* There are five acrocentric chromosomes (see Fig. 2-1) among the 23 pairs (chromosomes 13, 14, 15, 21, and 22), and all are commonly seen in translocations. *Robertsonian translocations are the most common chromosomal rearrangement.* In Down syndrome, the translocation always involves chromosome 21, of course, often fused to chromosome 14. Initially, breaks occur in the two chromosomes in the region of the centromere. Then, the two long arms of broken chromosomes 14 and 21 become joined together at the centromere. This newly formed, relatively large chromosome is referred to as a 14/21 translocation chromosome; it is written more precisely as t(14q;21q). This large translocation chromosome carries the essential genes of chromosomes 14 and 21. The two small arms, containing tandemly arrayed ribosomal RNA genes, are lost.

When all genetic material is present, the chromosomes are said to be in a *balanced rearrangement* and the carrier is typically asymptomatic. The loss of 14p and 21p in the 14/21 translocation is inconsequential, since ribosomal RNA genes represent middle repetitive sequences repeated many times in the genome on several chromosomes (Chapter 1).

Translocation is without clinical consequence to the mother, inasmuch as redundant copies of ribosomal RNA genes occur in other acrocentric chromosomes. However, the consequences for her children can be significant, since the woman carrying the t(14q;21q) translocation chromosome can produce several kinds of eggs. Eggs with only three chromosomal complements are viable, or capable of being fertilized (Fig. 2-13). Specifically, the three types of viable

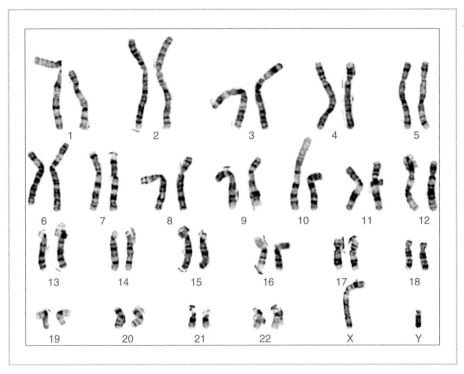

Figure 2-12. Reciprocal translocation: 46,XY, t(1p;10p). (Courtesy of Dr. Linda Pasztor, Sonora Quest Laboratories.)

eggs, when fertilized by normal sperm, result in three possible outcomes: (1) a completely normal child with a normal chromosome set; (2) a normal child with the 14/21 translocation chromosome who potentially can transmit translocation-type Down syndrome; and (3) a Down syndrome child with three copies of chromosome 21, one of which is fused to chromosome 14.

The t(14q;21q) translocation event is not confined to the mother. Cases are known in which the father has been the carrier. Curiously, when the father carries the translocation, the empirical chance of having a Down child is only about one in 20. This may reflect a lack of viability of chromosomally unbalanced sperm cells.

BIOCHEMISTRY

rRNAs

Ribosomal RNAs are an integral part of ribosomes. There are four rRNAs: 5.8S, 18S, 28S, and 5S, which are transcribed by RNA polymerase I. The 45S precursor gives rise to 5.8S, 18S, and 28S. 5S is transcribed from separate clusters of genes and requires RNA polymerase III for transcription. Each genome has 150 to 200 45S genes, located in clusters of 30 to 40 tandem repeats on the p12 band of each acrocentric chromosome: 13, 14, 15, 21, and 22. There are about 200 to 300 5S functional genes and many nonfunctional pseudogenes.

The nucleolus forms around the tandemly repeated rRNA genes, and this combination of a nucleolus and rRNA genes is called the "nucleolar-organizing region" (NOR). These regions are responsible for rRNA transcription and for assembly of components for ribosome synthesis.

In trisomy 21 caused by nondisjunction, recurrence of Down syndrome in a given family is a rare event. Most of the cases of nondisjunction Down syndrome are isolated occurrences in an otherwise normal family. In sharp contrast, translocation Down syndrome runs in families. When a parent is a balanced carrier for a robertsonian translocation that involves chromosome 21, the risk of an affected, translocation Down syndrome child among those developing to term is one chance in three. This is the theoretical expectation. Empirically, from studies of actual family pedigrees, the chance is nearer to one in ten, the difference reflecting decreased viability of the trisomic embryo. Nevertheless, the situation is very different from nondisjunction trisomy, in which the risk of giving birth to an affected child is about one in 700. About 5% of all Down syndrome children have the translocation type abnormality.

Another example of a balanced translocation occurs between the terminal regions of chromosome 22 and chromosome 9. The new chromosome 22 is referred to as the Philadelphia chromosome, reflecting where it was originally described. The translocation event is dramatic because a new gene is created! The new fusion gene consists of a sequence of DNA from the original chromosome 22 known as breakpoint cluster region (BCR) plus a gene from chromosome 9, called ABL which becomes attached to bcr (Fig. 2-14). The fusion gene, BCR-ABL, codes for an abnormally large chimeric product of this composite gene that is fundamental to the pathogenesis of chronic myelogenous leukemia (CML). The ABL gene is an oncogene, which is fairly innocuous in its normal location on chromosome 9. When associated with an unfamiliar DNA sequence (in this case, BCR), the ABL gene fosters an uncontrolled proliferation of white blood cells. The ABL gene has

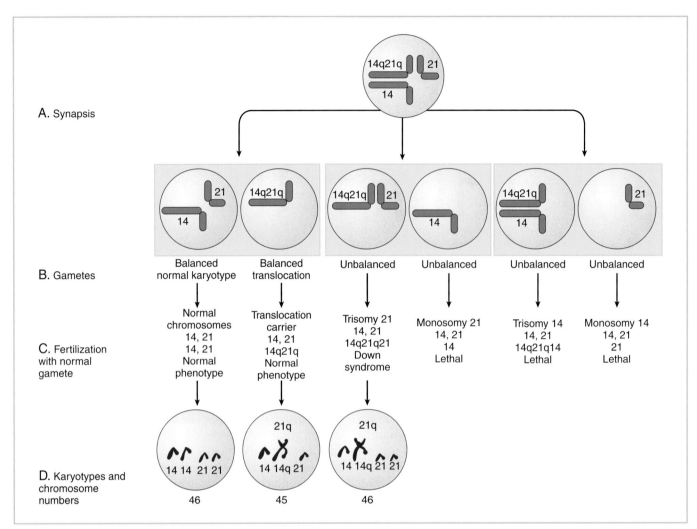

Figure 2-13. Possible gametes produced by an individual with translocation Down syndrome and the consequences of these gametes becoming fertilized. **A**, Synapsis of the translocation chromosome 14q21q and normal chromosomes 21 and 14; 14p and 21p have been lost. **B**, Six types of gametes are possible; three of these are viable. **C**, Fertilization with a normal gamete will produce one normal genotype, one translocation carrier with a normal phenotype, one translocation Down syndrome zygote, and three lethal zygotes.

potent tyrosine kinase activity. Cell proliferation is enhanced as activated tyrosine kinase results in autophosphorylation of a number of sites on the fusion protein and phosphorylation of other proteins (see Chapter 5).

PATHOLOGY

Chronic Myelogenous Leukemia (CML)

CML is a myeloproliferative disease of bone marrow characterized by an increased proliferation of the granulocytic cell line that does not lose the capacity to differentiate. The blood profile has increased granulocytes and immature precursors, including occasional blast cells. CML is responsible for 20% of all adult leukemias. There are three phases of disease: chronic, blast, and accelerated. Splenomegaly is the most common physical finding.

Deletion Errors

Sometimes a piece of chromosome breaks off, resulting in a deletion of genetic material. The effects of the loss of a portion of a chromosome depend on the particular genes lost. One of the earliest deletions noted with staining techniques was the loss of a portion of the short arm of chromosome 5. Affected infants have a rounded, moonlike face and utter feeble, plaintive cries described as similar to the mewing of a cat, and the disorder was named cri du chat (French, "cat cry") syndrome. The cry disappears with time as the larynx improves and is rarely heard after the first year of life. The facial features also change with age, and the moon-shaped face becomes long and thin. Most patients survive beyond childhood, but they rank among the most profoundly retarded (IQ usually < 20). Cri du chat syndrome is one of the most common deletions found in humans, occurring with a frequency of 1 in 500,000 live births (Table 2-2).

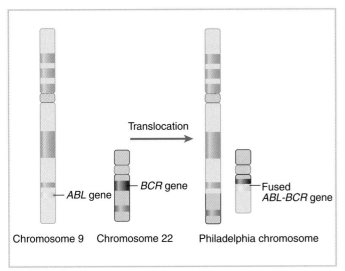

Figure 2-14. A reciprocal translocation occurs between the *ABL* gene of chromosome 9 and the *BCR* gene on chromosome 22 to create an altered gene and protein.

TABLE 2-2. Some Deletion Syndromes

Syndrome	Deletion	Clinical Presentation
Angelman	15q11-13	Mental retardation, ataxia, uncontrolled laughter, seizures
Velocardiofacial	22q11	DiGeorge anomaly, characteristic facies, cleft palate, cardiac defects
Miller-Dieker	17p13.3	Lissencephaly, characteristic facies
Prader-Willi	15q11-13	Mental retardation, hypotonia, obesity, short stature, small hands and feet
Smith-Magenis	17p11.2	Mental retardation, hyperactivity, dysmorphic features, self-destructive behaviors
Williams	7q1	Developmental disability, characteristic facies, supravalvular aortic stenosis

Deletions of varied types, notably interstitial and terminal, have played a role in delineating the segment of chromosome 21 responsible for Down syndrome. Deletions of different segments of one of the long arms of chromosome 21 in trisomy 21 individuals (resulting in *partial trisomy*) have made it possible to identify the chromosome region responsible for the phenotypic features of Down syndrome. The "Down syndrome critical region" has been identified as a 5- to 10-Mb region of the chromosome and encompasses bands 21q22.2 to 21q22.3.

Duplication and Inversion Errors

Duplication of genetic material results from errors in replication. These may occur when a segment of DNA is copied more than once or when unequal exchange of DNA occurs between homologous chromosome pairs. The results may be a direct, or tandem, repeat or an inverted repeat of the DNA. Unequal exchange, or recombination, occurs in meiosis when homologous chromosomes do not align properly. The recombination results in a deletion for one chromosome and a duplication for the other. In either case, DNA content has been changed in both chromosomes and consequences of an unbalanced expression may occur in progeny cells.

Genetic material may also be moved from one location to another without the loss of any material. Such movements may occur within a chromosome or between chromosomes. The latter is recognized as a translocation and has been discussed. Within a chromosome, movements are usually seen as inversions (Fig. 2-15). Inversions either include the centromere (pericentric inversion) or are in one arm of the chromosome (paracentric inversion). These changes provide significant

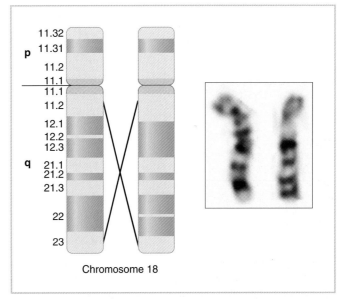

Figure 2-15. Paracentric inversions of chromosome 18: 46,inv(18), (q11.2;q23).

challenges to the chromosome during meiosis. Proper alignment of homologous chromosomes is impossible. If recombination is attempted, distribution of genetic material to gametes becomes unbalanced; some gametes may receive duplicate copies of DNA segments while others are missing these DNA segments.

Mechanisms of Inheritance   3

CONTENTS

One of the most remarkable characteristics of chromosomes is the ability to sort precisely the genetic material represented in homologous pairs of chromosomes into daughter cells and gametes, as previously discussed. This assortment is recognized through the many visible characteristics of individuals. This *phenotype*, or visible presentation of a person, is influenced by the expression of alleles at different times during development, at different efficiencies, and in different cells or tissues. Observed differences are the result of a cell's *genotype*, or molecular variation in alleles.

Mechanisms of inheritance generally refer to traits resulting from a single factor or gene, called *unifactorial inheritance*, or from the interaction of multiple factors or genes, called *multifactorial inheritance*. Because it is the simplest inheritance pattern, unifactorial inheritance is the best understood. Gregor Mendel first investigated this type of inheritance in his famous studies of garden peas in 1865. Because the underlying principles of Mendel's work became hallmarks to understanding inheritance, mechanisms of unifactorial inheritance are often called *mendelian inheritance* and the other mechanisms are referred to as *nonmendelian inheritance*.

Multifactorial inheritance is more complex because of the variation of traits within families and populations. Individual genes within a disease demonstrating multifactorial inheritance may have a dominant or recessive inheritance pattern; but when numerous nongenetic factors and genes interact to cause the disease, the mechanisms can be difficult to interpret and explain.

●●● MENDELIAN INHERITANCE

Genes are found on autosomes and sex chromosomes, and evidence for the existence of genes prior to the molecular revolution was based on measurable changes in phenotype. These changes resulted from allelic variation. Observing variation depends on the relationship of one allele to another. The terms used to describe this relationship are dominant and recessive. If only one allele of a pair is required to manifest a phenotype, the allele is *dominant*. If both alleles must be the same for a particular phenotypic expression, the allele is *recessive*. This is described by the notation AA, Aa, aa, where "A" is dominant and "a" is recessive. The AA condition is called *homozygous dominant*, Aa is called *heterozygous*, and aa is called *homozygous recessive*.

Sex chromosomes also have alleles with dominant and recessive expression. However, this situation is different because for males all X chromosome genes are expressed from the same single chromosome. Females have two X chromosomes, but the scenario is different from that of autosomes because of lyonization.

Variation in alleles results from mutations. The effects of any mutation may influence the character and function of the protein formed. Many times the mutation will create a protein with a recessive nature, but this is not always the case. Several mechanisms through which an allele can affect a function are shown in Table 3-1. These mechanisms are independent of mode of inheritance.

Autosomal Dominant Inheritance

Mendelian inheritance is classified as autosomal dominant, autosomal recessive, and X-linked (Box 3-1). A diagram representing family relationships is called a *pedigree* and can be informative about inherited characteristics. Figure 3-1 shows conventional symbols used in pedigree construction.

The family pedigree shown in Figure 3-2 has features suggesting autosomal dominant inheritance. It can be noted

TABLE 3-1. Selected Mechanisms of Allele Action

Mechanism		Example
Loss-of-function	Gene product or activity is reduced.	Waardenburg syndrome results from mutations in PAX3, a DNA binding protein important in regulating embryonic development.
Gain-of-function	Gene product is increased. Gene expression occurs at the wrong place or time. Gene product has increased activity.	Charcot-Marie-Tooth disease results from the overexpression of PMP22 (peripheral myelin protein) caused by gene duplication.
Protein alteration	Normal protein function is disrupted.	Kennedy disease results from CAG (polyglutamine) expansion at the 5′ end of the androgen receptor. The mutant protein misfolds, aggregates, and interacts abnormally with other proteins, leading to toxic gain of function and alteration of normal function.
Dominant effects of recessive mutation	Alleles are recessive at the molecular level but show a dominant mode of inheritance.	Retinoblastoma is inherited as a recessive allele. A mutation in the second, normal allele (also known as the two-hit hypothesis) results in tumor formation.

Box 3-1. EXAMPLES OF INHERITED DISORDERS

Mendelian	Nonmendelian
Autosomal dominant	Triplet repeats
Achondroplasia	Fragile X syndrome
Marfan syndrome	Myotonic dystrophy
Neurofibromatosis type 1	Spinocerebellar ataxia
Brachydactyly	Friedreich ataxia
Noonan syndrome	Synpolydactyly
Autosomal recessive	Genomic imprinting
Albinism	Prader-Willi syndrome
Cystic fibrosis	Angelman syndrome
Phenylketonuria	Mitochondrial
Galactosemia	LHON
Mucopolysaccharidoses	MERRF
X-linked dominant	MELAS
Hypophosphatemic rickets	
Orofaciodigital syndrome	
X-linked recessive	
Duchenne/Becker muscular dystrophies	
Hemophilia A and B	
Glucose-6-phosphate dehydrogenase deficiency	
Lesch-Nyhan syndrome	

senting a homozygous condition, are stillborn or die in infancy; heterozygous individuals surviving to adulthood produce fewer offspring than normal. This observation underscores an important point for many autosomal dominant disorders—two mutated alleles often have severe clinical consequences.

Characteristics of Autosomal Dominant Inheritance

Guidelines for recognizing autosomal dominant inheritance in humans may be summarized as follows:

1. The affected offspring has one affected parent, unless the gene for the abnormal effect was the result of a new mutation.
2. Unaffected persons do not transmit the trait to their children.
3. Males and females are equally likely to have or to transmit the trait to males and females.
4. The trait is expected in every generation.
5. The presence of two mutant alleles generally presents with a more severe phenotype. Detrimental dominant traits are rarely observed in the homozygous state.

Autosomal Recessive Inheritance

A gene can exist in at least two allelic forms. For the sake of simplicity, two will be considered—A and its alternative (mutant) allele, a. From these two alleles, there are three

that each affected person has at least one affected parent. Moreover, the normal children of an affected parent, when they in turn marry normal persons, have only normal offspring. In this particular instance, the mutant allele is dominant and the normal allele is recessive. In nearly all instances of dominant inheritance, as exemplified by the pedigree, one parent carries the detrimental allele and shows the anomaly, whereas the other parent is normal. The affected parent will pass on the defective dominant allele, on average, to 50% of the children. Normal children do not carry the harmful dominant allele, hence their offspring and further descendants are not burdened with the dominant trait.

There are numerous examples in humans of defective genes that are transmitted in a dominant pattern. *Achondroplasia*, a form of dwarfism, is inherited as an autosomal dominant trait. Achondroplasia is a *congenital disorder*, a defect present at birth. Affected individuals are small and disproportionate, with particularly short arms and legs. With an estimated frequency of 1 in 15,000 to 40,000 live births, achondroplasia is one of the more common mendelian disorders. Most infants affected by achondroplasia with two mutated alleles, repre-

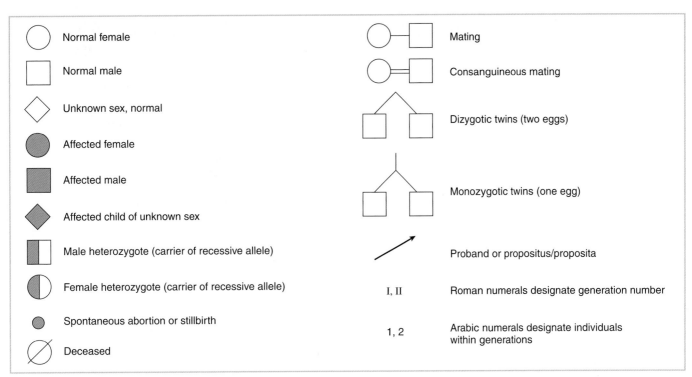

Figure 3-1. Conventional symbols used in pedigrees.

Normal female	Mating
Normal male	Consanguineous mating
Unknown sex, normal	Dizygotic twins (two eggs)
Affected female	
Affected male	Monozygotic twins (one egg)
Affected child of unknown sex	
Male heterozygote (carrier of recessive allele)	Proband or propositus/proposita
Female heterozygote (carrier of recessive allele)	I, II Roman numerals designate generation number
Spontaneous abortion or stillbirth	1, 2 Arabic numerals designate individuals within generations
Deceased	

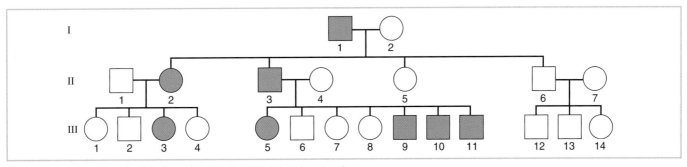

Figure 3-2. Pedigree of a family with an autosomal dominant trait.

different genotypes, AA, Aa, and aa, that can be arranged in six types of marriages. These genotypes and their offspring are listed in Table 3-2. The outcome of each type of marriage follows the mendelian principles of segregation and recombination.

In the vast majority of cases of recessive inheritance, affected persons derive from marriages of two heterozygous carriers; affected individuals receive a mutant allele from each parent and represent homozygous recessive expression. In other words, recessive disorders in family histories tend to appear only among siblings and not in their parents. This is demonstrated by the family pedigree in Figure 3-3. This pedigree shows that a normal male marries a normal woman. Apparently, both were heterozygous carriers, since one of the four children (the first child, designated II-1) exhibited the recessive trait. This son, although affected, had two normal offspring (III-1 and III-2). These two children must be carriers (Aa), having received the a allele from their father (II-1) and

the A allele from their unaffected mother (II-2). The genetic constitution of the mother (II-2) cannot be ascertained; she may be either homozygous dominant (AA) or a heterozygous carrier (Aa). The marriage of first cousins (III-3 and III-4) increases the risk that both parents of IV-1 and IV-3 have received the same detrimental recessive gene through a common ancestor. In this case, the common ancestors are the parents in generation I.

It can be deduced from this pedigree that the daughter (II-6) of the first marriage was a carrier (Aa). Her two children were normal, but it is noted that her first child (III-4) married a first cousin (III-3), and from this marriage affected children (IV-1 and IV-3) were born. Accordingly, the daughter of the third generation (III-4) must have been heterozygous, and in turn, her mother (II-6) was most likely heterozygous (or else she married a heterozygous man). Similarly, the male involved in the cousin marriage (III-3) must have been heterozygous, as was his father (II-3).

TABLE 3-2. Possible Combinations of Genotypes and Phenotypes in Parents and the Possible Resulting Offspring

| Mating Type | | Gametes | | | | Offspring | |
| | | First Parent | | Second Parent | | | |
Genotype	Phenotype	50%	50%	50%	50%	Genotype	Phenotype
AA x AA	Normal x normal	A	A	A	A	100% AA	100% Normal
AA x Aa	Normal x normal	A	A	A	a	50% AA 50% Aa	100% Normal
Aa x Aa	Normal x normal	A	a	A	a	25% AA 50% Aa 25% aa	75% Normal 25% Abnormal
AA x aa	Normal x abnormal	A	A	a	a	100% Aa	100% Normal
Aa x aa	Normal x abnormal	A	a	a	a	50% Aa 50% aa	50% Normal 50% Abnormal
aa x aa	Abnormal x abnormal	a	a	a	a	100% aa	100% Abnormal

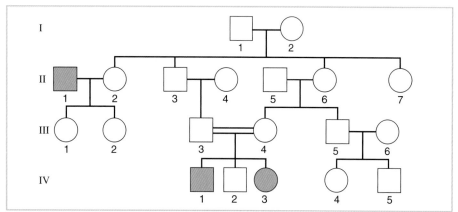

Figure 3-3. Pedigree of a family with an autosomal recessive trait.

Pedigrees of the above kind typify the inheritance of such recessively determined traits in humans as *albinism*, *cystic fibrosis*, and *phenylketonuria*. Special significance is attached to the *heterozygous carrier*—the individual who unknowingly carries the recessive allele. It is usually difficult to tell, prior to marriage, whether the individual bears a detrimental recessive allele. Thus, a recessive allele may be transmitted without any outward manifestation for several generations, continually being sheltered by the dominant normal allele. The recessive allele, however, becomes exposed when two carrier parents happen to mate, as seen in Figure 3-3. This explains cases in which a trait, absent for many generations, can suddenly appear without warning.

Often only one member in a family is afflicted with a particular disorder. In such an event, it would be an error to jump to the conclusion that the abnormality is not genetic solely because there are no other cases in the family. Without a positive family history, and sometimes the corroboration of diagnoses, the occurrence of a single afflicted individual may represent a new, sporadic mutation.

Characteristics of Autosomal Recessive Inheritance

Guidelines for recognizing autosomal recessive inheritance may be summarized as follows:

1. Most affected individuals are children of phenotypically normal parents.
2. Often more than one child in a large sibship is affected. On average, one fourth of siblings are affected.
3. Males and females are equally likely to be affected.
4. Affected persons who marry normal persons tend to have phenotypically normal children. (The probability is greater of marrying a normal homozygote than a heterozygote.)
5. When a trait is exceedingly rare, the responsible allele is most likely recessive if there is an undue proportion of marriages of close relatives among the parents of the affected offspring.

Consanguinity and Recessive Inheritance

Offspring affected with a recessive disorder tend to arise more often from consanguineous unions than from marriages of unrelated persons (see Chapter 12). Close relatives share more of the same alleles than persons from the at-large population. If a recessive trait is extremely rare, the chance is very small that unrelated marriage partners would harbor the same defective allele. The marriage of close relatives, however, increases the risk that both partners have received the same defective allele through some common ancestor. Not all alleles are equally detrimental. Stated in another way, identical alleles may produce an extreme phenotype, whereas two different alleles of the same gene may appear mild or even normal.

With increasing rarity of a recessive allele, it becomes increasingly unlikely that unrelated parents will carry the same recessive allele. With an exceedingly rare recessive disorder, the expectation is that most affected children will come from cousin marriages. Thus, the finding that the parents of Toulouse-Lautrec, a postimpressionist artist who documented bohemian nightlife, particularly at the Moulin Rouge in Paris, were first cousins is the basis for the current view that the French painter was afflicted with *pycnodysostosis*, characterized by short stature and a narrow lower jaw. This condition is governed by a rare recessive allele unlike achondroplasia, another form of short stature that is determined by a dominant allele. Thus, it was more likely that Toulouse-Lautrec suffered a rare disorder expressed as a result of his parents' relatedness rather than a common disorder that could only be explained by a new mutation.

Codominant Expression

In some heterozygous conditions, both the dominant and recessive allele phenotypes are expressed. From a molecular viewpoint, the relationship between the normal allele and the mutant allele is best described as *codominant*. This means that, at the molecular level, neither allele masks the expression of the other. An example of codominance is sickle cell anemia. In this example, two types of hemoglobin are produced: normal type hemoglobin A and a mutant form, called hemoglobin S. Another example is the expression of both A and B antigens on the surface of red blood cells in individuals with type AB blood.

The terms dominant and recessive have little, if any, utility when both gene products affect the phenotype. Dominance and recessiveness are attributes of the trait, or phenotype, *not* of the gene. An allele is *not* intrinsically dominant or recessive—only normal or mutant.

X-Linked Recessive Inheritance

No special characteristics of the X chromosome distinguish it from an autosome other than size and the genes found on the chromosome, but these features distinguish all chromosomes from each other. X chromosome inheritance, often called X-linked or sex-linked, is remarkable because there is only one X chromosome in males. Most of these alleles are therefore *hemizygous*, or present in only one copy, in the male because there is no corresponding homologous allele on the Y chromosome. Presence of a mutant allele on the X chromosome in a male is expressed, whereas in the female a single

BIOCHEMISTRY & PHYSIOLOGY

Hemoglobin

Hemoglobin is composed of *heme,* which mediates oxygen binding, and *globin,* which surrounds and protects the heme. Hemoglobin is a tetramer of globin chains (two α-chains and two β-chains in adults), each associated with a heme. There are many variants of hemoglobin. In sickle cell, the β-globin chain is a mutation and is known as hemoglobin S (HbS). A missense mutation causes valine to be placed in the protein in place of glutamic acid.

The mutation that causes HbS produces oxygenated hemoglobin that has normal solubility; however, deoxygenated hemoglobin is only about half as soluble as normal HbA. In this low-oxygen environment, HbS molecules crystallize into long fibers, causing the characteristic sickling deformation of the cell. The deformed cells, which can disrupt blood flow, are responsible for the symptoms associated with sickling crises such as pain, renal dysfunction, retinal bleeding, and aseptic necrosis of bone, and patients are at an increased risk for anemia owing to hemolysis of the sickled cells.

IMMUNOLOGY

ABO Blood Groups

There are 25 blood group systems that account for more than 250 antigens on the surface of red blood cells. The ABO blood group is one of the most important, and the antigens expressed are produced from alleles of one gene. There are three major alleles—A, B, and O—but more than 80 have been described.

The ABO gene encodes glycosyltransferases, which transfer specific sugars to a precursor protein known as the H antigen. The H antigen is a glycosphingolipid consisting of galactose, *N*-acetylglucosamine, galactose, and fructose attached to a ceramide. In the absence of sialic acid, it is a globoside rather than a ganglioside. The A allele encodes α1, 3-*N*-acetylgalactosamyl transferase, which adds *N*-acetylgalactosamine to the H antigen to form the A antigen. The B allele produces α1,3-galactosyltransferase, which transfers galactose to the H antigen, thus forming the B antigen. The O allele produces the H antigen, but it has no enzyme activity.

mutant allele may have a corresponding normal allele to mask its effects, as expected in the situation of dominance versus recessiveness.

The special features of X-linked recessive inheritance are seen in the transmission of hemophilia A (Fig. 3-4). This is a blood disorder in which a vital clotting factor (factor VIII) is lacking, causing abnormally delayed clotting. Hemophilia exists almost exclusively in males, who receive the detrimental mutant allele from their unaffected mothers. Figure 3-4 shows part of the pedigree of Queen Victoria of England. Queen Victoria (I-2) was a carrier of the mutant allele that

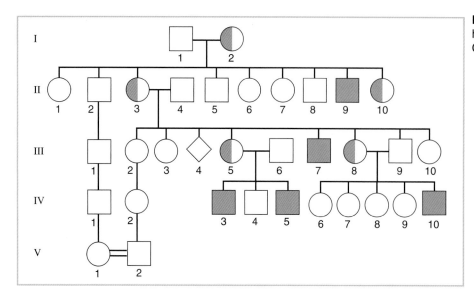

Figure 3-4. X-linked inheritance of hemophilia A among descendants of Queen Victoria (I-2) of England.

occurred either as a spontaneous mutation in her germline or was a mutation in the sperm of her father, Edward Augustus, Duke of Kent. Queen Victoria had one son (II-9) with hemophilia and two daughters (II-3 and II-10) who were carriers. The result of these children marrying into royal families in other countries spread the mutant factor VIII allele to Spain, Russia, and Germany. The children of II-3 have hemophilia in two more generations (III-7, IV-3, IV-5, and IV-10). The families of II-9 and II-10 also revealed hemophilia through two more generations (not shown). Though the grandson of III-2 married V-1, no hemophilia allele was introduced back into the family of the first son of Queen Victoria, Edward VII, and the royal family of England has remained free of hemophilia. Generation V is represented by Queen Elizabeth and Prince Philip.

For alleles on the X chromosome, each son of a carrier mother has a 50% chance of being affected by hemophilia, and each daughter has a 50% chance of being a carrier. Hemophilic females are exceedingly rare, since they can only derive from an extremely remote mating between a hemophilic man and a carrier woman. A few hemophilic women have been recorded in the medical literature; some have married and given birth to hemophilic sons.

Characteristics of X-Linked Recessive Inheritance

Guidelines for recognizing X-linked recessive inheritance may be summarized as follows:

1. Unaffected males do not transmit the disorder.
2. All the daughters of an affected male are heterozygous carriers.
3. Heterozygous women transmit the mutant allele to 50% of the sons (who are affected) and to 50% of the daughters (who are heterozygous carriers).
4. If an affected male marries a heterozygous woman, half their sons will be affected, giving the erroneous impression of male-to-male transmission.

X-Linked Inheritance and Gender

As noted, X-linked inheritance is distinguished by the presence of one chromosome in males but two in females. To explain the appearance of a condensed body in female cells, known as a *Barr body*, and to justify the possibility of twice as many X chromosome gene products in females as in males, the Lyon hypothesis was proposed. This hypothesis, which has been become well established, recognizes the Barr body in female cells as an inactivated X chromosome. Through inactivation, dosage compensation occurs in a female that generally equalizes the expression between males and females.

In general, lyonization suggests that (1) alleles found on the condensed X chromosome are inactive, (2) inactivation occurs very early in development during the blastocyst stage, and (3) inactivation occurs randomly in each blastocyst cell. Lyonization is more complicated than this simplistic presentation because some alleles are expressed only from the inactive X chromosome, other alleles escape inactivation and are expressed from both X chromosomes, and still other alleles are variably expressed. It is easiest to understand X inactivation as a random event, or that about 50% of cells have the maternal X chromosome inactivated and about 50% of cells have the paternal X chromosome inactivated; however, this situation does not always occur. It is possible to have *skewed inactivation*, whereby the X chromosome from one parent is more or less likely to become inactivated. Depending on the degree of skewing, a clinical presentation will be affected. The more extreme the skewing in favor of keeping the mutant X active, the poorer the prognosis for the individual.

The onset of X inactivation is controlled by the *XIST* gene. This gene is expressed only from the inactive X chromosome and is a key component of the X inactivation center (XIC) found at the proximal end of Xq. The cell recognizes the number of X chromosomes by the number of XICs in the cell. In the presence of two X chromosomes, *XIST* is activated and

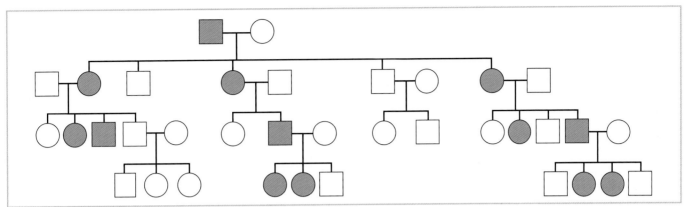

Figure 3-5. Inheritance of an X-linked dominant trait. Note that daughters always inherit the trait from an affected father whereas sons of an affected father never inherit the trait.

RNA molecules are produced that bind to regions of the X chromosome, rendering it inactive. It is not known how some genes escape the influence of the RNA molecules and remain active.

X-Linked Dominant Inheritance

Disorders resulting from X-linked dominant inheritance occur far less frequently than other forms of inheritance. As noted, X-linked recessive inheritance can occur, and males are almost always the affected gender although in very rare cases it is possible for females to acquire two mutant alleles or express milder phenotypes as carriers. With X-linked dominant inheritance, *there are no carriers;* expression of the disease occurs in both males and females, and only one mutant allele is required. As might be expected, heterozygous females may be less affected than males because of the presence of a normal, nonmutated allele. The distinguishing feature between an X-linked dominant and an autosomal disorder is that an autosomal mutation is transmitted from males and females to male and female offspring. When a mutation is located on the X chromosome and expressed in a dominant manner, females transmit the mutant allele to both male and female offspring; however, *males can only transmit it to females* (Fig. 3-5). In addition, affected females may only transmit the mutant allele to 50% of offspring; males will transmit the mutant allele to 100% of females.

Penetrance and Expressivity

Not every person with the same mutant allele necessarily manifests the disorder. When the trait in question does not appear in some individuals with the same genotype, the term *penetrance* is applied. Penetrance has a precise meaning— namely, the percentage of individuals of a specific genotype showing the expected phenotype. If the phenotype is always expressed whenever the responsible allele is present, the trait is *fully penetrant.* If the phenotype is present only in some individuals having the requisite genotype, the allele expressing the trait is *incompletely penetrant.* For a given individual, penetrance is an all-or-none phenomenon; i.e., the

phenotype is present (penetrant) or not (nonpenetrant) in that one individual. In penetrant individuals, there may be marked variability in the clinical manifestations of the disorder. When more than one individual is considered, such as a population of individuals, a percentage is usually applied to the proportion of individuals likely to express a phenotype. To illustrate this point, if a trait occurs with 80% penetrance, expression is expected in 80% of individuals with the trait.

Nonpenetrance is a cul-de-sac for clinicians and genetic counselors. Figure 3-6 demonstrates a pedigree with an autosomal dominant trait in which nonpenetrance is pervasive. Individual II-2 most likely carries the disease allele, unless offspring III-2 arose from a new dominant mutation. The future offspring III-4 is at risk for the dominant disease. The calculated mathematical risk would take into consideration the empirical penetrance percentage for the trait (say, 60%) and the probability that a person from the general population (spouse II-6) would harbor the disease allele.

Expressivity is the term used to refer to the range of phenotypes expressed by a specific genotype. This is much more frequent than nonpenetrance. A good example of expressivity is seen in neurofibromatosis (NF). NF consists of two disorders, NF1 and NF2, caused by mutations in different genes. NF is an autosomal dominant disorder, and in both

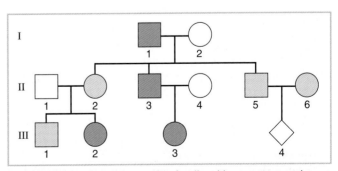

Figure 3-6. Nonpenetrance in a family with an autosomal dominant disorder. The light-colored boxes indicate individuals who do not express the phenotype for the disorder.

forms over 95% of affected individuals have café-au-lait spots. Café-au-lait spots are flat, coffee-colored macules. The expressivity of these spots, which resemble birthmarks, is variable and differs in number, shape, size, and position among individuals.

Late-Acting Genes

Proper interpretation of penetrance and expressivity may be complicated when the genes involved are expressed in the adult rather than the child. These late-acting genes include many genes involved with aging but may also include certain disease genes. *Huntington disease* is an inherited disorder characterized by uncontrollable swaying movements of the body and the progressive loss of mental function. The mutation in the gene is present at birth in all cells of the individual, but the effect of the protein is not evident until much later. The symptoms usually develop in an affected person between the ages of 30 and 45 years. Penetrance is 100%, there is no cure, and the progress of the disease is relentless, leading to a terminal state of helplessness. No therapy can significantly alter the natural progression of the disease, and there are no states of remission. Death occurs typically 12 to 15 years after the onset of the involuntary, jerky movements.

●●● NONMENDELIAN INHERITANCE

Some clinical presentations do not fit the classical patterns of mendelian inheritance and represent examples of nontraditional or nonmendelian inheritance (see Box 3-1). These include triplet repeats, genomic imprinting, mosaicism, and mitochondrial inheritance.

Triplet Repeats

The expansion of short tandem arrays of di- and trinucleotides from a few copies to thousands of copies demonstrates a new type of mutation with the potential of having profound effects on the phenotype of offspring through an unusual mode of inheritance. First demonstrated with fragile X syndrome, the expansion of triplet repeats is found in several neurologic disorders. The expansion probably occurs as a result of faulty mismatch repair or unequal recombination in a region of instability. The proximity of the region of instability to an allele is of paramount importance. Trinucleotide repeats can be found in any region of gene anatomy: the 5'-untranslated promoter region, an exon, an intron, or the 3' untranslated region of the gene. Interestingly, trinucleotide expansions in any of these regions can also result in disease (Table 3-3). The effects of location may result in a *loss of function*, as seen with fragile X syndrome. A *gain of function* is seen with amplification of CAG, resulting in polyglutamine tracts that cause neurotoxicity in several other neurodegenerative diseases. Finally, RNA can be detrimentally affected if the expansion occurs within a noncoding region. In myotonic dystrophy, the expanded transcript is unable to bind RNA proteins correctly for splicing and remains localized in the nucleus (see Chapter 8).

During normal replication, when the double helix separates into small, single-stranded regions, secondary structures can form with complementary and repeated sequences. These structures, represented as loops and hairpins, hinder the

TABLE 3-3. Neurologic Disease Due to Triplet Repeat Amplification

Location/Disorder	Chromosome Locus	Repeat	Normal Range (repeats)	Disease Range (repeats)
In the 5' Untranslated Region				
Fragile X-A	Xq27.3	CGG in *FMR*1 gene	6–54	50–1500
Fragile X-E	Xq28	CGG/CCG in *FMR2* gene	6–25	200+
Within the Translated Region of the Gene				
Spinobulbar muscular atrophy (Kennedy disease)	Xq21.3	CAG in androgen receptor gene	13–30	30–62
Huntington disease	4p16.3	CAG in *HD* gene	9–37	37–121
Spinocerebellar ataxia type 1	6p24	CAG in ataxin-1 gene	25–36	43–81
Spinocerebellar ataxia type 3 (Machado-Joseph disease)	14q	CAG in undescribed gene	13–36	68–79
Dentatorubropallidoluysian atrophy (DRPLA)	12p13.31	CAG of atrophin gene	7–23	49–88
In the 3' Untranslated Region				
Myotonic dystrophy	19q13.3	CTG of cAMP-dependent muscle protein kinase	5–37	44–3000
In an Intron				
Friedreich ataxia	9q13	GAA in the first intron of the *FRDA* gene	7–20	200–900

progression of replication by DNA polymerase. An example is (GAA)$_n$/(TTC)$_n$ expansions that bind to each other. As a result, the polymerase may dissociate either slightly or completely. If its realignment or reassociation does not occur at the exact nucleotide where it should, *DNA has slipped.* Consequently, synthesis continues, but it may "resynthesize" a short region, resulting in amplification. This amplified region distorts the helical structure of DNA—a distortion under the surveillance of mismatch repair proteins. Ordinarily, proteins stabilize the DNA not matching the template strand into a loop that can be excised followed by repair and ligation of any correct nucleotides inserted with the DNA strand. Mismatch repair is the mechanism responsible for slippage repair. Failure of the mismatch repair mechanism to remove the extra DNA does not imply a mutation of any of the repair proteins but rather an inability to adequately repair all regions involved in slippage. This suggests that triplet repeat amplification may occur through events of large slippage that overwhelm the repair system, through unequal recombination, or both. The mechanism by which DNA avoids repair during amplification is unknown.

A process known as unequal crossing-over, or recombination, may further amplify duplications. In this process, there is physical exchange of genetic material between chromosomes. During meiosis, homologous chromosomes may mispair with each synapsis. Should a crossover event occur, the DNA breaks, an exchange occurs, and the DNA ends are ligated. The resulting chromatids have gained or lost genetic material if the exchange is unequal (Fig. 3-7). For amplifications, the result is a gain of triplet repeats for one chromatid.

The presence of triplet repeats is not an abnormal condition. It is when the number of repeats reaches a threshold

Hairpin Structure

Hairpins are fundamental structural units of DNA. They are formed in a single-stranded molecule and consist of a base-paired stem structure and a loop sequence with unpaired or mismatched nucleotides. Hairpin structures are often formed in RNA from certain sequences, and they may have consequences in DNA transcription such as causing a pause in transcription or translation that results in termination.

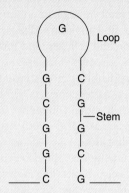

number that disease is expressed (see Table 3-3). When the number of repeats remains stable in the absence of amplification, or with limited amplification below a threshold number, a *normal* condition exists. Once amplification begins to occur, a *premutation* may exist in which some individuals, but not all, may express some symptoms. At this stage, amplification can proceed in the gametes of a premutation individual to a *full mutation* in which all individuals are

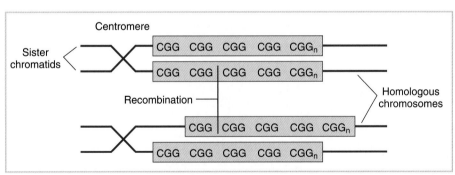

A

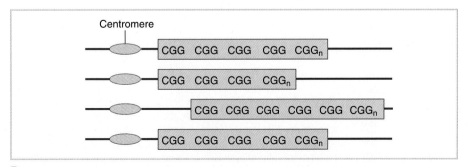

B

Figure 3-7. Unequal crossover and sister chromatid exchange. **A**, One chromatid of sister chromatids incorrectly pairs with its corresponding sister chromatid. **B**, The outcome shows one chromosome gained DNA, one lost DNA, and two remained the same.

affected. Depending on the gene affected and its chromosomal location, a triplet repeat disease may demonstrate autosomal dominant, autosomal recessive, or X-linked expression.

Unlike most X-linked or recessive disorders, the premutation phenotype presents a different clinical image than expected. Neither males nor females show any outward signs of fragile X syndrome. However, male carriers of the fragile X premutation are at a high risk for fragile X associated tremor/ataxia syndrome (FXTAS), an adult-onset neurologic disorder characterized by ataxia, intention tremor, short-term memory loss, atypical Parkinson's disease, loss of vibration and tactile sensation and reflexes, and lower limb weakness. Penetrance of this disorder increases with age. With the appearance of these features in this group of males (premutation males occur at a frequency of 1 in 813), the premutation presentation is a more common cause of tremor and ataxia in men over age 50 (1 in 3000) than are other ataxia-tremor associated disorders.

Females with premutations are also reported with FXTAS although the incidence is lower. Two additional effects seen in these females is premature ovarian failure occurring before age 40 and an increased incidence of dizygotic twins. Women with full mutations do not experience these features, just as men with full mutations have a different constellation of physical features. Approximately 22% to 28% of women in this group experience premature ovarian failure. Some studies suggest the increase in twinning may be linked more closely to premature ovarian failure than to the premutation itself.

A particularly interesting feature of triplet repeat amplification is that, in many disease presentations, the amplification is parental-specific during gametogenesis. This is the underlying cause of confusion about its mode of inheritance. For fragile X syndrome, two elements contribute to the expression of trinucleotide repeats and disease expression. First, expansions tend to occur through female meiosis I gamete formation. Second, males are more often affected than carrier females due to X chromosome inactivation. This explains why in fragile X syndrome the sons of carrier females are more affected than daughters and why offspring of carrier males do not express the disorder. The risk of mental retardation and other physical features depends on the position of an individual in a pedigree relative to a transmitting male. The daughters of normal transmitting males inherit the same regions of amplification as are present in the transmitting father.

During oogenesis in the daughter of a normal transmitting male, further amplification occurs that is inherited by sons and daughters. Because males carry only a single X chromosome, the effect is more pronounced than in females carrying two X chromosomes, one of which presumably is normal. Females are therefore obligate carriers. The reverse occurs in Huntington's disease, in which amplification occurs preferentially in meiotic transfer from the father. In either situation, a molecular explanation now exists for the observation in some neurologic disorders of an increase in disease severity through successive generations. Referred to as *genetic anticipation*, repeat amplification provided a scientific explanation to allay fears in an affected family that the disease was occurring earlier and with greater severity in successive generations because the mothers were worrying during pregnancy and beyond and somehow contributing to the disease etiology.

Genomic Imprinting

For most autosome genes, one copy is inherited from each parent and generally both copies are functionally active. There are some genes, however, whose function is dependent on the parent from whom they originated. Stated another way, allelic expression is parent-of-origin specific for some alleles. This phenomenon is known as *genomic imprinting*. Genomic imprinting differs from X chromosome inactivation in that the latter has a somewhat random nature and involves most of the chromosome. Genomic imprinting involves specific alleles on a particular chromosome.

DNA is imprinted through methylation, though the signal for initiating this process is unknown. It is a reversible form of allele inactivation. During gametogenesis, most DNA is demethylated to remove parent-specific imprints in germ cells. Remethylation then occurs on alleles specific to the sex of the parent (Fig. 3-8); some alleles are methylated specifically in the copy inherited from the father, inactivating that

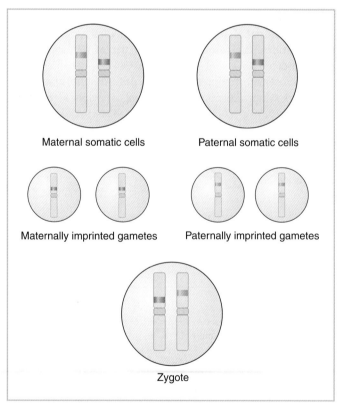

Figure 3-8. Genomic imprinting. Somatic cells have methylated alleles from a specific parent. At gamete formation, the imprint is removed and all alleles are imprinted for the sex of the parent. When gametes form a zygote, parent-specific alleles are present. Blue is a paternal imprint and pink is a maternal imprint.

copy of the gene, while others are methylated specifically in the maternally inherited copy. In females, methylation occurs prior to ovulation when oocyte development resumes. In males, imprinting in spermatogonia is less clear but probably occurs at birth when spermatogonia resume mitosis. However, it is clear that DNA methyltransferase expression in the nucleus correlates with maternal and paternal imprinting. Methylation remains throughout embryogenesis and postnatally. *The consequence of imprinting is that there is only one functional allele for these imprinted genes.* This has significant clinical implications if the functionally active allele is inactivated by mutation.

A number of clinically important genetic diseases are associated with imprinting errors. The first recognized genomic imprinting disorder was Prader-Willi syndrome. It is also the one of the most common microdeletion syndromes and involves at least 12 genes at the chromosome 15q11.2-q13 locus. At least two of these are imprinted genes depending on the parent of origin and hold special importance for Prader-Willi and Angelman syndromes: *SNRPN* and *UBE3A*, respectively. The *SNRPN* gene, producing small nuclear ribonucleoprotein N, is methylated during oogenesis but not spermatogenesis. The *UBE3A* gene, producing ubiquitin-ligase, is methylated during spermatogenesis but not oogenesis (Fig. 3-9). As a common microdeletion, or contiguous gene, syndrome, deletion of a region of the paternal chromosome 15 results in Prader-Willi syndrome because no SNRPN protein is expressed from the imprinted maternal chromosome 15 *SNRPN* allele. Likewise, deletion of the same region from the maternal chromosome 15 yields Angelman syndrome and not Prader-Willi syndrome. SNRPN protein is produced in

BIOCHEMISTRY

DNA Methylation

DNA methylation occurs by the addition of a methyl group to cytosine. With the presence of "CpG islands," or regions of adjacent cytosines and guanines in promoter regions, methylation of these cytosines is an important aspect of gene regulation. Promoter regions that are highly methylated provide fewer readily available target sites for transcription factors to bind. Therefore, methylation is associated with down-regulation of gene expression and demethylation is associated with up-regulation of gene regulation. Methylation occurs in the presence of DNA methyltransferase, which transfers a $-CH_3$ group donated by S-adenosylmethionine. The $-CH_3$ group is added to carbon 5 of cytosine and becomes 5-methylcytosine (m^5C).

Barr bodies, the physical presentation of inactive X chromosomes, are heavily methylated. Aberrant DNA methylation can lead to disease.

Angelman syndrome, but UBE3A protein is not expressed from the imprinted paternal chromosome.

Prader-Willi and Angelman syndromes occur from microdeletions in 75% to 80% of cases and can be detected by FISH analysis. However, as seen in Figure 3-9, other mechanisms exist including the possibility of mutations within the individual genes. These represent the major mutation mechanisms. Gross deletion of the promoter and exon 1 of *SNRPN* has been reported; most mutations reported in the *UBE3A* gene are nonsense mutations

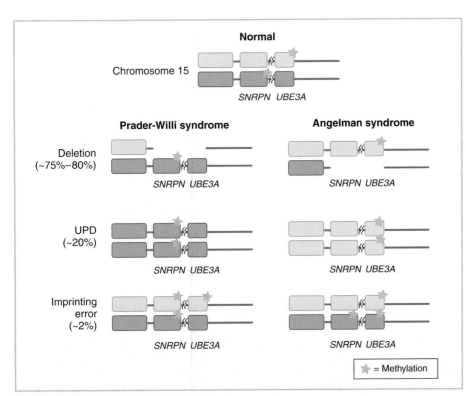

Figure 3-9. Differences between Prader-Willi and Angelman syndromes. The genes *SNRPN* and *UBE3A* are shown to demonstrate the effect of parent-specific methylation. Prader-Willi and Angelman syndromes may occur selectively from a microdeletion of chromosome 15q11.2-q13, uniparental disomy, or an imprinting error. Deletion areas contain several genes (e.g., contiguous gene sign/microdeletion). Not represented are individual gene mutations.

resulting in a nonfunctional protein. Molecular analysis with restriction enzymes can reveal changes in methylation sites. Not all chromosomes have imprinted genes. In fact, only nine chromosomes with imprinted alleles have been reported. Most of the genes that are imprinted occur in clusters and probably number only a few hundred.

Uniparental disomy (UPD) is responsible for approximately 20% of Prader-Willi and Angelman syndromes and occurs when two copies of one chromosome originated from one parent by nondisjunction. This differs from a complete hydatidiform mole, which receives an entire complement of chromosomes from one parent and is incompatible with life. When a homologous pair of chromosomes is inherited from a single parent, consequences may arise if some genes on the chromosome are imprinted and thus not expressed (see Fig. 3-9). As seen in Prader-Willi and Angelman syndromes, UPD is a factor in a significant number of cases.

Uniparental disomy occurs in Prader-Willi and Angelman syndromes when a gamete has two of the same chromosome from nondisjunction of chromosome 15. Upon fertilization, trisomy 15 occurs but fetal demise is avoided through "rescue" and loss of one of the three copies. Most of the time, normal disomy is restored. However, about a third of the time uniparental disomy occurs. Most nondisjunction occurs in maternal meiosis I. Therefore, the resulting UPD is a *heterodisomy*, or the presence of two different homologous chromosomes from a parent, rather than an *isodisomy*, or the presence of two chromosomes with identical alleles. If genomic imprinting exists on these chromosomes, genetic disease occurs. The fetus may have escaped the consequences of trisomy but not the necessity of fine regulation of gene expression.

Clinically, Prader-Willi and Angelman syndromes present quite differently. Angelman's syndrome is characterized by microcephaly, severe developmental delay and mental retardation, severe speech impairment with minimal or no use of words, ataxia, and flapping of the hands. Symptoms become apparent beginning around age 6 months and are fully evident by age 1. Because affected individuals often have a laughing, smiling facies, the term "happy puppet" was used in the past to describe them.

Prader-Willi syndrome may first be apparent in utero, where the fetus is hypotonic and displays reduced move-

ments. This hypotonia is apparent at birth; feeding may be difficult owing to a poor sucking reflex, and nasogastric feeding may be required. Between the ages of 1 and 6 years, the child develops hyperphagia, leading to morbid obesity. Individuals have short stature. Children have cognitive learning disabilities but are generally only mildly mentally retarded. Their behaviors are distinctive and characterized by tantrums, stubbornness, manipulative behaviors, and obsessive compulsiveness, such as picking at sores. Both males and females demonstrate hypogonadism and incomplete pubertal development with a high incidence of infertility. Other features include small hands and feet, almond-shaped eyes, myopia, hypopigmentation, and a high threshold for pain. Obesity can be managed by diet and exercise to yield a more normal appearance.

Mosaicism

The presence of cells with different karyotypes in the same individual is mosaicism. It arises from a mutation occurring during early development that persists in all future daughter cells of the mutated cell. If the mutation occurs early in development, more cells as well as tissues will be affected; thus, clinical presentations are generally more pronounced the earlier a mutation occurs.

Mosaicism may either be *chromosomal mosaicism* or *germline mosaicism*. With chromosomal mosaicism, the presence of an additional chromosome or the absence of a chromosome from nondisjunction will create some trisomic or monosomic cells. Monosomic cells are likely to die, but trisomic cells may persist, yielding a clinical presentation less severe than complete trisomy in which all cells have an extra chromosome. This underscores an important concept about chromosomal mosaicism: the more cells with an extra chromosome, the more severe the clinical presentation. Mosaicism may also result from a less dramatic event than nondisjunction. A new mutation may occur on a particular chromosome in some cells that persists in some tissues but not necessarily all. If the expression of the mutated gene or region of chromosome adversely affects the cells or tissues in which it is located, a more discrete effect will occur. If germ cells are not affected by chromosomal mosaicism, gametes will be normal and offspring will be unaffected. A minority of Down syndrome cases as well as many types of cancers are examples of somatic mosaicism affecting chromosomes.

In germline mosaicism, the mutation is not in somatic cells and an individual is unaware of the mutation until an affected offspring is born. All cells of the affected offspring will carry the mutation. Parental testing will not reveal the mutation unless germ cells are tested. With one affected child, the occurrence of a de novo mutation in the child or gamete cannot be distinguished from a germline mosaicism. De novo mutations are also called *spontaneous mutations*. However, the occurrence of the same mutation or condition in more than one offspring is suggestive of a parental germline mutation (Fig. 3-10). Germline mosaicism is suspected in

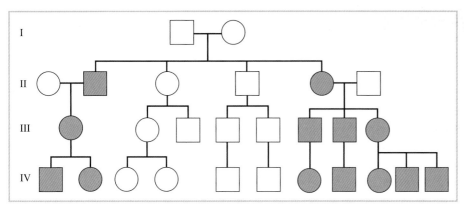

Figure 3-10. Pedigree suggesting a germline mutation in individual I-1 or I-2.

about one third of young males developing Duchenne type muscular dystrophy (see Chapter 7).

Mitochondrial Inheritance

All inheritance models, with the exception of mitochondrial inheritance, involve genes found on chromosomes in the nucleus. These genes are contributed to offspring through gametes from each parent. Mitochondria also contain DNA (mtDNA) that contributes genes to the process of cellular energy production. Mitochondria, however, are contributed to the zygote only from the maternal gamete and thus represent a maternal inheritance pattern. Females always pass mitochondrial mutations to both sons and daughters, but males never pass these mutations to their offspring (Fig. 3-11).

Human mtDNA is a circular molecule that encodes 37 gene products on 16.5 kb of DNA. There may be a few to thousands of mitochondria per cell. If all copies within a cell are the same, the cell is *homoplasmic*. In part owing to a very high sequence evolution rate, some mtDNAs may become mutated while others remain normal within the same cell. This situation in which normal and mutated mtDNAs exist in the same cell is termed *heteroplasmy*. Segregation of mtDNA during cell division is not as precise as chromosomal segregation, and daughter cells may accumulate different proportions of mutated and normal mtDNA. The random

segregation of mtDNA during mitosis may yield some cells that are homoplasmic or cells with variable heteroplasmy. For this reason, many members of the same family may have different proportions of mutated mtDNAs. Unlike nuclear chromosomal allele mutations demonstrating autosomal dominant, autosomal recessive, or X-linked inheritance, *a threshold of mutated mtDNAs is generally required before a disease results*. Typically, clinical manifestations result when the proportion of mutant mtDNA within a tissue exceeds 80%. This threshold is tissue- and mutation-dependent. As a result, there is variability in symptoms, severity, and age of onset for most mitochondrial diseases. Stated another way, both penetrance and expressivity are dependent on the degree of heteroplasmy within an individual with a mitochondrial disease.

Mitochondria are extremely important in producing ATP through oxidative phosphorylation. It may then be intuitive that those tissues with the highest energy requirements might be the most highly affected by mtDNA mutations. This also suggests that those tissues with the greatest energy demands may also have a lower threshold for mtDNA mutations (i.e., a lower proportion of heteroplasmy will result in disease). Mitochondrial diseases often involve muscle, heart, and nervous tissues and present with CNS abnormalities with or without neuromuscular degeneration. Examples of mitochondrial disease are Leber's hereditary optic neuropathy

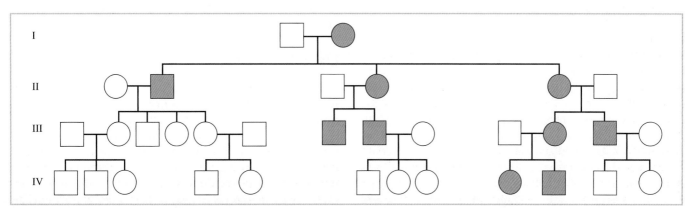

Figure 3-11. Mitochondrial inheritance. mtDNA is inherited from females only.

Box 3-2. EXAMPLES OF MULTIFACTORIAL INHERITANCE

Congenital Malformations	Adult-Onset Diseases
Cleft lip/palate	Diabetes mellitus
Congenital dislocation of the hip	Epilepsy
Congenital heart defects	Hypertension
Neural tube defects	Manic depression
Pyloric stenosis	Schizophrenia

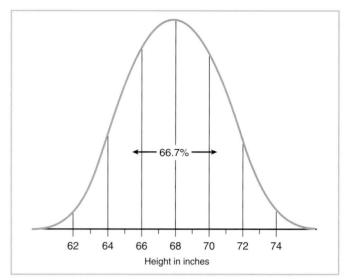

Figure 3-12. Height in adult males demonstrates a bell-shaped curve as expected for multifactorial, polygenic traits.

(LHON), mitochondrial encephalomyopathy with lactic acidosis and stroke-like episodes (MELAS), and myoclonic epilepsy and ragged red fibers (MERRF) (see Chapter 7).

It is important to point out that mitochondrial diseases have two different origins. Mutations within mtDNA lead to mitochondrial disease dependent on the degree of heteroplasmy in cells containing the mutation and exhibiting a maternal inheritance pattern. A second type of mitochondrial disease results from mutations in nuclear genes affecting the expression and function of proteins required in mitochondria. There are approximately 3000 of these proteins, and not all have been identified. The criterion for distinguishing between the two forms of mitochondrial disease is that one is maternally inherited and the other demonstrates mendelian patterns of inheritance, the latter reflecting nuclear chromosome expression. Risk to families with mitochondrial disease is different with the two modes of inheritance.

MULTIFACTORIAL INHERITANCE

Many conditions are represented by a complex interaction of several to many genes, and environmental factors may also influence their expression. Individual alleles in this complex interaction may individually demonstrate any of the mendelian or nonmendelian inheritance patterns previously discussed. However, the expression of these individual alleles is dependent on other alleles and factors. Therefore, the understanding of these types of interactions and the diseases demonstrating *multifactorial inheritance* is quite complex (Box 3-2). Several examples will be discussed briefly to demonstrate the principles of multifactorial inheritance. A more detailed discussion of diabetes will ensue to illustrate a disease with genetic and nongenetic influences that affects millions of individuals each year.

Phenotypic Distribution

Many genes influence phenotypes such as height and weight. As a result, the distribution of the many phenotypes demonstrated by multifactorial inheritance is expected to form a bell-shaped curve. For example, the normal curve of distribution of heights of fully grown males is shown in Figure 3-12. The average, or *mean*, is 68 inches, with a *standard deviation* of 2.6 inches. Standard deviation (SD) is a measure of the variability of a population. Briefly, if a given population is normally distributed, then approximately two thirds of the population lies within 1 SD on either side of the mean—in this case, 68 − 2.6 and 68 + 2.6, or between 65.4 and 70.6 inches. Ninety-five percent of the individuals, or 19 in 20, may be expected to fall within the limits set by 2 SD on either side of the mean. Exceptionally short people (<62.8 inches) and exceptionally tall people (>73.2 inches) occupy the extreme limits of the curve.

The bell-shaped distribution characterizes traits such as height and weight in which there is *continuous variation between one extreme and the other*. In regard to height, those at the extremes of the curve—the exceedingly short and the exceptionally tall—are not generally recognized as having a disorder. An exceptionally tall person is not judged as having a clinical condition! In certain other situations, however, those individuals at the tail of the distribution curve are potential candidates for a congenital disorder such as spina bifida. The point in the distribution curve beyond which there is a risk that a particular disorder will emerge is called the *threshold level* (Fig. 3-13). All individuals to the left of the threshold level are not likely to have the disorder and those to the right of the threshold value are predisposed to the disorder.

Liability and Risk

The term liability expresses an individual's genetic predisposition toward a disorder and also the environmental circumstances that may precipitate the disorder. As an analogy, in the case of an infectious disease, an individual's susceptibility to a virus or bacterium depends on inherent immunologic defenses, but the liability includes also the degree of exposure to the infective agent. In the absence of exposure to an infectious virus or bacterium, the genetically vulnerable person does not become ill. Likewise, in spina

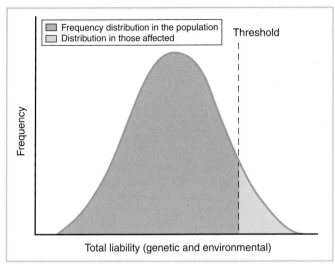

Figure 3-13. The threshold level is shown for the continuous variation of a multifactorial, polygenic trait.

bifida, a strong genetic predisposition renders the fetus susceptible or at a risk, but the intrauterine environment may turn the risk into the reality of the disorder. Environmental influences are thus superimposed on the polygenic determinants for high risk. A condition such as spina bifida or cleft palate is often referred to as a *multifactorial trait*, since it results from the interaction of both genetic factors involving multiple genes and environmental agents.

The greater the number of risk genes possessed by the parents, the greater the probability that they will have an affected child. It also follows that the larger the number of risk genes in an affected child, the higher the probability that a sib will be affected. As a general rule, the closer the relationship, the greater the number of genes that are shared. Table 3-4 shows the proportion of genes that relatives have in common. A parent and child share 50% of their genes, since the child receives half of his or her genes from a single parent.

TABLE 3-4. Family Relationships and Shared Genes

Relationship to a Given Subject	Proportion of Genes in Common (Coefficient of Relationship, *r*)
Identical twin	1
Fraternal twin	1/2
First-degree relatives	1/2
Parent-child	
Siblings	
Second-degree relatives	1/4
Grandparent-grandchild	
Uncle-nephew	
Aunt-niece	
Third-degree relatives	1/8
First cousins	

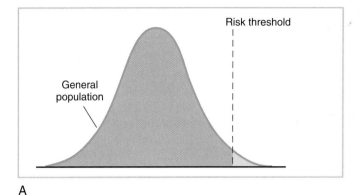

A

B

C

D

Figure 3-14. Risk factors and therefore the risk threshold for relatives increase with degree of relatedness.

Figure 3-14 illustrates the liabilities of a disorder determined by many genes, with a population incidence of 0.005, for relatives; the risk factors for relatives are respectively 1, 5, and 10 times the general incidence. On average, 50% of the genes of first-degree relatives (parents, children, and siblings) are shared with the affected individuals. The mean of the distribution for first-degree relatives is shifted to the right. Thus, first-degree relatives have more risk genes than does the general population, and the incidence of the disorder among first-degree relatives can be expected to be higher than in the general population. The distribution of second-degree relatives is also shifted to the right, but in a direction less than that of first-degree relatives. Third-degree relatives exhibit a distribution curve that tends to approximate that of the general population. Although first cousins do not share as many genes as first-degree relatives, the risk of a polygenically determined disorder is higher when the parents are first cousins than when they are unrelated.

Risk and Severity

The risk to relatives varies directly with the severity of the condition in the proband. Individuals with the more severe cases possess a higher number of predisposing genes and accordingly tend to transmit greater numbers of risk genes. For example, for cleft lip, if the child has unilateral cleft, the risk to subsequent siblings is 2.5%. If the child has bilateral cleft lip and palate, the sibling risk rises to 6%. In the most severe cases, the individual is at the extreme tip of the tail of the curve, having inherited a vast number of predisposing genes.

Gender Differences

Both anencephaly and spina bifida occur more frequently in females than in males. Anencephaly has a male to female ratio of 1 to 2, while spina bifida approximates a male to female ratio of 3 to 4. This suggests that there are sex-specific thresholds.

Children of affected females with pyloric stenosis are more likely to be born with the pyloric stenosis than children of affected males. The threshold value for the *female who is affected* is shifted to the left, with the consequence that the affected female possesses a large quantity of predisposing genes required for the expression of the disorder. The affected female imposes a greater risk to relatives, particularly to the male child or sibling, because of the larger number of predisposing genes. The threshold level of the male is closer to the population mean than that of the female. Strange as it may seem, the less frequently affected sex, or the female, in the case of pyloric stenosis, transmits the condition more often to the more frequently affected sex, or the male in this example.

Environmental Factors

Neural tube defects are multifactorial traits, reflecting a genetic predisposition that is polygenic, with a threshold beyond which individuals are at risk of developing the malformation if environmental factors also predispose. We are largely ignorant of the predisposing environmental triggers. We do know that the dietary intake of folic acid by women tends to protect their fetuses against neural tube defects.

BIOCHEMISTRY

Folic Acid

Folic acid is a vitamin, a water-soluble precursor to tetrahydrofolate. It plays a key role in one-carbon metabolism and the transfer of one-carbon groups. This makes it essential for purine and pyrimidine biosynthesis as well as for the metabolism of several amino acids. It is also important for the regeneration of S-adenosylmethionine, known as the "universal methyl donor."

Folate deficiency is also the most common vitamin deficiency in the United States. The classic deficiency syndrome is megaloblastic anemia. However, the group most likely to be deficient in folate is women of childbearing age, whose deficiency should be treated. Folic acid prevents neural tube defects and is recommended for all women prior to conception and throughout pregnancy in doses ranging from 0.4 to 4.0 mg per day.

Characteristics of Multifactorial Inheritance

The unique characteristics of multifactorial inheritance as they pertain to certain congenital conditions are as follows:

1. The greater the number of predisposing risk genes possessed by the parents, the greater the probability that they will have an affected child.
2. Risk to relatives declines with increasingly remote degrees of relationship.
3. Recurrence risk is higher when more than one family member is affected.
4. Risk increases with severity of the malformation.
5. Where a multifactorial condition exhibits a marked difference in incidence with sex, the less frequently affected sex has a higher risk threshold and transmits the condition more often to the more frequently affected sex.

Diabetes

Diabetes mellitus (DM) is an example of a complex disease that is not a single pathophysiologic entity but rather several distinct conditions with different genetic and environmental etiologies. Two major forms of DM have been distinguished: insulin-dependent diabetes mellitus (IDDM), or type 1, and non-insulin-dependent diabetes mellitus (NIDDM), or type 2. A difference between these types is whether endogenous insulin is available to reduce glucose and prevent ketoacidosis, as in NIDDM, or whether exogenous insulin is required, as in IDDM.

IDDM has been referred to by obsolete expressions such as "juvenile-onset diabetes," "ketosis-prone diabetes," and "brittle diabetes." NIDDM has been called "maturity-onset diabetes," "ketosis-resistant diabetes," and "stable diabetes." NIDDM is the more prevalent type, comprising 80% of the cases. IDDM is predominantly a disease of whites or populations with an appreciable white genetic admixture. In the United States, the prevalence of IDDM is about 1 in 400 by age 20. The mean age of onset is approximately 12 years.

BIOCHEMISTRY

Insulin

Insulin is produced by the β-cells of the pancreatic islets of Langerhans, which are found predominantly in the tail of the pancreas. Insulin is translated as preproinsulin and cleaved to proinsulin in the endoplasmic reticulum. During Golgi packaging, proteases cleave the proinsulin protein, yielding C peptide and two other peptides that become linked by disulfide bonds. This latter structure is mature insulin. C peptide has no function but is a useful marker for insulin secretion, since these should be present in a 1:1 ratio. Because the liver removes most insulin, measurements of C peptide reflect insulin measurements.

Insulin secretion is initiated when glucose binds to GLUT2 glucose transporter receptors on the surface of β-cells and the glucose is transported into the cell, thereby stimulating glycolysis. The increase in ATP or ATP/ADP inhibits the ATP-sensitive membrane K^+ channels, causing depolarization and leading to the activation of voltage-gated Ca^{++} membrane channels. Calcium influx leads to exocytosis and release of insulin from secretory granules into the blood.

In addition to this primary pathway, the phospholipase C and adenyl cyclase pathways can also modulate insulin secretion. For example, glucagon stimulates insulin via the adenylyl cyclase pathway by elevating cAMP levels and activating protein kinase A. Somatostatin, however, inhibits insulin release by inhibiting adenylyl cyclase.

PHARMACOLOGY

Insulin Therapy

First-line therapy for type 2 diabetes (NIDDM) are "insulin sensitizers" such as the thiazolidinediones and metformin. Insulin is used when this first approach fails to completely resolve the situation. Exogenous insulin, used for type 1 diabetes mellitus (IDDM) and NIDDM, can be administered intravenously or intramuscularly. For long-term treatment, subcutaneous injection is the predominant method of administration.

Several aspects of subcutaneous injection of insulin differ from its physiologic secretion. The kinetics of the injected form of insulin does not parallel the normal response to nutrients. Insulin from injection also diffuses into the peripheral circulation instead of being released into the portal circulation. Preparations are classified by duration of action: short, intermediate, or long-acting.

- Short: lasts 4 to 10 hours (insulin lispro/insulin aspart, regular)
- Intermediate: lasts 10 to 20 hours (insulin)
- Long-acting: lasts 20 to 24 hours (insulin glargine)

The two broad categories of DM are separable on the basis of several observations, such as mean age of onset, the association with certain genes within the major histocompatibility complex (MHC), the presence of circulating islet-cell antibodies, and the predisposition of β-cells to destruction by certain viruses and chemicals. Evidence supports the view that early-onset IDDM is a genetic autoimmune disease in which insulin-producing β-cells of the pancreas are ultimately and irreversibly self-destroyed by autoreactive T lymphocytes. NIDDM and IDDM are genetically distinct, inasmuch as NIDDM is not known to be associated with any particular HLA haplotype.

Family Studies

NIDDM tends to be familial—i.e., it "runs in families." Most studies show that at least one third the offspring of NIDDM parents will exhibit diabetes or abnormalities in glucose intolerance in late life. Specifically, the prevalence of NIDDM among children of NIDDM parents is 38%, compared with only 11% among normal controls. *In sharp contrast*, familial aggregation of IDDM is *uncommon*. The usual finding in family studies is that 2% to 3% of the parents and 7% of the siblings of a proband with IDDM have diabetes (Table 3-5). Stated another way, the likelihood that a parent with IDDM will have a child with IDDM is only 2% to 3%. If one child has IDDM, the average risk that a second child will have IDDM is only 7%.

Children of a diabetic father have a greater liability to IDDM than children of a diabetic mother. By the age of 20, 6.1% of the offspring of diabetic fathers had diabetes, whereas only 1.3% of the offspring of diabetic mothers had the disease. Hence, IDDM is transmitted less frequently to the

TABLE 3-5. Lifetime Risk of IDDM in First-degree Relatives*

Relative	Risk (%)
Parent	2.2 ± 0.6
Children	5.6 ± 2.8
Siblings	6.9 ± 1.3
HLA nonidentical sib	1.2
HLA haploidentical sib	4.9
HLA identical sib	15.9
Identical twin	30–40
General population	0.3

Data from Harrison LC. Risk assessment, prediction and prevention of type 1 diabetes. *Pediatr Diabetes*. 2001;2(2):71–82.
*When diagnosed in the proband before age 20 years.

ANATOMY

Pancreas

The pancreas is a retroperitoneal organ except for the tail, which projects into the splenorenal ligament. It is an exocrine gland and produces digestive enzymes. It is also an endocrine gland and produces insulin and glucagon. The main pancreatic duct joins the bile duct, which runs through the head of the pancreas, to form the hepatopancreatic ampulla that enters the duodenum.

offspring of diabetic mothers than to those of diabetic fathers. The mechanism responsible for the preferential transmission is not clear.

In essence, the low incidence of hereditary transmission of IDDM suggests the intervention of one or more critical environmental insults. One hypothesis suggests that IDDM requires two hits, analogous to the two hits required in the development of some cancers. The first hit is an infection, and the second hit is the selection of self-reactive T cells, which is influenced genetically through the MHC. The incisive questions are: What are the nongenetic (environmental) factors that trigger IDDM, and how do they interact with the genetic factors?

Monozygotic Twin Studies

To elucidate the role of genetic and environmental factors in the etiology of diabetes, pairs of identical (monozygotic) twins have been studied. Theoretically, if diabetes is influenced strongly by inherited factors and one identical twin manifests the disease, the other would be expected to display the disease. The extent of genetic involvement is estimated from the degree of *concordance* (both twins developing diabetes) as opposed to *discordance* (only one twin developing diabetes).

In a study of 100 pairs of identical twins for NIDDM, it was found that when one twin of a pair developed diabetes after age 50, the other twin developed the disease within several years in 90% of cases. Thus, older (i.e., > 50 years) identical twins are usually concordant for NIDDM. The very high concordance rate for late-onset NIDDM is impressive in that the diabetic condition arises at a time when twins usually live apart and ostensibly share fewer environmental factors than during early childhood. The twin studies support the hypothesis that NIDDM is determined primarily by genetic factors.

On the other hand, when one twin developed the disease before age 40, the other twin developed the disease in only half the cases. Accordingly, younger (i.e., <40 years) identical twins are 50% discordant for IDDM—i.e., if one has IDDM, the other does not and shows no signs of becoming so in half the cases. These findings demonstrate that genetic factors are predominant in NIDDM, and additional factors, presumably environmental, are required to trigger IDDM.

HLA Studies

Studies in several laboratories have revealed a strong association between IDDM and HLA antigens at the DR locus of the MHC. The major antigens conferring enhanced risk to IDDM are DR3 and DR4. Indeed, 95% of white patients with IDDM express either DR3 or DR4, or both. Individuals who express both DR3 and DR4 antigens are at the highest risk, whereas DR2 and DR5 expression is uncommon in IDDM. The DR3 and DR4 alleles are *not in themselves* diabetogenic but, rather, are *markers* for the true susceptibility allele in the HLA region.

The DQ locus consists of two tightly linked genes: DQA1 and DQB1. These encode α- and β-chains. Both loci are highly polymorphic. There are 8 and 15 major allelic variations in DQA1 and DQB1, respectively. Alleles at both loci demonstrate susceptibility to IDDM. Certain DQ alleles that are usually inherited in conjunction with DR3 and DR4 are recognized as prime susceptibility alleles. In white patients, DR3 and DR4 are almost universally associated with the DQB1*0302 and DQB1*0201 antigens.

It is clear that both HLA-DQA1 and HLA-DQB1 alleles are important in establishing a susceptibility to diabetes. DQA1*0501-DQB1*0201 and DQA1*0301-DQB1*0302 haplotypes, representing closely linked markers that are inherited together, confer the highest risk for IDDM. In combination, their effect is even stronger than that observed for individuals homozygous for DQA1*0501-DQB1*0201 or DQA1*0301-DQB1*0302, suggesting that heterodimers formed from gene products in *trans* conformation (i.e., DQA1*0501 and DQB1*0302) may be particularly diabetogenic. Other DQ haplotypes conferring a high risk for IDDM include DQA1*0301-DQB1*0201 among blacks, DQA1*0301-DQB1*0303 in the Japanese, and DQA1*0301-DQB1*0401 in the Chinese. The DQA1*0102-DQB1*0602

ANATOMY & EMBRYOLOGY

Twins and Fetal Membranes

Monozygotic (MZ) twins are identical twins that originate from one zygote, a process that usually begins during the blastomere stage. Dizygotic (DZ) twins are fraternal twins that originate from two zygotes.

The type of placenta depends on when twinning occurs. Most MZ twins have monochorionic-diamniotic placentas (65% to 70%). If twinning occurs later (9 to 12 days after fertilization), then monochorionic-monoamniotic placentation may occur, but this is rare (1%). In this latter case, twin-to-twin transfusion syndrome can occur. If twinning occurs after day 12, separation is incomplete and conjoined twins are the result.

DZ twins have dichorionic-diamniotic placentas, most of which are separate (60%). If implantation sites are close, placentas may fuse (40%). Since DZ twins occur more frequently than MZ twins, the most prevalent placentation is dichorionic-diamniotic.

IMMUNOLOGY

Human Leukocyte Antigens

Human leukocyte antigens (HLAs) are alloantigens important for maintaining tolerance, and they serve as antigen-presenting receptors for T lymphocytes. HLA genes are clustered on chromosome 6p. Class I proteins such as HLA-A, HLA-B, and HLA-C are each independent allele products. Class II proteins such as HLA-D (DP, DQ, DR) are formed from admixing maternal and paternal allele products. Each person has one haplotype from each parent.

haplotype is protective and is associated with a reduced risk for IDDM in most populations.

Autoimmunity

IDDM is an autoimmune disease. Sera from newly diagnosed IDDM patients contain an antibody that reacts with the β-cells in the islets of Langerhans taken from normal, nondiabetic individuals. IDDM represents the culmination of a slow process of immune destruction of insulin-producing β-cells (Fig. 3-15) and is also classified as an HLA-associated autoimmune disease.

What triggers the production of antibodies against the pancreatic β-cells? A promising hypothesis is that the antibody is the remnant of an immune response to components of the islet cells that were altered or damaged by viruses. An intriguing association suggests a viral triggering event from the observation that 20% of all children with congenital rubella—primarily those who are DR3-positive or DR4-positive—become diabetic later in life. This form of diabetes may be a consequence of the widespread effects of congenital rubella on the immune system.

Whatever triggering event may be operative, it is clear that destruction of insulin-producing cells is a slowly developing process, not an acute one. There is definitive evidence that T lymphocytes are the major determinants of this process. Essentially then, the current popular theory of the pathogenesis of IDDM encompasses β-cell damage by a foreign viral antigen, activation of the immune system, and the subsequent induction of autoimmunity directed against the β-cells.

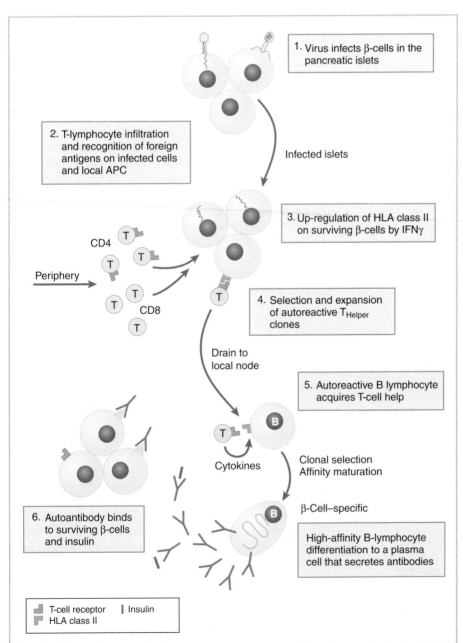

1. Virus infects β-cells in the pancreatic islets

2. T-lymphocyte infiltration and recognition of foreign antigens on infected cells and local APC

Infected islets

3. Up-regulation of HLA class II on surviving β-cells by IFNγ

CD4

Periphery

CD8

4. Selection and expansion of autoreactive T_Helper clones

Drain to local node

5. Autoreactive B lymphocyte acquires T-cell help

Cytokines

Clonal selection
Affinity maturation

β-Cell–specific

6. Autoantibody binds to surviving β-cells and insulin

High-affinity B-lymphocyte differentiation to a plasma cell that secretes antibodies

T-cell receptor   Insulin
HLA class II

Figure 3-15. Process depicting destruction of insulin-producing β-cells in a hypothetical model of viral-induced islet cell autoimmunity. Infection of the pancreatic islet by a virus (e.g., coxsackie B4 or cytomegalovirus) may lead to a robust intra-islet T lymphocyte-mediated response. As a result of T lymphocyte infiltration, local inflammation, and/or IFN secretion, induction of HLA class II expression on the β cell is enhanced, leading to the selection of T lymphocyte clones. Through mimicry, reactivation of these T lymphocyte clones occurs when antigen-presenting, auto-reactive B lymphocytes capture and present specific β-cell antigens released from the damaged islet. The specific B/T lymphocyte interaction provides co-stimulation and avoids anergic deactivation of auto-reactive B cells. As these clones survive and expand, islet-specific auto-antibodies accumulate in the circulating immunoglobulin pool. This view is supported by studies of high-risk subjects showing that antibodies to candidate auto-antigens may exist long before disease develops. The presence of islet immunity, however, does not necessarily imply loss of β-cell function. (Courtesy of Dr. Ronald Garner, Mercer University School of Medicine.)

Several studies have identified susceptibility genes for diabetes. As noted, IDDM is associated with the HLA region of chromosome 6. For NIDDM, which is the most prevalent form of diabetes, several susceptibility genes have been identified in different groups including Mexican Americans, an isolated Swedish population living in Bosnia, Pima Indians in the southwest United States, and Utah families of European descent. Each of these studies identified different genes specific to that population. These data suggest that different combinations of susceptibility genes have different effects within populations and increase the incidence of disease within individuals and populations.

Molecular Mimicry

There is evidence that a defect in the expression of HLA-directed class II molecules may establish the conditions for autoimmune disease. Class II molecules, which enable T cells to perceive antigen, are normally expressed on antigen-presenting cells that interact with helper T cells—namely, dendritic cells, macrophages, and B cells. The usual inability of nonlymphoid cells, such as pancreatic cells, to express class II surface markers apparently serves as protection against autoimmunity, preventing nonlymphoid cells from presenting

their own proteins as antigens. If pancreatic cells were to express class II molecules inadvertently, they could cause an autoimmune response via T cells.

What triggers the expression of class II antigens in the pancreatic cells? A promising hypothesis is that the production of class II molecules is the consequence of an immune response to pancreatic cells, specifically to islet β-cells, that have been altered or damaged by viruses. A viral infection insult activates, in some manner vaguely understood, the pancreatic cells to express class II molecules (see Fig. 3-15). A plausible scenario is that a viral protein shares appreciable amino acid sequences with a pancreatic islet protein—an instance of molecular mimicry.

When the pancreatic cells are abnormally triggered to express class II molecules, they can then present their antigens to helper T cells, just like macrophages. Stated another way, the pancreatic cell protein receptor alongside the class II molecule forms a functional unit capable of interacting with helper T cells. The outcome is a large-scale activation of T cells and a cascade of effects that include the production of circulating antibodies by plasma cells specifically directed against the surface receptors on the pancreatic B cells and other components.

Viruses may be only one of many triggering agents of IDDM. Other environmental insults such as drugs and toxic chemicals might similarly damage β-cells and give rise to diabetes. In experimental animals, drugs such as alloxan and streptozotocin can induce diabetes by destroying β-cells. In 1975, a rodent poison known as Vacor, which has a molecular structure resembling that of streptozotocin, was introduced in the United States. It was accidentally ingested by a number of people, several of whom developed acute diabetes with clear evidence of β-cell destruction. Not all of these people developed diabetes, indicating that the environmental insult interacts with a complex genetic background, which can be protective.

NIDDM

As stated earlier, NIDDM has a greater genetic component than does IDDM in that concordance for IDDM among monozygotic twins approaches 100%. Yet environmental factors also play a role; ironically, environmental factors are better known in IDDM than in NIDDM.

NIDDM most often occurs in individuals who are over age 40 and overweight. Obesity facilitates expression of the genetic predisposition to NIDDM. The changes in lifestyle that result in both obesity and NIDDM are vividly exemplified by the urbanization of the Pima Native Americans of Arizona. The exceptionally high prevalence of NIDDM among the Pima (affecting 50% of the adult population) reflects a modern change in dietary pattern from low caloric intake, in which both obesity and diabetes were rare, to caloric abundance, in which both clinical conditions are common.

The susceptibility gene among the Pima Indians is calpain-10, a protease that regulates the function of other proteins. It is composed of 15 exons and undergoes differential splicing

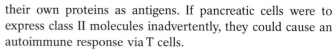

to form at least 8 different proteins expressed in a tissue-specific manner. Calpain-10 is found only in pancreatic islet cells. A specific A-to-G mutation in an intron 3, referred to as UCSNP-43 (for University of Chicago single nucleotide polymorphism 43), increases the risk for diabetes. Two other mutations, UCSNP-19 in intron 6 and UCSNP-63 in intron 13, also affect risk. Two mutated UCSNP-43 alleles and two different alleles at the other two sites are associated with the greatest risk for developing diabetes. The presence of two different DNA sequences at three sites in the same gene allows for eight different combinations of sequences. It is hypothesized that these alterations affect expression in different tissues: the UCSNP-43 alleles alter calpain-10 expression in the pancreas and the other alleles affect expression in muscle or fat cells.

Pima Indians with two UCSNP-43 mutations but without diabetes produced 53% less calpain-10 mRNA in muscle. These same individuals have a lower metabolism and increased insulin resistance suggestive of mild diabetes, characteristics that also increase obesity. Calpain-10 itself does not cause diabetes, but it does interact with other factors such as diet and exercise to cause diabetes. These mutations have also been found in other populations and when present increase the risk for diabetes.

Restriction endonuclease analyses of the insulin gene and an adjacent large, "hypervariable" region proximal (5′) to the gene itself have revealed an array of mutational events, but thus far it has been difficult to associate most known nucleotide changes with specific physiologic mechanisms. It can be asserted that the risk for transmission of NIDDM is greater than that for IDDM because of the need of an environmental stress or insult to the B cells. For first-degree relatives, the risk is 10% to 15%; the risk of impaired glucose tolerance, which is the usual precursor of NIDDM, is 20% to 30%. A good case can be made for periodic screening of first-degree relatives with oral glucose tolerance tests: those with impaired tolerance should be advised to maintain ideal body weight. In a minority, but significant percentage, of families, NIDDM occurs without the precondition of obesity. In those families, NIDDM is probably caused by a different mechanism.

Maturity-onset Diabetes of the Young

A small subset, representing about 2% to 5% of individuals with diabetes, have maturity-onset diabetes of the young (MODY). As the oxymoronic name suggests, this form of disease resembles "normal" NIDDM but can be present in young adulthood, usually occurring before age 25 as opposed to after age 40. MODY is transmitted as an autosomal dominant disease with high penetrance; 50% of the offspring of an affected parent exhibit at the least impaired glucose tolerance, which usually progresses to frank, but often mild, diabetes. The symptoms of MODY are quite variable, reflecting its genetic heterogeneity.

MODY, characterized by defects in pancreatic β-cell function, is caused by mutations in at least six genes representing six MODY types (Table 3-6). Five of these are transcription factors, and mutations in all six genes are loss-of-function mutations. Seventy-five percent of cases of MODY are caused by transcription factor mutations. The most common form, MODY3, representing 69% of cases, is caused by mutations in a transcription factor (TCF1) gene that regulates expression of several liver genes, including the hepatic nuclear factor–1α (HNF-1α) protein. The second most common presentation is MODY2, caused by mutations in the glucokinase (GCK) gene. For these individuals, glucose levels may be elevated to twice normal, whereas patients with mutations in HNF-1α may have glucose levels increased up to five times normal (Fig. 3-16).

Gestational Diabetes

Finally, diabetes may also develop during pregnancy from an unknown cause. Gestational diabetes occurs in approximately 4% of all pregnancies and usually resolves after pregnancy. Insulin resistance is thought to occur as a result of hormone levels during pregnancy. Symptoms generally occur in the second half of pregnancy and are characterized by fatigue resulting from a lack of glucose in tissues.

If untreated, maternal hyperglycemia is harmful to the developing fetus. Since insulin does not cross the placenta and glucose does, the fetal pancreas responds by increasing insulin secretion. Extra glucose is stored and is responsible for the large size of newborns, a condition known as *macrosomia.*

TABLE 3-6. Comparison of MODY Types

MODY Type	Gene	Protein	Protein Function*	Mutation Effect	Prevalence
1	HNF4α	Hepatocyte nuclear factor–4α	Transcription factor		
2	GCK	Glucokinase	Phosphorylates glucose		Common
3	TCF1	Hepatic nuclear factor–1α	Transcription factor		Most common
4	IPF1	Insulin promoter factor–1	Transcription factor	Loss of function	
5	TCF2	Hepatic nuclear factor–1β	Transcription factor		
6	NEUROD1	Neurogenic differentiation factor–1	Transcription factor		

*Each of these transcription factors is involved in the regulation of the insulin gene through a complex process affecting the gene directly or through regulation of each other. Thus, mutations decrease transcription, leading to increased blood glucose. Ultimately, complete β-cell failure occurs.

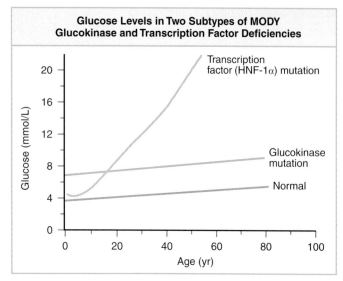

Figure 3-16. MODY3 (HNF-1α) and MODY2 (glucokinase) cause more than 80% of maturity-onset diabetes of the young. Glucose is elevated in both types but may be dramatically increased in MODY3. (Redrawn with permission of The American Diabetes Association from Pearson ER, Velho G, Clark P, et al. β-Cell genes and diabetes: quantitative and qualitative difference in the pathophysiology of hepatic nuclear factor-1α and glucokinase mutations. *Diabetes* 2001;50(1):S101–S107.)

Newborns subsequently suffer from hypoglycemia because of elevated insulin and have an increased risk of perinatal mortality and morbidity. This must be corrected to prevent mental retardation and other signs of failure to thrive. These infants are at an increased risk for breathing problems. They also have an increased risk of later developing obesity and NIDDM. Similarly, up to 50% of the mothers of these infants will develop NIDDM. In addition, the risk of a mother experiencing gestational diabetes in future pregnancies is 67%. Clearly, there are many aspects to diabetes that result from a complex interaction between genetic factors and nongenetic factors.

Genetics of Metabolic Disorders 4

CONTENTS

It is an accepted tenet that an inheritable change of an allele reveals itself as a modification in the structure and function of that specific allele product. Often these products are proteins, but modifications can also affect mRNAs in ways that are not reflected in the protein; they may also occur in tRNAs, rRNAs, and other less well recognized RNAs. Modifications in protein structure result from any of the mechanisms presented in Chapter 1, with effects ranging from benign to an inactive or absent protein. Even a single amino acid replacement in a protein may have important clinical consequences, as evidenced by sickle-cell hemoglobin (see Chapter 6). Both structural proteins and enzymes are subject to these alterations; however, many of the earliest described inherited anomalies were biochemical defects, or *inborn errors of metabolism*, resulting from enzymatic deficiencies. The consequence of an enzyme deficiency is the direct impairment of a specific metabolic pathway. Many of these have been characterized and are responsible for the appearance of metabolic disease.

Metabolic disorders represent an expansive literature. There are several logical ways to group these disorders. Although most metabolic diseases are rare, this chapter presents selective disorders that are most familiar to students and practitioners because they represent classical studies of disease or disorders commonly tested for in newborn screening. They include selected amino acidopathies, a carbohydrate metabolic disorder, and several organic acidemias. Additional disorders, such as lysosomal storage disorders and cystinuria, are presented in other chapters more appropriate to the defect or clinical presentation.

● ● ● HISTORICAL PERSPECTIVE

The first example of recessive inheritance occurred in patients excreting "black urine." From an analysis of family histories, Archibald Garrod concluded that this anomaly, known as *alkaptonuria*, appeared when affected children inherited one defective gene from each parent. He later theorized that the defective gene prevented the formation of a particular enzyme. As seen in Figure 4-1, the normal allele specifies the synthesis of the enzyme that converts homogentisic acid to acetoacetic acid. In an alkaptonuric individual, the enzyme is absent or deficient and homogentisic acid accumulates, since its conversion to acetoacetic acid is blocked or reduced. The excess homogentisic acid is then eliminated in urine. Urine containing homogentisic acid, on exposure to air, gradually darkens.

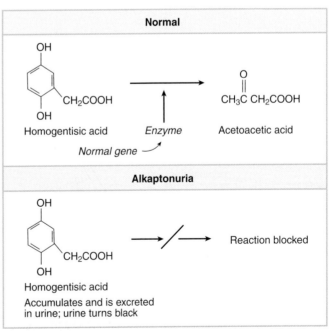

Figure 4-1. Alkaptonuria. The inability of homogentisic acid to form acetoacetic acid because of deficient or defective enzyme results in alkaptonuria.

Subsequently, it became clear that each gene controls the formation of a single enzyme and therefore a single metabolic reaction. This *one gene–one enzyme* thesis was reinforced and expanded. It was extended to include all cellular proteins and was, at the time, more precisely defined as the *one gene–one polypeptide* principle. However, as the mechanisms of genetic variability have become further clarified, it has become even more amazing to find that the mechanisms of alternative splicing may provide different protein products per gene and allele.

●●● MODEL OF BLOCKED METABOLIC REACTIONS

The consequences of an alteration of a single enzyme are shown in Figure 4-2, which depicts the model reaction sequence A→D and the relevant genes for each step. In this model, it is assumed that each gene acts independently and each is responsible for the formation of a specific enzyme. Substrate A is converted to end product D through a series of

metabolic steps that are each catalyzed by a separate enzyme. As illustrated, a number of consequences may arise if enzyme "c" is not formed because gene "c" is mutated and transcription does not occur. One effect would be the lack of formation of product D, which could lead to a clinical disorder. In addition, the immediate precursor of the blocked reaction could accumulate in abnormal amounts. For example, it has already been shown that homogentisic acid accumulates in alkaptonuria because its conversion to acetoacetic acid is blocked. The outcome is an increase in urinary excretion of homogentisic acid along with a blue-black discoloration of connective tissue including bone, cartilage, and skin caused by deposits of ochre-colored pigment—a condition known as *ochronosis*. The block between C and D may also cause increased use of other pathways, resulting in greater production of alternative products. For example, in phenylketonuria (PKU), a single enzymatic block results not only in the accumulation of phenylalanine (product C) but also in gross overproduction of phenylpyruvic acid (product Z). This provides a general orientation to *inborn errors of metabolism* in humans.

An important consideration in the development of disease is the period of gene expression. Those genes important for early development will have earlier consequences if mutated than will genes not expressed until puberty or after. These genes are *differentially* expressed; they are expressed at some periods but not at other periods. Some genes are expressed continually and are called *constitutively* expressed genes. A different group of genes may be expressed only in a particular tissue. These *tissue-specific* genes may be either differentially or constitutively expressed (Table 4-1).

A different consideration is the type of mutation and the location of the mutation within the affected allele. As recognized in Chapter 1, there are several types of mutations. In addition to mutations altering structure and function, other mutations may cause a modification in the rate of

---

BIOCHEMISTRY

Alternative Splicing

Alternative splicing is the differential joining of exons to form more than one variant from the same gene. The significance of this mechanism is that it increases the diversity of gene products. A prominent example at the DNA level is immunoglobulin class switching. At the RNA level, this is demonstrated at the dystrophin, the gene mutated in Duchenne and Becker muscular dystrophies. Dystrophin has seven promoters that are used to generate specific, cell-type expression.

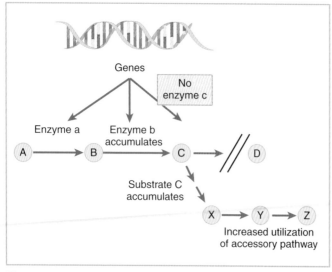

Figure 4-2. Model of metabolic disease. Genes altered by different forms of mutations may cause altered enzymes that prevent the conversion of a substrate to a product. In some cases, substrate may be converted to alternative metabolites by a different pathway.

TABLE 4-1. Types of Gene Expression

Type of Gene Expression	Expression Product	Nature of Expression Product
Constitutive	tRNAs rRNAs Cell membrane enzymes Some transcription factors	Non-tissue-specific
	Insulin Cytochrome P-450 G protein–coupled receptor	Tissue-specific
Differential	Receptors Transcription factors	Non-tissue-specific
	Cortisol Globins Dystrophins	Tissue-specific

synthesis, posttranslational mechanisms, or transporting of proteins out of the cell. Even if these changes produce products at normal or near-normal levels, a modification may alter the function, efficiency, or half-life of the protein and result in a disease condition.

Heterogeneity of disease among different individuals can occur if any of these situations occur; i.e., mutations occurring in different locations may affect expression, structure, or function. For example, a particular mutation within the promoter region may abolish transcription of an allele critical for a cellular function. A different mutation within an exon may result in the incorporation of a different amino acid in the protein that will reduce, but not abolish, its function. Another mutation may have no consequence for expression of the protein. These differences result from *allelic variation*, or *allelic heterogeneity*. Alleles differ in their expression because they are defined by different mutations and thus result in different versions of the same protein. Some alleles may present the same clinical phenotype within a population (see Achondroplasia in Chapter 7). However, for many diseases, a continuum of symptoms may be seen in individuals from mild to very severe because of the differences between alleles. In reality, variable expressivity is not a peculiarity of a few disorders. It is what should be expected and is seen in the vast majority of genetic diseases. This variability is not only the effect of specific mutations but also a consequence of the temporal interaction of gene products with the environment of the cell. This is readily seen in individuals with cystic fibrosis, a condition caused by a mutation in the cystic fibrosis transmembrane conductance regulator gene (*CFTR*). Over 1000 mutations have been reported in this gene, which is composed of over 300,000 bp spanning 27 exons. The severity of cystic fibrosis is associated with specific mutations. For example, the deletion of three base pairs coding for phenylalanine (referred to as the ΔF508 mutation) results in a severe presentation when present in two copies. An insertion of 7 polythymidines is asymptomatic when present on both alleles but may present as a mild or classical phenotype when present with a different mutation (see also Cystic Fibrosis in Chapter 9).

NEWBORN SCREENING

Newborn screening programs in the United States and other countries have proved invaluable in the detection of serious metabolic disorders. The goal is to identify infants with genetic conditions that can be helped by early intervention programs. Mass screening of metabolic disorders became feasible as rapid, cost-effective assays, such as the Guthrie test, became available. All states screen for PKU, congenital hypothyroidism, galactosemia, and sickle cell disease (only selected populations in some states). Most countries, reporting tests, performed tests for PKU and hypothyroidism. Screening tests for other disorders may include maple syrup urine disease, homocystinuria, biotinidase deficiency, congenital adrenal hyperplasia, cystic fibrosis, and human immunodeficiency virus. With the advent of newer technologies, such as tandem mass spectrophotometry and DNA-based technologies, newborn screening tests are expanding in most states to better identify infants at risk for metabolic disorders.

Inborn errors of metabolism should be considered in all critically ill infants. Frequently, these infants are normal at birth. Good health deteriorates over a period of hours to weeks with symptoms such as poor feeding, failure to thrive, developmental delay, or delayed milestones. Older undiagnosed children may have recurrent problems such as vomiting, lethargy, ataxia, or seizures. Failure to diagnose these conditions may often lead to dysmorphologies, mental retardation, or even death. Sometimes older children with mild or subtle disorders may actually have undiagnosed metabolic disorders that went undetected at birth.

There are several considerations for determining which disorders should be screened routinely in newborns. Although many of the disorders currently tested for are not frequently seen, the clinical value of screening tests must be established (Table 4-2). Enough individuals should be affected that

BIOCHEMISTRY

Posttranslational Modification

Posttranslational modification leads to the formation of 100 or more different amino acids derivatives from the basic 20. Modifications may be permanent or reversible. Examples include converting a protein to a functional form, directing a protein to a specific site, aiding in protein secretion, or altering protein activity or stability.

Proteins are frequently modified at the ends. At the amino terminus, modifications may include formylation, acetylation, aminoacylation, and glycosylation. At the carboxyl terminus, modifications may include methylation, glycosyl-phosphatidylinositol anchor formation, and ADP-ribosylation. An example is insulin that is modified by cleavage in the Golgi, where disulfide bonds link two of the fragments. Another example occurs with the addition of oligosaccharides to proteins that form the glycoproteins. Most proteins that are secreted or bound to the cell membrane are modified by the attachment of various carbohydrates.

TABLE 4-2. Considerations for Newborn Screening Tests

Guideline	Justification
Incidence	The incidence of the disorder must warrant screening
Benefit	The test must provide a potential benefit to the infant
Treatment	A treatment must be available for newborns
Cost	The cost-benefit ratio should favor screening over not screening for the infant
Feasibility	The test must be practical for population screening with minimal false-negative results

screening is valued. The infants should benefit from the test by having an effective treatment available, and early treatment should be more beneficial than delayed treatment. Treatment should also be significantly less expensive than treating an affected individual with the disorder. Finally, it should be feasible to screen large numbers of individuals, and the number of false negatives should be minimal.

●●● AMINOACIDOPATHIES

Inborn errors of amino acid metabolism generally are the outcome of enzyme deficiencies that result in the accumulation of a substrate. More than 70 disorders have been described. Most of these are autosomal recessive single-gene defects in amino acid synthesis or catabolism. Some amino acids are synthesized within the cell, whereas others require dietary intake. However, having amino acids in the diet does not guarantee a healthy state unless levels are carefully monitored. The dietary amino acid may become a substrate for another important product, as seen with leucine, isoleucine, and valine, also known as branched-chain amino acids. Most of the resulting conditions are rare but clinically important because of the debilitating consequences to the homozygous individual with two defective alleles and the extreme financial and psychological burdens on their family. Disorders are named for the amino acid that accumulates in the blood or urine.

Phenylalanine Metabolism and Hyperphenylalaninemia

Phenylalanine is the starting point for a series of reactions essential in metabolism. Reflected in this pathway of reactions are several inherited defects: phenylketonuria, albinism, tyrosinemia, and alkaptonuria (Fig. 4-3). Each of the four metabolic disorders results from a block at a different point. All are recessive, and the heterozygote typically produces sufficient enzyme and thus is "normal."

Classic *phenylketonuria* is recognized as a deficiency of phenylalanine hydroxylase. Shortly after birth, the affected infant has an unusually high concentration of phenylalanine, an "essential" dietary amino acid, in the blood. Some phenylalanine is incorporated into various body proteins. Most, however, is normally converted to tyrosine, which is involved in several metabolic pathways, including the formation of pigment and neurotransmitters. The deficiency of the enzyme phenylalanine hydroxylase (PAH) results in the accumulation of phenylalanine in fluids and tissues. The increased concentration of phenylalanine leads, in turn, to an increased rate of formation of phenylpyruvic acid, which is excreted in the urine (Fig. 4-4). Excess phenylpyruvic acid in sweat accounts for the unusual "mousy" body odor of PKU patients. Phenylpyruvic acid is a competitive inhibitor of the pyruvate dehydrogenase complex, which is important in glucose metabolism and subsequently in synthesis of fatty acids and cholesterol. This may contribute to the lack of myelin formation and mental retardation in these individuals. Phenylalanine will also interfere with hydrophobic amino acid transport across the blood-brain barrier. It also competes for the same active transport system, as does leucine, an important component of myelin. Postmortem studies of PKU infants with microcephaly suggest that the decreased brain size is due to a decreased amount of myelin and a reduction in other protein components of the brain.

BIOCHEMISTRY

Amino Acids

Amino acids are classified as essential (those that must be derived from the diet) and nonessential (those synthesized by the body). The essential amino acids include histidine, isoleucine, leucine, lysine, methionine, phenylalanine, threonine, tryptophan, and valine. The nonessential amino acids include alanine, arginine, asparagine, aspartic acid, glutamine, glycine, proline, serine, and tyrosine.

In extended periods of stress, the biosynthetic pathways cannot fulfill the requirement for certain nonessential amino acids. These amino acids then become *conditionally essential*, and dietary supplementation is required. Cysteine and glutamic acid are examples of two amino acids that become essential during periods of stress.

PATHOLOGY

Changes in Urinary Amino Acids Associated with Clinical Presentations

Condition	Examples
Inherited metabolic disorders	PKU, tyrosinemia, homocystinuria, cystinuria, other hyperaminoacidurias
Malnutrition	Dietary protein malabsorption, extreme metabolic crises such as fasting, starvation, or muscle wasting. Hydroxyproline excretion is associated with celiac disease and malabsorption disease.
Decreased protein ingestion	Recent dietary insufficiency demonstrates decreased amino acid excretion
Alcoholism	Nutritional anemia and alcoholic gastritis demonstrate altered amino acid excretion
Cushing disease	Increased cystine
Chronic fatigue syndrome	Strongly associated with β-alanine; increased ratio of tryptophan to branched-chain amino acids
Muscle catabolism	3-Methylhistidine indicates excessive muscle catabolism
Osteoporosis	Elevated hydroxyproline with increased osteocalcin secretion indicates high bone turnover

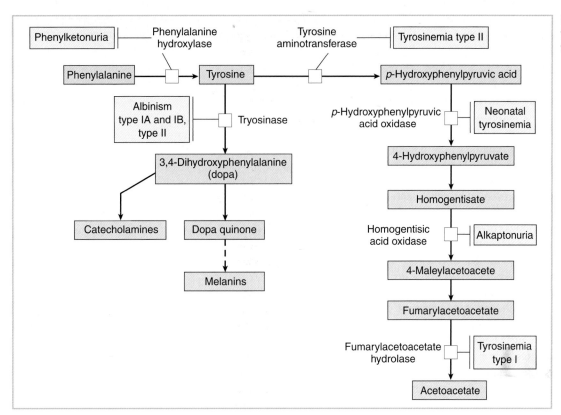

Figure 4-3. Disorders of the phenylalanine-tyrosine pathways.

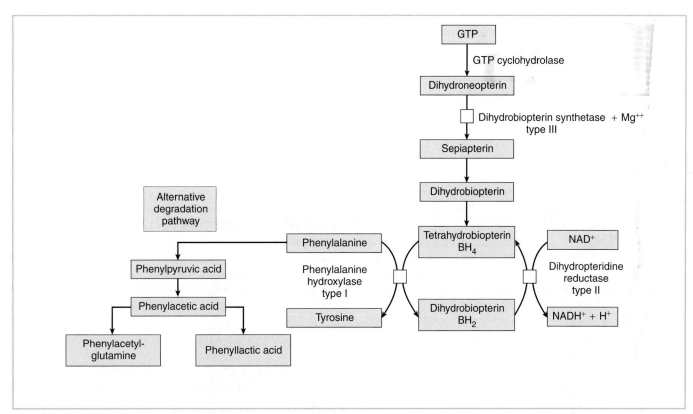

Figure 4-4. Different forms of hyperphenylalaninemia. Defects in the ability to produce tetrahydrobiopterin efficiently will lead to PKU types II and III. PAH may be normal, but without tetrahydrobiopterin synthase (BH_4), there is excess phenylalanine and a decrease in tyrosine.

Nearly 500 mutations have been described in the PAH gene. Most mutations result in hyperphenylalaninemia owing to reduced enzyme activity. Mutations have been described in each of the 13 exons; however, five mutations are present at a higher frequency than expected and account for approximately 60% of mutations in Europeans. These "hot spots" for mutations provide a better understanding to allelic heterogeneity. Stated another way, if 60% of PAH mutations are represented by only 5 of 500 mutations, the phenotypical expectation among individuals with PKU and hyperphenylalaninemia is more likely to be based on these 60% rather than phenotypes that may be represented by other mutations.

Both the excessive amount of phenylalanine and the lack of tyrosine produce the abnormal consequences of PKU (see Fig. 4-3). High levels of phenylalanine are damaging to rapidly developing brain tissues in the developing infant. Brain damage in the untreated patient occurs after birth rather than before because the placenta produces phenylalanine hydroxylase. Therefore, the placenta converts excess phenylalanine to tyrosine for the developing fetus. Production of this enzyme in the infant's liver begins after birth.

Figure 4-4 also demonstrates that a deficiency of tyrosine can occur in other ways that result in elevated levels of phenylalanine and decreased levels of tyrosine. These forms of *hyperphenylalaninemia* are often referred to as type II and type III PKU to distinguish them from classic, or type I, PKU. Each form can be detected with the Guthrie test or with amino acid profiling of urine or plasma. However, the choice, and ultimately the success, of treatment depends on which enzyme is affected. Individuals with classic PKU are treated with a phenylalanine-restricted diet; however, in type II and type III hyperphenylalaninemia, phenylalanine is elevated but these individuals are not spared the effects of progressive neurologic deterioration by a phenylalanine-restricted diet (Table 4-3). Defects in dihydrobiopterin synthetase and dihydropteridine reductase resulting in deficiencies of tetrahydrobiopterin and dihydrobiopterin block or reduce the conversion of phenylalanine to tyrosine, leading to inadequate neurotransmitter formation.

When relying on the Guthrie screening test, the physician must be cautious about positive results. Elevated tyrosine associated with low birth weight, seen in infants on high protein diets, and with vitamin C deficiency may also cause a positive Guthrie test. Liver disease and galactosemia can cause a positive test. Two additional tests can be used to detect elevated levels of phenylalanine and other amino acids. A fluorometric assay is an automated test that produces fewer false positives than does the Guthrie test. Tandem mass spectrometry is used to identify numerous metabolic defects. This test is extremely sensitive to trace metabolites. Its biggest drawback for routine screening is cost-effectiveness. In spite of the cost factor, the use of tandem mass spectrometry screening is increasing in newborn screening programs.

An excessively high phenylalanine level during pregnancy is of particular concern because of its toxicity to the developing fetus. *Maternal PKU* results from the lack of PAH in the liver and placenta that ordinarily would convert excess

TABLE 4-3. Comparison of Hyperphenylalaninemias

Type	Enzyme Affected	Percentage of All Hyperphenylalaninemias
I	Phenylalanine hydroxylase, <1% activity	60%
I (mild, persistent)	Phenylalanine hydroxylase 2, ≤ 35% activity	35%
II	Dihydropteridine reductase	3%
III	Dihydrobiopterin synthetase	1% to 3%

MICROBIOLOGY

Guthrie Test

The Guthrie test is a bacterial inhibition assay. β_2-Thienylalanine is placed in the medium and normally causes the inhibition of *Bacillus subtilis* growth. However, in the presence of excess of phenylalanine, this inhibition is overridden and bacterial growth occurs. This test is the least expensive screening method available for determining excess phenylalanine in the blood, but other tests are used to confirm findings.

phenylalanine to tyrosine. This situation may occur when the mother fails to inform the physician that she has PKU or she forgets (often repressing the memories) the special diet she had as a child. When the PHE-restricted diet is no longer maintained, PHE levels rise but may have less dramatic effects than seen during early infant and childhood development. Failure of the mother's enzyme to convert excess phenylalanine to tyrosine subsequently leads to malformations in an infant who may be genetically normal but is affected by the mother's abnormal PAH. Malformations include intrauterine growth retardation (IUGR), microcephaly, heart abnormalities, and mental retardation (Table 4-4). It is important that the mother's phenylalanine levels be monitored, since the earlier phenylalanine levels are maintained within normal limits the less prevalent malformations will be in the infant. A corollary is that tyrosine levels must not be too low, since this will affect the level of neurotransmitters formed in the fetus.

Tyrosine Metabolism

Many genes are involved in the production of pigment of skin and hair. The best-described condition affecting pigment production is *classic albinism*, which results from a lack of tyrosinase (see Fig. 4-3). Individuals with classic PKU may demonstrate pale skin and hair coloration that might suggest albinism. However, once diagnosed, these individuals receive

TABLE 4-4. Clinical Features of Classic Phenylketonuria at Different Periods

Appearance	Symptoms
Newborn	*Usually no symptoms immediately* Lethargy Feeding difficulty Reduced pigmentation of hair, skin, eyes Eczema
Child	*Irreversible after about 6 months* Seizures Nausea Vomiting Hyperactivity Aggressive behavior Poor coordination Ataxia Abnormal posturing Self-injurious behavior "Mousy" odor of body and urine Mental retardation
Pregnant female with untreated PKU	Spontaneous miscarriage
Infant of mother with untreated maternal PKU	IUGR Microcephaly Psychomotor retardation Congenital heart defects Postnatal growth retardation Abnormal neurologic findings Mild craniofacial dysmorphology

tyrosine in their diet, which bypasses the metabolic deficiency of PKU and allows pigment formation.

Classic albinism is also known as oculocutaneous albinism type I. *Type IA is tyrosinase negative, whereas type IB has reduced tyrosinase activity.* In patients with albinism, the body is incapable of synthesizing the pigment melanin, which is a metabolite of tyrosine. Albinism does not vary with race or age and is commonly characterized by nystagmus, photophobia, and reduced visual acuity. Oculocutaneous albinism *type II is tyrosinase positive* and is the most common form of albinism throughout the world. This albinism also results from mutations in the tyrosinase gene. Type II differs from type IB clinically. In type IB, there is a general reduction in pigmentation. Type II is also distinguished by pigmented nevi, suggesting that it is more difficult to identify in blacks, who have pigmented spots but also yellow hair. In some regions, such as South Africa, type II is the most common recessive disorder.

Tyrosine is essential for protein synthesis, catecholamine production, melanin production, and thyroid hormone synthesis. Though tyrosine is available from the diet, a large percentage is formed during phenylalanine metabolism. Accumulation of tyrosine due to a metabolic disorder is rare, with the exception of *neonatal tyrosinemia*, which results from delayed synthesis or stability of *p*-hydroxyphenylpyruvic acid oxidase. Normal newborns, especially those of low-birth

weight, tend to have unusually high levels of tyrosine in their blood. This transient form of tyrosinemia is benign and rarely presents with symptoms. Blood tyrosine levels usually become normal (< 4 mg/100 mL) within a few weeks. Infants with neonatal tyrosinemia have a positive Guthrie screening test; hence, care must be exercised when diagnosing PKU in a newborn. Positive Guthrie tests are typically followed by more detailed investigations including serum phenylalanine and tyrosine levels.

Tyrosinemia types I and II are rare but can be detected by molecular analysis. Type I, also known as hepatorenal tyrosinemia, is potentially fatal. Present in either acute or chronic form, it is associated with liver failure or with liver dysfunction and renal nephropathy. Type II, also known as oculocutaneous tyrosinemia, usually presents during the first year as eye irritations in the form of photophobia, conjunctivitis, or pain resulting from tyrosine crystals within the cornea. Skin lesions begin as blisters on fingertips and toes; later keratotic plaques appear on palms and soles. Both types result from the accumulation of tyrosine. Mental retardation may occur in these individuals, but it is unclear whether it

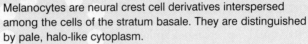

HISTOLOGY

Melanocytes

Melanocytes are neural crest cell derivatives interspersed among the cells of the stratum basale. They are distinguished by pale, halo-like cytoplasm.

Melanocytes possess organelles known as melanosomes that produce melanin. The melanin-containing melanosomes are transported to and take up location covering the nuclei in keratinocytes, protecting them from ultraviolet radiation. Hence, skin color depends on activity of melanocytes rather than their number.

NEUROSCIENCE & PHARMACOLOGY

Catecholamines

Catecholamines serve as neurotransmitters and circulating hormones. They are derived from tyrosine and include dopamine, epinephrine, and norepinephrine. The rate-limiting step in this pathway, which begins with the essential amino acid phenylalanine, is tyrosine hydroxylase.

After release from chromaffin cells of the adrenal gland and sympathetic axons, catecholamine reuptake primarily occurs at synaptic clefts although non-neuronal uptake also occurs. This mechanism is sodium dependent but not ATP-dependent; transporters are therefore referred to as Na^+-dependent transporters. An example is the Na^+-dependent norepinephrine transporter (NET). After uptake, catecholamines are either stored or catabolized by monoamine oxidase (MAO) and catechol-*O*-methyltransferase (COMT).

Catecholamine receptors are specific for ligands. Dopamine effects are mediated by D1 and D2 receptor subfamilies. Norepinephrine and epinephrine act via two broad families of receptors (α and β) or five classes (α_1, α_2, β_1, β_2, and β_3).

results from elevated tyrosine or is secondary to the enzyme deficiency.

Homocystinuria and Hyperhomocystinuria

Methionine is an essential amino acid that is converted to cysteine. These amino acids are the only two sulfur-containing amino acids in protein synthesis. Therefore, the roles they play in synthetic pathways are critical. For example, an important methionine derivative is S-adenosylmethionine (SAM), which serves as an endogenous methyl donor. Methionine is also important in the synthesis of carnitine, taurine, phosphatidylcholine, and phospholipids. Cysteine is critical in the production of heparin, coenzyme A, biotin, and glutathione.

An intermediate in the methionine to cysteine pathway is homocysteine, a thiol compound required to regenerate methionine. Classic homocystinuria is a recessive metabolic disorder due to deficiency of cystathionine β-synthase (CBS) that produces increased urinary homocystine and methionine. About 50% of homocysteine is recycled to methionine. As shown in Figure 4-5, two other enzymes may result in hyperhomocystinuria: methionine synthase and 5,10-methylenetetrahydrofolate reductase.

Clinical manifestations of homocystinuria include lens dislocation (ectopia lentis), excessive height, and length of limbs, and vascular abnormalities that may lead to myocardial infarction, stroke, or pulmonary embolism. Developmental and mental delay may be present, but a third of individuals with homocystinuria may have normal intelligence. In many ways, homocystinuria resembles Marfan syndrome (see Chapter 7) including the phenotypes mentioned above plus arachnodactyly, pectus excavatum, and scoliosis. Phenotypic differences between the two are normal intelligence in Marfan syndrome and upward lens dislocation in Marfan syndrome versus downward in homocystinuria. Lens dislocation is the primary symptom leading to diagnosis in 80% of patients

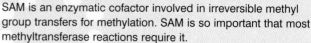

BIOCHEMISTRY

S-Adenosylmethionine (SAM)

SAM is an enzymatic cofactor involved in irreversible methyl group transfers for methylation. SAM is so important that most methyltransferase reactions require it.

Many targets of methylation are in the brain. In particular, catecholamines are degraded by the actions of monoamine oxidase (MAO) and catechol-O-methyltransferase (COMT). COMT transfers a methyl group from SAM to catecholamines, initiating a degradation process. In the absence of sufficient SAM, COMT, or other degradation enzymes, accumulations in degradation products occur and are seen in several neurologic disorders.

BIOCHEMISTRY

Homocysteine, Homocystine, and Homocysteine-cysteine

Homocysteine, homocystine, and homocysteine-cysteine are sulfur-containing thiols. Homocysteine can form a disulfide with another homocysteine or cysteine to form homocystine or a mixed disulfide, respectively. The disulfides are the component that is primarily measured in standard amino acid analysis, since this form accounts for about 98% of homocysteine. Of this about 75% is bound to protein, such as albumin, and the remainder occurs in a non-protein-bound form as homocystine, homocysteine-cysteine disulfide, and other minor forms. Normally, only about 1% to 2% occurs as the homocysteine thiol; however, in homocystinuria, the thiol homocysteine may represent 10% to 25% of the total concentration.

PHYSIOLOGY

Hyperaminoaciduria

Hyperaminoacidurias, or the increased plasma concentration of an amino acid, are explained by several mechanisms: (1) a defect may occur before the kidney, as seen in hyperargininemia, where the defect causes increased plasma arginine; (2) competition for the same transporter may occur when the same transporter is used for more than one amino acid and the high filtering load of one amino acid inhibits the others; and (3) a defective transporter may occur and result in decreased reabsorption by the kidney. Finally, a generalized proximal tubule dysfunction may occur from inherited or acquired conditions affecting the proximal tubule cells. In this type of hyperaminoaciduria, also called Fanconi syndrome, the kidney fails to appropriately reabsorb the particular amino acids as well as Na^+, Cl^-, HCO_3^-, glucose, and water.

with undiagnosed homocystinuria; it is usually diagnosed between ages 4 and 6.

There are two forms of homocystinuria: vitamin B_6-responsive and vitamin B_6-nonresponsive. Pyridoxine (B_6) responsiveness is the ability to enhance transsulfuration of homocysteine upon pyridoxine administration. B_6-responsive homocystinuria is typically milder than the nonresponsive form. Pyridoxine responsiveness determined by a challenge test is defined as a decrease of total homocysteine below 50 μmol/L, whereas nonresponsiveness is no change in plasma total homocysteine after a dose of up to 10 mg/kg of pyridoxine per day administered for at least 2 weeks. About 40% of homocystinuria patients respond to B_6 supplementation. Those who fail to respond require a diet restricted in methionine.

Most of the 132 mutations found in the CBS gene are missense mutations with the majority being unique mutations. However, among these the two most frequent mutations are I278T and G307S both of which are found in exon 8 of the gene. The I278T, in which isoleucine is replaced by threonine at codon 278, accounts for about 25% of all homocystinuric alleles. G307S, in which glycine replaces serine, is the leading cause of homocystinuria in Ireland, where it accounts for

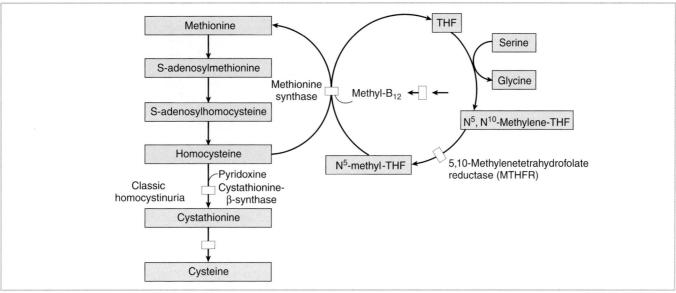

Figure 4-5. Classic homocystinuria results from a deficiency of cystathionine β-synthase. Other mutations can affect the pathway but have less damaging effects.

BIOCHEMISTRY & PATHOLOGY

Pyridoxine

Pyridoxine is also known as vitamin B_6 and is an essential cofactor for many transamination reactions, including gluconeogenesis. It is also involved in the synthesis of niacin (vitamin B_3) from tryptophan, the synthesis of several neurotransmitters, and the synthesis of δ-aminolevulinic acid, a precursor of heme. Deficiencies in this vitamin are usually seen along with deficiencies of other water-soluble vitamins. Characteristics of a deficiency include stomatitis, angular cheilosis, glossitis, irritability, and depression; in moderate to severe deficiencies, confusion may occur.

Deficiencies are often associated with microcytic, hypochromic anemia because sideroblastic anemias are much more common than inherited forms. Sideroblastic anemias have diverse etiologies but have the common association of nonheme iron "encrustations" of the mitochondria of erythroid precursors. Mitochondria are the site where heme biosynthesis begins. Some drugs, toxins, or nutritional deficiencies may antagonize B_6 metabolism, thereby producing a reversible sideroblastic anemia.

PATHOLOGY

Pyridoxine Challenge Test

B_6-responsiveness is determined by a pyridoxine challenge. Baseline amino acids are determined during a normal diet. Pyridoxine is then given orally (100 mg), and amino acid concentrations are determined 24 hours later. A 30% reduction in homocysteine or methionine or both suggests B_6 responsiveness. If no change is observed in amino acids, pyridoxine is increased to 200 mg and 500 mg. No significant decrease following these challenges indicates B_6-nonresponsiveness.

more than 70% of the mutations, suggesting that at least in this population a founder effect for this allele may exist. The I278T mutation is almost always B_6 responsive, whereas the G307S mutation is almost always B_6 nonresponsive. This type of information is necessary for knowing which tests to perform and similarly which therapies might be effective.

As noted, there are several causes of hyperhomocystinuria in addition to the classical form (see Fig. 4-5). These may be benign or associated with mental retardation. Liver disease due to hepatitis or tyrosinemia type I will cause elevated serum methionine. A deficiency of folic acid or vitamin B_{12} resulting in methylmalonic acidemia will also cause homocystinuria if vitamin B_{12} deficiency is sufficient to also affect homocysteine to methionine recycling. Metabolic disorders of B_{12} synthesis result in the same biochemical presentation but with different symptoms. Similarly, a deficiency of methionine synthase will mimic a deficiency of folic acid as a result of the inability to convert homocysteine to methionine.

A deficiency of 5,10-methylenetetrahydrofolate reductase (MTHFR) is the most common inborn error of folate metabolism. It results in homocystinuria and *hypomethioninemia*. These disorders present in infancy or adolescence with developmental delay, motor dysfunction, seizures, psychiatric disturbances, and other neurologic abnormalities. Patients also have an increased risk for coronary artery disease.

●●● A CARBOHYDRATE METABOLISM DISORDER

Galactosemia

Galactosemia is an extraordinary metabolic disorder in which affected infants are unable to utilize galactose found in milk. Galactose is important beyond its ability to provide glucose. It is also a component of cerebrosides, gangliosides, and

PATHOLOGY & PHYSIOLOGY

Homocysteine (HCY)

Elevated HCY causes oxidative stress and injury to vascular cells through the auto-oxidation of HCY, formation of HCY mixed disulfides, interaction of HCY thiolactones, and protein homocysteinylation. Oxidation of HCY produces reactive oxygen species (ROS), primarily superoxide, hydroxyl radicals, and peroxynitrites. These lead to the formation of peroxide and hypochlorous acid. All are toxic to tissues and cause damage to lipids, nucleic acids, and proteins.

The formation of mixed disulfides leads to the formation of additional ROS. In addition, HCY may undergo rearrangements to form HCY thiolactones that will acylate lysines in proteins. These homocysteinylate proteins initiate further ROS damage and loss of biological activity. In particular, low-density lipoproteins may be affected, leading to inflammation and the formation of foamy cells associated with atherosclerosis. The ability to inactivate these ROS is the function of antioxidants. However, even with up-regulation of glutathionine peroxidase and superoxide dismutase, there is evidence that they are depleted in chronic situations.

Vascular cells do not express cystathionine β-synthase (CBS), so they are more vulnerable to elevated HCY. These cells are therefore more dependent on the methionine synthase and methyl-B_{12} remethylation pathway.

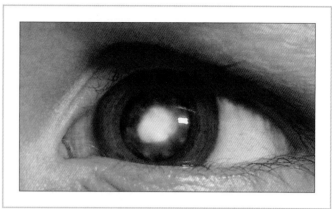

Figure 4-6. Galactosemia cataract. The accumulation of galactose in the lens leads to the production of galactitol. This sugar alcohol exerts increased osmotic pressure within the lens because it diffuses very slowly. The induced swelling is not solely responsible for subsequent cataract formation; however, evidence supports its role in cataract formation rather than galactose-1-phosphate because a galactokinase deficiency in which galactose-1-phosphate is absent will still yield cataracts. (From Kanski J. *Clinical Ophthalmology: A Systemic Approach,* 4th ed. London, Butterworth Heinemann, 1999, p 177.)

glycoproteins. These are constituents of cell membranes, and cerebrosides and gangliosides are a significant portion of brain lipid. Galactose ordinarily is converted to glucose and, eventually, oxidized to provide energy. In affected infants, galactose is not transformed and accumulates in various tissues. The infant suffers from malnutrition, becomes severely retarded mentally, and develops cataracts (Fig. 4-6). Characteristically the liver becomes grossly enlarged. Untreated, the infant usually dies.

Classic galactosemia, an autosomal recessive disorder, results from a block in the conversion of galactose-1-phosphate to glucose-1-phosphate by *galactose-1-phosphate uridyltransferase* (Fig. 4-7). As a result of the defect, galactose-1-phosphate and galactose metabolites accumulate in tissues and are elevated in the blood and urine. Galactose-1-phosphate competes with the UTP-dependent glucose-1-phosphate to reduce UDP glucose production. Two known mutations account for 62% of the mutations identified: Q188R (54%) and S135L (8.4%). Twenty-nine percent of the mutations are either private (unique to a specific family) or unknown.

In a nonclassical form of galactosemia, *galactokinase* is deficient. This rare form demonstrates elevated levels of galactose but does not have deposition of galactose-1-phosphate in tissues. Excess galactose is metabolized by alternative pathways to metabolites that are normally present in only trace amounts. Both forms of galactosemia result in cataract formation from galactitol, the reduced sugar alcohol of galactose, by aldose reductase. Galactitol accumulates in

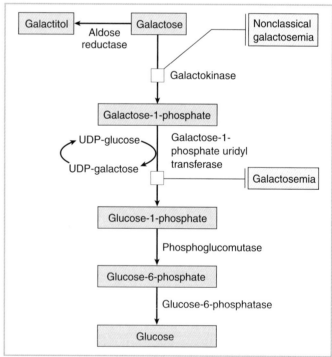

Figure 4-7. Pathway of glucose formation from galactose. A defect in galactokinase or the galactose-1-phosphate uridyl transferase results in the formation of galactitol from aldose reductase.

the lens, causing a change in osmotic pressure as water is absorbed and swelling occurs.

If the diagnosis of galactosemia is made before the disease is too far advanced, nearly all the symptoms will disappear if galactose is excluded from the infant's diet. The liver returns to normal size, vomiting ceases, and nutrition and growth improve markedly. Unfortunately, unless a galactose-free diet is instituted promptly at birth, there is usually no recovery from the mentally retarded state. Damage to the liver, brain, and eyes occurs in the very first days of life. Accordingly, if a newborn infant is a first-degree relative of an individual with galactosemia, pre- or perinatal testing can identify the condition. Estimates for the prevalence of galactosemia vary widely, from 1 in 18,000 to 1 in 70,000 infants.

ORGANIC ACIDEMIAS

During normal degradation of many amino acids, intermediate metabolites known as organic acids are formed. Enzyme deficiencies causing the accumulation of organic acids can lead to severe metabolic acidosis. Failure to recognize the underlying cause of metabolic acidosis can have serious consequences to the individual. Typically, infants appear normal during the first few days prior to the onset of symptoms. Clinical symptoms of organic acid disorders may include vomiting, metabolic acidosis, ketosis, dehydration or coma, hyperammonemia, lactic acidosis, hypoglycemia, failure to thrive, hypotonia, global developmental delay, sepsis, and hematologic disorders.

Maple Syrup Urine Disease

Maple syrup urine disease (MSUD) was one of the earliest and best known of the inborn errors of amino acid metabolism, primarily because it was associated with an odor in the urine strongly reminiscent of maple syrup. It represents a disturbance of metabolism of the branched-chained amino acids (BCAAs) leucine, isoleucine, and valine (Fig. 4-8). The normal degradation of these three essential amino acids is initiated in muscle and yields NADH and $FADH_2$ that can be utilized for ATP generation. *Branched-chain keto acid decarboxylase* is involved in each of these reactions. This enzyme

PHYSIOLOGY

Metabolic Acidosis

Metabolic acidosis, one of four major acid-base disorders, is a sign of an underlying problem and occurs when total body acid increases because of an imbalance between acids and alkali. Clinically, this can occur with a decrease in urinary secretion of H^+ from renal failure, ketoacidosis from diabetes, lactic acidosis seen in shock, or HCO_3^- loss occurring with severe diarrhea. These lead to decreases in pH and HCO_3^-. Metabolic response to acidosis occurs by extracellular buffering, especially by hemoglobin, intracellular and bone buffering, respiratory compensation, and renal excretion of H^+.

is a complex of four enzymes suggesting that mutations in several genes can affect the overall activity of the complex. Enzyme deficiencies result in the accumulation of high concentrations of both BCAAs and α-keto acids in the blood and urine.

Infants with MSUD appear normal at birth but quickly demonstrate failure to thrive. Because essential amino acids are involved, the goal of dietary management is normalizing concentrations rather than restricting concentrations. Infants who survive usually demonstrate neurologic damage due to cerebral edema and degeneration. Symptoms begin 3 to 4 days after birth in infants with the classical form of this disease. If it is not detected, severe acidosis and hypoglycemia occur; clinical progression is rapid, and death can occur. Neurologic deterioration is apparent with flaccidity, hypertonicity, a high-pitched voice, and opisthotonic posturing.

Milder forms of MSUD may also occur with a later onset after the neonatal period. These individuals are usually only mildly retarded and have elevated plasma levels of BCAAs. Periodic ketoacidosis may occur with mild MSUD after infections or high protein diets. As might be expected, many diagnoses of mild MSUD are made during an illness. As with

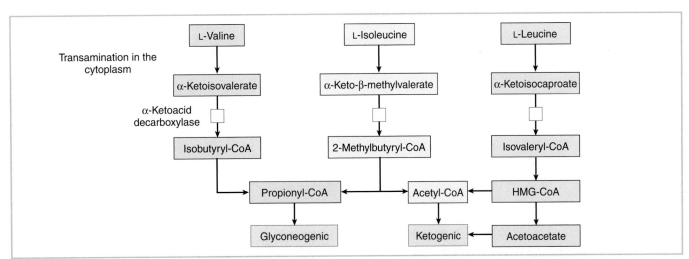

Figure 4-8. Branched-chain amino acid metabolism. A mutation in the α-ketoacid decarboxylase enzyme complex results in the accumulation of valine, isoleucine, leucine and the α-keto analogs of these branched-chain amino acids in the urine, resulting in maple syrup urine disease.

most diseases, the nature of the mutation will probably be displayed in variable degrees of severity depending on the percentage of activity in the enzyme complex.

As with all the organic acidemias listed in Table 4-5, MSUD is inherited in an autosomal recessive manner. In the general population, MSUD is not the most common organic academia; however, among the Mennonites, it is quite common with a general incidence of 1 in 1000. Some isolated populations of Mennonites with a high incidence of consanguinity have an incidence as high as 1 in 176.

Biotinidase Deficiency

Biotin is a water-soluble vitamin that acts as a prosthetic group for four carboxylases required for the degradation of several branched-chain amino acids, the first step of gluconeogenesis, and fatty acid synthesis. Biotinidase is responsible for cleaving biocytin in food to form biotin and lysine. It is also necessary for the recycling of biotin from the enzymes.

The carboxylases dependent on biotin are pyruvate carboxylase, propionyl-CoA carboxylase, 3-methylcrotonyl-CoA carboxylase, and acetyl-CoA carboxylase. Without biotin, the functions of these enzymes are dramatically reduced because biotin normally forms a transient covalent bond to the COO^- group to be transferred and thus facilitates the carboxylase activity.

Individuals with profound biotinidase deficiency have less than 10% enzyme activity. Those with a partial deficiency have enzymatic activity of 10% to 30%. Most affected individuals have profound biotinidase deficiency and become biotin deficient during infancy or early childhood. Biotinidase deficiency can occur from two different gene mutations. Mutations in the biotinidase gene are usually referred to as the late-onset form while the early-onset form is attributed to a mutation in the holocarboxylase synthetase gene. Both are similar in presentation, although the early-onset form generally appears before 3 months of age and the late-onset form after 3 months of age. Symptoms may occur independently or in concert, including neurologic and cutaneous symptoms. Among the neurologic symptoms, seizures and hypotonia are the most common although mental retardation and coma may also occur. Some cases of sudden infant death have been attributed to biotinidase deficiency. Cutaneous symptoms are striking and include alopecia and an eczematous, scaly, perioral or facial rash. As a metabolic disorder the symptoms do not respond to dermatologic treatments. Other symptoms may include breathing difficulties, ataxia, hearing loss, and developmental delay. As an autosomal

TABLE 4-5. Features of Organic Acidemias

Disorder	Incidence	Amino Acid Pathway Affected	Defective Enzyme	Ketosis	Acidosis	Other
Maple syrup urine disease (MSUD)	1 in 150,000 (general population) 1 in 1000 (Mennonites)	Leucine, isoleucine, valine	Branched-chain ketoacid dehydrogenase	Yes		Maple syrup odor to urine
Propionic acidemia	1 in 20,000	Isoleucine, methionine, threonine	Propionyl-CoA carboxylase	Yes	Yes	Neutropenia
Methylmalonic acidemia (MMA)	1 in 20,000	Isoleucine, valine, methionine, threonine	Methylmalonyl-CoA mutase	Yes	Yes	Neutropenia
Isovaleric acidemia	1 in 150,000	Leucine	Isovaleryl-CoA dehydrogenase		Yes	Sweaty feet odor
Biotin-unresponsive 3-methylcrotonyl-CoA carboxylase deficiency	1 in 15,500	Leucine	3-Methylcrotonyl-CoA carboxylase		Yes	Hypoglycemia
3-Hydroxy-3-methylglutaryl-CoA (HMG-CoA) lyase deficiency	Unknown	Leucine	Hydroxymethylglutaryl-CoA lyase	No		Reye's syndrome, hypoglycemia
Ketothiolase deficiency	Unknown	Isoleucine	Mitochondrial acetoacetyl-CoA thiolase	Yes	Yes	Hypoglycemia
Glutaric acidemia type I (GA I)	1 in 150,000	Lysine, hydroxylysine, tryptophan	Glutaryl-CoA dehydrogenase		No	Basal ganglia injury with movement disorder

recessive disorder, biotinidase deficiency can be diagnosed prenatally or with newborn screening.

Propionyl-CoA carboxylase and 3-methylcrotonyl–CoA carboxylase deficiencies result in organic acidemias (see Table 4-5). These conditions, however, are caused by mutations in enzymes within a pathway and not by availability of biotin. In fact, treatment with biotin has little effect in these disorders but is very effective in biotinidase deficiency. *Biotinidase deficiency results in the deficiencies of multiple carboxylases* rather than one. Ketoacidosis, organic aciduria, and mild hyperammonemia may occur with biotinidase deficiency, but in partial deficiency these symptoms may occur only during metabolic stress. Partial biotinidase deficiency, in particular, is associated with metabolic stresses such as illness, fever, and fasting. Urinary organic acid analysis will distinguish between isolated and multiple carboxylase deficiencies.

●●● TREATMENT OF GENETIC DISEASE

The essential principles underlying treatment of many inherited metabolic disorders are avoidance of the harmful environmental factors that exacerbate the condition and restoration of a normal internal metabolism by modifications of the diet. In the examples described, the environmental factor is often a component of the diet. Removing this component removes the substrate that accumulates because of the defective enzyme. However, it is important to remember that products downstream of the defective enzyme may be critical to health. Early recognition is important to minimize effects of the disease.

Treatments for inborn errors of metabolism are generally found in one or more of several categories: dietary restriction of substrate, replacement of end product, depletion of storage substrate, amplification of mutant protein, replacement of mutant protein, organ or bone marrow transplantation, and surgical removal (Table 4-6). As discussed in this chapter, many of the disorders identified at birth can be treated by dietary restriction and supplementation. A classic example of dietary restriction is PKU. Phenylalanine should be restricted soon after birth to achieve normal growth and cognitive development. Special formulas are used and adjusted as the infant grows. Early in the history of PKU treatment, many patients were taken off the diet in childhood or as teenagers. Likewise, other individuals lacked continual compliance with the diet as they got older. Adherence to a low-phenylalanine diet should be life-long and particularly so for women of childbearing age. A range of plasma phenylalanine levels from 2 to 6 mg/dL is recommended until age 12 years. Afterward, the suggested range is from 2 to 15 mg/dL.

Some inborn errors of metabolism may not present symptoms until months to years after birth even though the

TABLE 4-6. Strategies of Treatment for Inborn Errors of Metabolism

Strategy	Examples	Treatment
Dietary restriction of substrate	Galactosemia Fructosemia Maple syrup urine disease Phenylketonuria Tyrosinemia	Restrict: Galactose Fructose Isoleucine, Leucine, Valine Phenylalanine Tyrosine
End-product replacement	Menkes syndrome Cystic fibrosis Familial goiters Orotic aciduria	Replace: Copper Pancreatic enzymes Thyroxine Uridine
Depletion of storage substance	Wilson disease Hypercholesterolemia Hemochromatosis	Deplete: Copper Cholesterol Iron
Replacement of mutant protein	Hemophilia Gaucher disease, type 1 Fabry disease Adenosine deaminase deficiency	Replace: Factor VIII Glucocerebrosidase Galactosidase Adenosine deaminase
Transplantation	Fabry disease Cystinosis Alport syndrome Mucopolysaccharidoses Tyrosinemia	Transplant: Kidney Kidney Kidney Bone marrow Liver
Surgical removal	Hereditary spherocytosis Multiple polyposis of the colon Medullary thyroid carcinoma syndrome	Remove: Spleen Colon Thyroid

genetic defect is present at birth. For example, infants normal at birth will begin to demonstrate the devastation of mucopolysaccharidoses (see Chapter 8) around age 2. Hemochromatosis (see Chapter 10) generally is not diagnosed until the ages of 30 to 50 years in men and beyond age 50 in women.

For many disorders, several treatment options may be available, but risks vary. For example, in maple syrup urine disease, liver transplantation has been successful in several patients. However, the risk and potential complications of this therapy are considerably higher than the low risk of dietary restriction, with which individuals have good outcomes.

Cancer Genetics 5

Over the last 30 years, it has become clear that cancer is a genetic disease. Under normal conditions, cells balance cell division and cell death, and these processes are accomplished and preserved by several biochemical "checkpoints" during the cell cycle. When these checkpoints are impinged, uncontrolled cellular proliferation and cancer can result. Because gene products regulate the life-death balance, mutations can destroy the checkpoints and promote cellular transformation into a neoplasia. Two general classes of cancer genes have been identified: oncogenes and tumor suppressor genes. Oncogenes facilitate tumor formation by directly accelerating cell division, whereas tumor suppressor genes work in the opposite manner to halt uncontrolled cell growth. When tumor suppressor genes suffer incapacitating mutations, the cell loses the capacity to guard against tumor formation.

Oncogenes and tumor suppressor genes can be activated or inactivated by various mutational mechanisms including point mutation, deletion, and chromosomal rearrangement, and each has a prominent role in sporadic and familial cancers.

Although small subsets of cancers are associated with inherited genetic mutations passed from generation to generation in a family, overall, cancer appears to result from an accumulation of such deleterious mutations in somatic tissues. While some mutations are found across multiple cancer types, other mutations are generally specific to certain cancer syndromes, demonstrating the importance of such genes to particular tissues. With the identification of an increasing number of cancer genes, attention has focused on molecular genetic screening for at-risk individuals. This has the advantage of providing early and presymptomatic detection, thus allowing appropriate cancer surveillance and treatment.

●●● GENETIC REGULATION OF THE CELL CYCLE

Many genes control the complex and critical balance between cell growth and the factors preventing unchecked growth. In general, these genes are involved in cell cycle regulation, cellular adhesion, contact inhibition, DNA repair and maintenance, and programmed cell death (known as apoptosis). Mutations in such genes can thereby initiate or perpetuate cancer. This is particularly true for those gene products involved in cell cycle regulation.

The eukaryotic cell cycle has four phases (Fig. 5-1). Three of these, G₁, S, and G₂, comprise interphase—the period between two successive mitoses. The cell spends the great majority of time in interphase, typically 16 to 24 hours. The fourth phase, M ("mitosis"), is relatively fast, taking 1 to 2 hours. During the G₁ ("gap 1") phase, the cell undertakes normal metabolic activities and prepares for DNA synthesis. Cells are diploid, and each chromosome consists of a centromere and a single chromatid. This phase generally shows the most variability in length, lasting only a few hours or for years. DNA replication occurs in the S ("synthesis") phase. At this point, the cell is diploid and each chromosome is represented as a bivalent, with two sister chromatids sharing a centromere. Here, it is important to note that the cell expends a considerable amount of resources to provide regulatory "checkpoints" at the G₁ to S transition. This is because the S phase represents a commitment to DNA synthesis and the subsequent cell division. During G₂ ("gap 2") phase, cells prepare for mitosis by manufacturing tubulin, necessary for microtubule formation as a component of the mitotic spindle apparatus. Mitosis concludes the cycle, with some cells

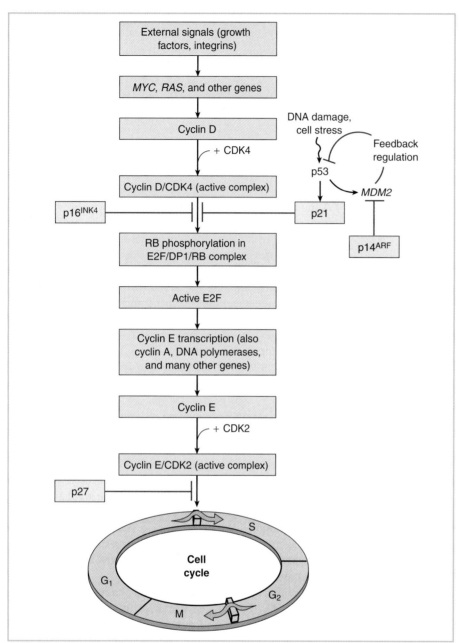

Figure 5-1. Movement from one phase of the cell cycle to another is dependent upon the regulating factors. *MYC* and *RAS* genes, activated by external factors, initiate the synthesis and stabilization of cyclin D. In the nucleus, the active cyclin D/CDK4 complex phosphorylates RB in the E2F/DP1/RB complex causing the activation of E2F. E2F is a transcription factor for cyclin E and cyclin A. The cell cycle can be blocked by p21 and p27 (CIP/KIP inhibitors) and by p16^{INK4A} and p14^{ARF} (INK4A/ARF inhibitors). In the event of DNA damage and cell stress, p53 causes cell arrest. (Redrawn from Kumar V, Abbas A, Fausto N. *Robbins & Cotran Pathologic Basis of Disease,* 7th ed. Philadelphia, WB Saunders, 2004, p 291.)

reentering the G_1 phase and recapitulating the cycle. Certain cells such as neurons, skeletal muscle, and erythrocytes, however, are postmitotic in that they do not divide again after they have differentiated. These cells are "frozen" in a perpetual G_1 state, sometimes termed G_0. Occasionally, such cells can be induced, for example by growth factor or hormone, to reenter the cycle.

Cells are provoked into cell division by the initiating actions of growth factors and hormones that permit transitions through the cell cycle. This process is typically begun at the cell membrane by receptor-ligand, or growth factor–receptor, interaction and is controlled by polypeptides called cyclins and their associated cyclin-dependent kinases (CDKs). Different cyclins are present within the cell at different stages of the cell cycle (Fig. 5-2). For example, at

the all-important transition from G_1 to S, which marks a commitment to DNA synthesis and mitosis, cyclin D is expressed following growth factor stimulation. Inhibitors of CDKs (CKI, cyclin kinase inhibitor) regulate cyclin-CDK complexes. Because they inhibit the action of cyclin-CDK complexes, CKIs also tend to slow cell cycle progression. Since the G_1 to S transition hallmarks a commitment to cell division, the molecular genetic events that regulate this transition will be examined in greater detail.

G_1 to S Cell Cycle Transition

For the cell to survive, all criteria for survival must be met before the cell enters S phase. Fundamentally, this means the genome must be prepared and ready to replicate. Otherwise,

HISTOLOGY

Mitotic Spindle

The mitotic spindle is a network of microtubules formed of α- and β-tubulin during prophase. Microtubular organizing centers, such as the mitotic spindle apparatus that includes basal bodies and centrioles, direct the assembly and disassembly of microtubules and organize them in such a fashion that they are oriented perpendicular to the plane of division.

Microtubules must attach to the kinetochore, a point within the centromere of the chromatids of the metaphase chromosome, for metaphase to proceed correctly. MAD proteins, which block the beginning of anaphase, remain attached to the kinetochore until microtubules attach. The kinesin spindle protein drives the formation of the spindle and enables chromosome segregation.

The mitotic spindle is a target for antimitotic drugs, such as paclitaxel (Taxol) and vinblastine.

BIOCHEMISTRY

Cyclins and Cyclin-dependent Kinases

The cyclin superfamily consists of proteins that bind to and activate cyclin-dependent-kinases (CDKs). Activation is required for progression through the cell cycle. The major cyclins controlling the cell cycle are:

- Cyclin D—G_1 phase
- Cyclins A and E—S phase
- Cyclins A and B—M phase

Major CDKs are:

- CDK4, CDK6—G_1 phase
- CDK2—S phase
- CDK1—M phase

damaging mutations are likely and the cell—if not the organ system—will either die or progress toward a pathology such as cancer. Thus, several "checkpoints," in the form of regulatory proteins, are in place. Principal among these are cyclin D, CDK4, and CDK6, the retinoblastoma gene product (pRB), and the E2F transcription factor (Fig. 5-3). Prior to transition to S phase, the pRB protein is "active" by virtue of its hypophosphorylated state and is bound to the E2F factor, thereby inhibiting the expression of genes necessary for DNA replication and cell proliferation. Here, the pRb protein acts as the "master brake" of the cell cycle progression. As the cell signals the time for replication, growth factors stimulate the expression of cyclin D. Cyclin D, in turn, is bound by CD4 and CD6, resulting in an activated protein kinase complex. An important target of this complex is the *Rb1* gene. When phosphorylated by the cyclin D-CDK complex, pRB is inactivated and unable to bind E2F. This allows the released E2F transcription factor to translocate to the nucleus, where it promotes the expression of genes important to DNA replication and cell growth.

Other cell cycle "brakes" exist besides pRB. As mentioned above, CKIs can regulate the cell cycle by inhibiting the activity of the cyclin-CDK complex. CKIs are classified into two groups: the Cip/Kip group and the INK4 group. Cip/Kip CKIs include the p21, p27, and p57 gene products and inhibit all cyclin-CDK complexes. INK4 members include the p15, p16, p18, and p19 gene products, and these proteins inhibit only the cyclin D-CDK4/6 complexes. In general, the CKIs act as cell cycle inhibitors by inactivating the cyclin-CDK complexes, which in turn keep pRB unphosphorylated and complexed to the E2F transcription factor. Interestingly, certain CKIs (p21, for example) can be expressed preferentially during times of cellular stress including DNA damage. This has the benefit of halting entrance into the S phase so that the cell has time to repair any genome damage prior to

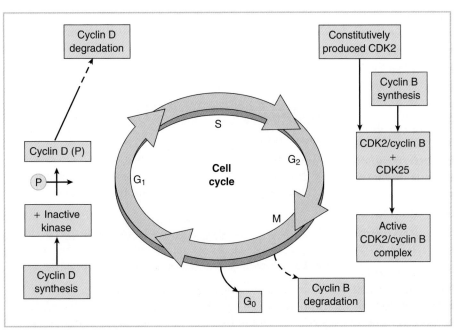

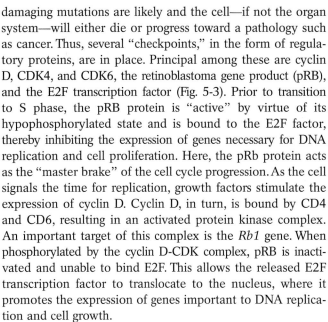

Figure 5-2. The cell cycle requires specific cyclins and cyclin-dependent kinases (CDKs) to progress through each stage. The transition from G_1 to S phase is regulated by cyclin D (D1-3) and cyclin E that are synthesized in G_1 and active when phosphorylated. Cyclins A and B1-2 control transition from G_2 to M. Cyclin B binds to CDK2, and this complex is activated by phosphorylation by CDK25 and other kinases.

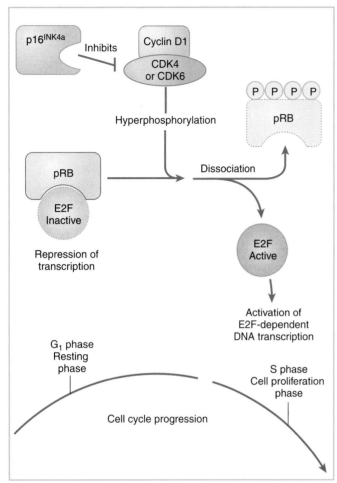

Figure 5-3. Control of cellular proliferation by retinoblastoma. When the retinoblastoma protein (pRB) exists in the underphosphorylated state, it can block exit from G$_1$ and progression of the cell cycle.

DNA replication. Stated differently, if a cell is stressed, p21 is expressed and cyclin CDK complexes remain inactive and thereby the phosphorylation of pRB is slowed. Since more pRB remains unphosphorylated and complexed to E2F, the E2F is unavailable as a transcription factor, slowing or halting the G$_1$ to S transition.

It can be appreciated now that tumors arise from alterations in the cell cycle resulting from abnormal proteins that dramatically alter the balance between cell growth and cell death. *The principal mechanisms for cell cycle perturbation are mutations in those genes that regulate it.* Predictably, the majority of genes associated with cancer are important in cell growth, proliferation, differentiation, death, and maintenance of the genome.

Genetic Paradigm for Cancer

Most of the time, cancer originates following genetic changes in a single cell; hence, cancers are monoclonal and all tumor cells are derived from a single progenitor. This cell exhibits altered physiologic properties that upset normal cellular

regulation of proliferation and death. Because daughter cells will carry the same mutation or mutations, the propensity for unchecked cellular growth is perpetuated during subsequent cell divisions. Thus, all cells in a tumor have a common origin.

Intense molecular genetic and family studies over the last two decades have revealed that the initial mutation leading to cancer either can occur spontaneously (de novo) in certain sporadic patients, or can be inherited, thus prescribing predisposition to heritable cancer. In either case, a single mutational event is rarely sufficient for neoplasia. Rather, a genetic paradigm has emerged in which cancer results from a progressive or sequential accumulation of mutations (Fig. 5-4). Often mutations may occur in genes necessary for DNA maintenance and repair. Such mutations may facilitate the process by increasing the likelihood of mutation within the cell. Accordingly, with each new mutational "step," cellular regulation of growth versus stasis or death diminishes, ultimately resulting in a cell lineage that divides without constraint. At this point, normal cell metabolism is profoundly altered, and cells may obtain the ability, through further genetic change, to infiltrate other tissues and metastasize to other organs, thus

BIOCHEMISTRY

Cyclin Kinase Inhibitors

Cyclin kinase inhibitors (CKIs) inhibit cyclin/CDK complexes. There are two classes of CKI: the INK4 family (p15/p16/p19) and the CIP/KIP family (p21, p27)

The INK4 family is specific for CDK4/cyclin D and regulates cell cycle entry in response to growth factors. Cyclin D activates CDK4, the kinase that phosphorylates RB. This phosphorylation inhibits the normal growth-suppressive function of RB and allows cell proliferation.

The CIP/KIP family is induced by p53 and can regulate all classes of CDK/cyclins by inhibiting all cell cycle regulatory kinases (CDKs). Thus, this inhibition prevents progression through the cell cycle. Therefore, the loss of p53 and CIP/KIP CDKs allows uncontrolled cell proliferation. These proteins may also mediate normal control and cell cycle response to damage.

PATHOLOGY

Types of Cancers

Major types of cancer can be described as:

- Carcinoma: (85% of all cancers) derived from epithelial tissues; includes cancers of glands, breast, skin, and most internal organs.
- Sarcoma: cancer of connective tissue origin, such as muscle, bone, adipose tissue, cartilage, blood vessels, or other connective or supportive tissue.
- Leukemia: uncontrolled proliferation of leukocytes by either lymphoid organs or bone marrow.
- Lymphoma: malignant cancer of lymphoid organs, particularly the spleen and lymph nodes.

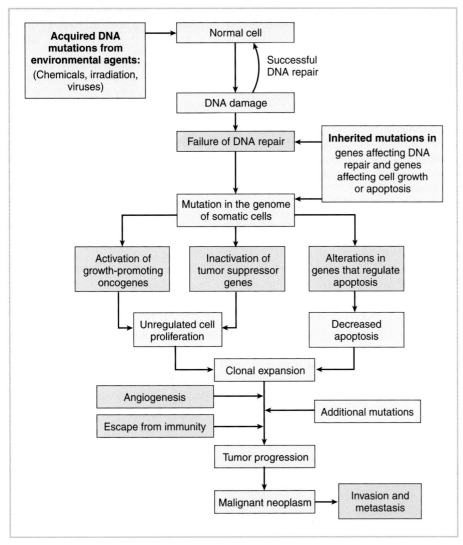

Figure 5-4. Simplified schematic for the molecular basis of cancer. (Redrawn from Kumar V, Abbas A, Fausto N. *Robbins & Cotran Pathologic Basis of Disease,* 7th ed. Philadelphia, WB Saunders, 2004, p 290.)

completing the transformation into a malignant neoplasm (see Fig. 5-4).

Although hundreds of genes regulate cell growth, death, and DNA repair, two general classes of cancer genes can be identified: oncogenes and tumor suppressor genes. In the broadest perspective, the actions of these gene products oppose each other; oncogenes typically stimulate cell growth while tumor suppressor genes inhibit proliferation. Accordingly, oncogenes are typically "activated" by a mutation in normal genes while tumor suppressor genes are generally "inactivated" by mutation. Below, the salient features of oncogenes and tumor suppressor genes are discussed along with examples of their role in cancer.

●●● ONCOGENES

Oncogenes ("cancer genes") are typically mutated genes that produce an aberrant protein that stimulates cell division, proliferation, or differentiation, even in the absence of proper growth signals. The majority of oncogenes are derived from proto-oncogenes, which are normal genes that participate in growth regulation. Because they regulate cellular proliferation, such genes are often growth factors, growth factor receptors, transcription factors, nuclear protein regulators, or cell signaling molecules. Mutations within proto-oncogenes occur either by spontaneous mutation or via a mutagen that promotes genetic change within the cell. Alternatively, a cell can undergo cancerous "transformation" from a normal to abnormal state through the introduction of an oncogene from a virus. Retroviruses, for example, are capable of transporting oncogenic versions of genes into human host cells via integration of their genome into the human chromosome. Even if a transforming retrovirus carries a proto-oncogene, it is quite possible that, given the high rate of mutation observed in retroviruses, a mutation will occur that alters the properties of the gene that turns it into an oncogene.

A large number of oncogenes have been identified (Table 5-1). They are named by three-letter abbreviations that indicate their origin and the type of resultant tumor. For example, the *RAS* oncogene was initially identified through retroviral studies of rat sarcomas. Normally, RAS functions as a G protein, a small protein that binds and hydrolyzes GTP. G proteins have a number of roles within the cell, including regulating cellular proliferation, morphogenesis, cell motility, and cytokinesis. These proteins act as cell regulators or switches via an intrinsic activation mechanism. They are activated to regulate cellular processes when bound to GTP, but these proteins slowly hydrolyze the GTP to GDP and P_i using an intrinsic GTPase activity (Fig. 5-5). In the activated (GTP-bound) state, G proteins are able to bind target proteins, but this capacity diminishes as GTP is slowly converted to GDP. Overall, the activities of G proteins are regulated by a number of G protein–related accessory proteins that serve to exchange GDP for GTP (GEF, or guanine nucleotide exchange factor), stimulate the rate of GTP hydrolysis (GAP, or GTPase activating proteins), thus inactivating the protein, or inhibit

MICROBIOLOGY

Retroviruses

Retroviruses give rise to transposable elements. There are usually three genes flanked by direct repeats. The genes of retroviruses include:

- *gag*: codes for core and structural proteins
- *pol*: codes for reverse transcriptase, protease, and integrase
- *env*: codes for viral coat proteins

Reverse transcriptase transcribes the viral RNA into DNA in the cytosol. The DNA then enters the nucleus and integrates into the genome, where it may cause insertional mutation. It may also translocate to another region (transposition) and carry additional genome sequences.

the dissociation of GDP from the protein (GDI, or GDP dissociation inhibitor), which is also an inactivating mechanism.

Specifically, RAS is located in the plasma membrane and is involved in regulation of cellular proliferation through interaction with growth factors (see Fig. 5-5). Normally, when RAS binds GTP, it undergoes a conformational change to its activated state and binds a protein kinase called RAF, a serine protein kinase also called MAPKKK (for mitogen-activated protein kinase kinase kinase), initiating the MAP kinase–mediated protein phosphorylation cascade that ultimately

TABLE 5-1. Examples of Oncogenes and Associated Cancers

Oncogene	Location	Function	Associated Cancers
Growth Factor Genes			
HST	11q13	Fibroblast growth factor	Stomach carcinoma
SIS	22q12	ß-Subunit of platelet-derived growth factor	Glioma
Growth Factor Receptor Genes			
RET	10q	Receptor tyrosine kinase	Multiple endocrine neoplasia, thyroid carcinomas
ERB-B	7p12	Epidermal growth factor receptor	Glioblastoma, breast cancer
ERB-A	17q11	Thyroid hormone receptor	Acute promyelocytic leukemia
NEU (ERB-B2)	17q21	Receptor protein kinase	Neuroblastoma, breast cancer
MET	7q31	Receptor tyrosine kinase	Hereditary papillary renal carcinoma, hepatocellular carcinoma
KIT	4q12	Receptor tyrosine kinase	Gastrointestinal stromal tumor syndrome
Signal Transduction Genes			
H-RAS	11p15	GTPase	Carcinoma of colon, lung, pancreas
K-RAS	12p12	GTPase	Melanoma, thyroid carcinoma, acute monocytic leukemia, colon carcinoma
B-RAF	7q34	Serine/threonine kinase	Malignant melanoma; colon cancer
ABL	9q34	Protein kinase	Chronic myelogenous leukemia; acute lymphocytic leukemia
CDK4	12q14	Cyclin-dependent kinase	Malignant melanoma
Transcription Factor Genes			
N-MYC	2p24	DNA-binding protein	Neuroblastoma, lung carcinoma
MYB	6q22	DNA-binding protein	Malignant melanoma, lymphoma, leukemia
FOS	14q24	Interacts with *JUN* oncogene to regulate transcription	Osteosarcoma

From Jorde LB, Carey CC, Bamshad MJ, White RL. *Medical Genetics*, 3rd ed. St. Louis, Mosby, 2003, p 236.

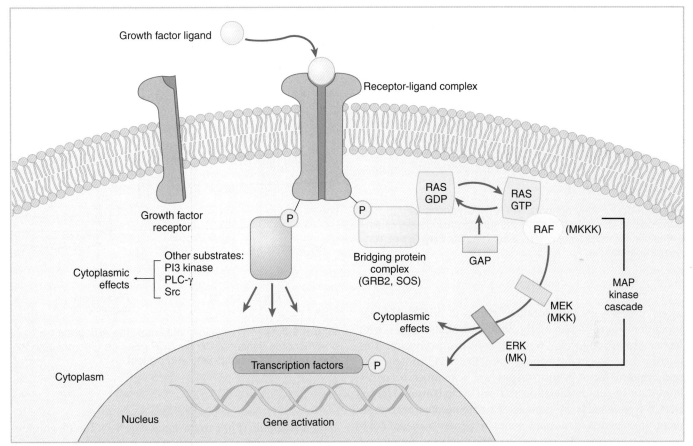

Figure 5-5. Tyrosine receptor signaling. Growth factor ligand causes the dimerization and autophosphorylation of tyrosines. Bridging proteins (BRB2/SOS) bring the receptor into the vicinity of RAS, where it catalyzes guanine exchange on RAS. The activated RAS associates with RAF1, a serine/threonine protein kinase, and RAF1 then activates and phosphorylates MEK. The MAP kinase cascade interacts with proteins that are translocated to the nucleus where transcription factors are activated. (Redrawn from Kumar V, Abbas A, Fausto N. *Robbins & Cotran Pathologic Basis of Disease*, 7th ed. Philadelphia, W.B. Saunders, 2004, p 99.)

results in the activation of at least one nuclear transcription factor that regulates the expression of genes important in cell proliferation. A mutation altering a single base pair in *RAS* is all that is necessary to produce an abnormal RAS that is constantly in the "active" conformation. In this case, the abnormal RAS protein would promote cellular growth and would not be constrained by normal cellular checkpoints, thus promoting tumor formation. In fact, RAS mutations have been found in many tumor types, including colon cancer, as will be discussed later.

Functionally, oncogenes exact their transforming capacity through dominant transmission, since only a single allele needs to be mutated in order to deregulate cell proliferation. Hence, oncogenes typically act as dominant, *gain-of-function mutations*. As discussed later, tumor suppressor genes do not share this genetic mechanism.

Oncogene Activation by Translocation

Burkitt Lymphoma

Burkitt lymphoma is a rare cancer of the jaw found in African children. Cytogenetic analysis has shown that the majority of patients have a balanced translocation involving the *myc*

proto-oncogene from chromosome 8q24 to chromosome 14q32 [t(8;14)(q24;q32)] (Fig. 5-6). Occasionally, the *MYC* gene is translocated to chromosome 2q11 or chromosome 22q11. In each of these three cases, the *MYC* gene is placed in a new genomic environment that features the genes for immunoglobulin heavy, κ light, and λ light chains, respectively. It is clear that this new genetic address results in uncontrolled *MYC* expression. Though *MYC* is constitutively expressed at low

BIOCHEMISTRY

G Proteins

G proteins are heterotrimers that bind GDP and GTP. These heterotrimers are found in all cells, and include three subunits: G_α, which has a binding site for nucleotide, G_β, and G_γ. Heterotrimers associate with the inner cell membrane surface as well as transmembrane receptors, such as receptors for polypeptide hormones.

GDP is bound to G_α in the inactive G protein state. Allosteric change occurs in G_α, and GTP replaces GDP. The activated G_α then activates an effector molecule.

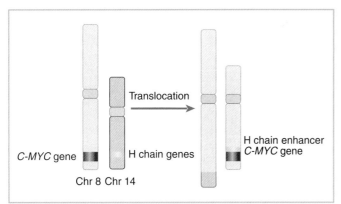

Figure 5-6. Burkitt lymphoma. The c-*MYC* gene is translocated downstream of the immunoglobulin heavy chain enhancer. Expression of c-*MYC* is up-regulated by its position near the enhancer.

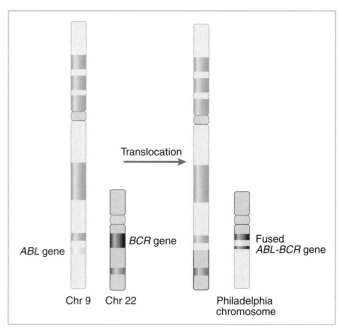

Figure 5-7. Chronic myeloid leukemia. The *ABL* gene on chromosome 9 inserts into the *BCR* gene on chromosome 22 and creates an altered gene and protein.

levels in cells, its translocation places it under different promoter control—that of the immunoglobulin genes with higher expression levels—resulting in its overexpression. This is critical to cancer formation, since the MYC protein is a transcription factor whose targets are a number of genes important in cell proliferation and cell cycle control. Hence, Burkitt lymphoma is an example of a chromosomal rearrangement that places a normal gene in a new genetic environment, altering its expression and thereby promoting cellular transformation.

Burkitt lymphoma is endemic in Africa and most people associate it with an African B-cell neoplasm involving the maxilla or mandible. However, there is also a sporadic form that usually does not involve the maxilla or mandible. This form involves the abdominal organs most frequently and presents with tumors causing swelling and pain. The distal ileum, cecum, or mesentery are more often involved than other abdominal organs, pelvic organs, or facial bones. Epstein-Barr virus is strongly implicated in the etiology of the African form, but this correlation is less clearly understood in the sporadic form.

Chronic Myeloid Leukemia

Chronic myeloid (myelogenous) leukemia (CML) is a form of leukemia hallmarked by a uniquely abnormal chromosome,

the Philadelphia (Ph) chromosome (Fig. 5-7). The Ph chromosome results from a translocation from the long arm of chromosome 9 to the long arm of chromosome 22. This t(9;22)(q34;q11) rearrangement is a balanced, reciprocal translocation that is found in 90% of patients with CML. The result of the translocation is a slightly longer chromosome 9 and a smaller chromosome 22. The translocation relocates the *ABL* proto-oncogene from 9q to 22q, where it is positioned within the "breakpoint cluster region 9," or *BCR*, consisting of genes of unknown function. Here, unlike Burkitt lymphoma, the genetic juxtaposition results in a novel fusion protein composed of *BCR*-encoded amino acids at the N-terminus and *ABL*-encoded amino acids at the C-terminus. This constitutively expressed BCR-ABL protein chimera is a 210-kd protein with an enhanced tyrosine kinase activity compared with the normal *ABL* gene product, a change in activity that promotes neoplasia. While the 210-kd chimera is the primary protein expressed, other forms may be expressed also depending on the exact breakpoint in *BCR* (Fig. 5-8). Product p230 is associated with chronic neutrophilic leukemia and thrombocytosis.

There are three phases of CML, which are progressive in symptomology as well as in increasing resistance to therapies. Understanding the tyrosine kinase activity of the chimeric protein led to the development of the first in a new class of pharmacologic agents specifically targeted to a cancer. Imatinib mesylate (Gleevec) is a specific and potent inhibitor of the BCR-ABL tyrosine kinase. Its efficacy has been demonstrated in different phases of CML disease (Box 5-1). It is also effective against other tyrosine kinases, such as ABL, platelet-derived growth factor receptor, and the stem cell factor receptor known as c-KIT.

PATHOLOGY

Hodgkin versus Non-Hodgkin Lymphomas

Hodgkin and non-Hodgkin lymphomas (NHLs) differ in several respects. Hodgkin lymphomas arise in a single or related nodes, spread continuously, and contain Reed-Sternberg cells.

Non-Hodgkin lymphomas may arise at extranodal sites and spread in an unpredictable manner. There are about 20 types of NHL, including Burkitt lymphoma.

Box 5-1. FEATURES OF CHRONIC MYELOID LEUKEMIA

Chronic Phase

Less than 10% to 15% blast cells
WBC $\geq 20 \times 10^3/\mu L$
Symptoms mild
25% to 40% progress directly to blast crisis
Average duration: 5 to 6 years

Accelerated Phase

10% to 15% blast cells (<30%)
Symptoms may include fever, bone pain, splenomegaly, hepatomegaly
Cytogenetic abnormalities increase—duplication of Ph chromosome, isochromosomes, trisomies
Average duration: 6 to 9 months

Blast Crisis

More than 30% blast cells
    50%—Myeloid blast crisis
    25%—Lymphoid blast crisis
    25%—Mixed
Symptoms may include anemia and infection, CNS disease, lymphadenopathy, bleeding
Poor prognosis
Average duration: 3 to 6 months

PHARMACOLOGY

Imatinib Mesylate (Gleevec)

Imatinib mesylate (Gleevec) is a specific inhibitor of tyrosine kinases, including BCR-ABL. It blocks the binding site for ATP on the kinase and prevents phosphorylation of tyrosines in proteins, which prevents signal transduction pathways leading to transformation in CML. It is metabolized by CYP3A4 of the P-450 enzyme system, and it is most effective in chronic phase of CML.

Gene Amplification

The phenomenon of gene duplication is another mechanism of altering the expression patterns of otherwise normal genes such that they become oncogenes. In gene amplification, certain regions of DNA are duplicated and amplified, resulting in as many as several hundred additional copies of genes contained within the amplified DNA. These changes are often visible at the microscopic level or are readily detected by modern cytogenetic techniques such as fluorescent in situ hybridization (FISH) or comparative genome hybridization (CGH) (Fig. 5-9).

Two general patterns of chromosomal alterations are observed with gene amplifications: multiple small chromosome-like structures called double minutes (*dms*) and homoge-

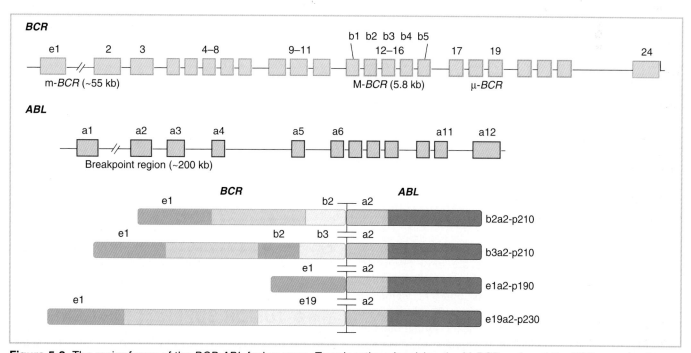

Figure 5-8. The major forms of the *BCR-ABL* fusion gene. Translocations involving the M-*BCR* region of the *BCR* gene lead to joining of the second or third exons of this region (b2,b3) with the second exon of the *ABL* gene (a2) to form the b2a2 or b3a2 transcripts and the p210 product. Breakpoints in the m-*BCR* region of the *BCR* gene result in fusion of the first exon of this gene (e1) with the second exon of the *ABL* gene (a2) to form the e1a2 *BCR-ABL* transcript that encodes the p190 hybrid protein. Breakpoints in the m-*BCR* region of the *BCR* gene juxtapose the exon 19 (e19) of this gene to the second exon of the *ABL* gene (a2) to produce the e19a2 transcript that encodes the p230 protein. (Redrawn courtesy of Rajyalakshmi Luthra, PhD, University of Texas MD Anderson Cancer Center, Houston, Texas.)

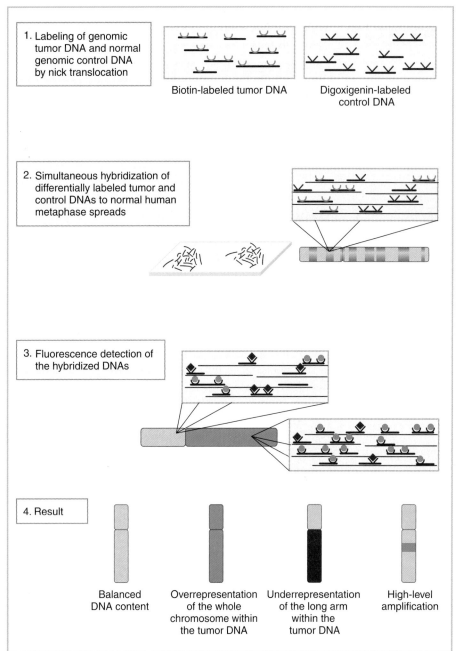

Figure 5-9. Comparative genomic hybridization (CGH). This cytogenetic technique demonstrates a change in DNA content of tumor cells. CGH can detect unbalanced chromosome changes only such as seen with double minutes (*dms*) and homogeneously staining regions (HSRs) by comparing the ratio of the intensities of the two fluorochromes along target chromosomes to indicate regions of DNA gain or loss. It will not detect balanced changes such as reciprocal translocations.

neously staining regions (HSRs). Together, *dms* and HSRs are seen in roughly 10% of tumors and are most frequently detected in the latter stages of cancer. The mechanism for *dms* formation is poorly understood. HSRs represent regions of amplification that do not label normally with chromosomal identification techniques; hence, they lack a normal banding pattern in karyotypic analysis. These amplified regions often contain proto-oncogenes such as *RAS* and members of the *MYC* family. For example, the n-*MYC* gene is amplified over 100-fold in 25% to 40% of late-stage neuroblastoma, a malignancy of neuroblasts found in infants or children that has widespread metastatic potential (Fig. 5-10). However, n-*MYC* amplification is rare in early-stage neuroblastoma. Hence, the appearance of amplified n-*MYC* appears to signify or promote an aggressive tumor and therefore predicts a poor prognosis.

TUMOR SUPPRESSOR GENES

Whereas oncogenes are typically dominant, gain-of-function mutations, tumor suppressor genes facilitate neoplastic transformation via a cellular recessive model where there is a *loss-of-function* in both alleles. In the normal state, these genes are active in "putting the brakes on" cellular proliferation. In this way, they function oppositely to growth-promoting oncogenes.

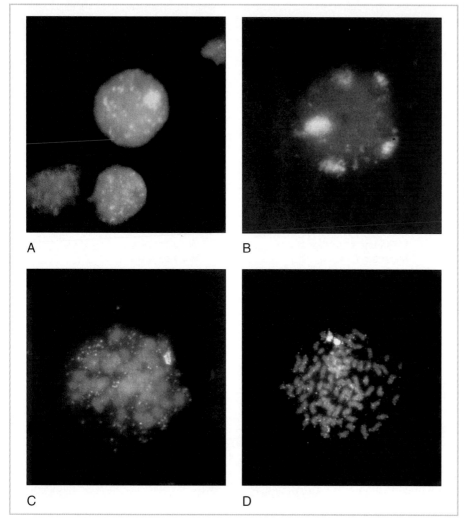

Figure 5-10. Fluorescence in situ hybridization with probe MYCN. **A**, Interphase nucleus with dms and one HSR from patient 1. **B**, Interphase nucleus with dms and five HSRs from the same patient. **C**, Metaphase cell with dms and one HSR from patient 2. **D**, Metaphase cell from the same case with dms and two HSRs. (From Yoshimoto M, de Toledo SRC, Caranet EMM, et al. MYCN gene amplification: identification of cell populations containing double minutes and homogeneously staining regions in neuroblastoma tumors. *Am J Pathol.* 1999;155:1439–1443. With permission from the American Society for Investigative Pathology.)

About 30 different tumor suppressor genes have been characterized (Table 5-2), and they can be subclassified into three general groups: genes that control cell division, genes that repair DNA, and genes that destroy cells. The first group is also referred to as "gatekeeper" genes that are actively and directly involved in cell cycle, cell growth, or contact inhibition regulation. The second group is also referred to as "caretaker" genes that are responsible for DNA repair and genomic maintenance; thus, when inactivated by mutation, these genes indirectly facilitate cancerous cellular change by enabling genetic change. If too much DNA damage accumulates within a cell, the cell undergoes apoptosis controlled by the third group of genes.

Cell Division–Controlling Genes

Retinoblastoma

Retinoblastoma (Rb) is a model for tumor suppressor genes in both inherited and sporadic cancer and is the most common intraocular tumor among early childhood with an incidence of 1 in 20,000 children. Unless treated, it is fatal. Retinoblastoma serves as the paradigm for tumor suppressor gene-related malignancies. Rb is caused by the genetic inactivation of the *RB1* gene on chromosome 13q14.3. *RB1* mutations inactivate the *RB1* gene product, a 110-kd phosphorylated protein that regulates the cell cycle at the point of the G_1 to S transition. Absence of pRB deconstrains this mitotic checkpoint, thus allowing cell proliferation. Because of its role in cell cycle control, the pRB protein provides an excellent example of a "gatekeeper" tumor suppressor gene.

TABLE 5-2. Examples of Tumor Suppressor Genes and Associated Cancers

Type of Tumor Suppressor Gene	Gene	Inherited Cancer	Noninherited Cancers
Cell division–controlling genes	RB1	Retinoblastoma	Many cancers
	VHL	Von Hippel–Lindau kidney cancer	Kidney cancers, hemangioblastomas of CNS, colon cancers
	NF1 NF2	} Nerve tumors, including brain	Colon cancers, melanomas, neuroblastoma
	APC	Familial adenomatous polyposis	Colorectal cancers
DNA repair genes	MLH1 MSH2 MSH6	} Colorectal cancer (without polyposis)	Colorectal, gastric, endometrial cancers
	BRCA1 BRCA2	} Breast and/or ovarian cancer	Rare ovarian cancers
Apoptosis genes	TP53	Li-Fraumeni syndrome	Many cancers
	INK4a (p16)	Melanoma	Many cancers
	HPC1 MSR	} Prostate cancer	Unknown

over 50% of leukocoria is associated with retinoblastoma (Fig. 5-11). Retinoblastoma originates from primitive retinal cells and may grow either over the retina and into the vitreous humor or under the retina, causing detachment. If undetected or untreated, the tumor may extend into the sclera, into the orbital lymphatics, or through the optic nerve (Fig. 5-12). It is the replacement of the vitreous humor with tumor that causes leukocoria. Another common presentation in children is strabismus.

The existence of inherited cancer syndromes such as Rb heralded the discovery of tumor suppressor genes. The relationship between the two was first elucidated in 1971 by A. G. Knudson, who observed the rare Rb tumor in patients with and without a family history of retinal tumors. Knudson proposed that two separate mutations were necessary for tumor development. One mutation might present in the germline cells and therefore was termed a "constitutional" mutation. This mutation would be present in every somatic cell in the body but would also be passed on to subsequent generations. The second mutational event would be a new mutation in the other, nonmutated RB1 allele. To affect Rb, this second mutation would occur within a retinal cell—a somatic cell. The combination of the first—inherited—"hit" and the second—somatic—"hit" would effectively eliminate the protein of both alleles of the RB1 gene in an individual and thus permit tumor formation. This paradigm of tumor suppressor gene action has come to be known as Knudson's "two-hit" hypothesis and serves as a model for cancers resulting from tumor suppressor genes.

With Rb as a model, it can now be seen how tumor suppressor genes are key etiologic factors in familial cancers. Rb can present as sporadic or familial cases (Fig. 5-13). In familial (or heritable) cases, a mutation of one RB1 allele is passed through generations in an autosomal dominant

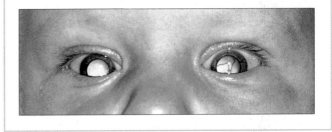

Figure 5-11. Leukocoria in a child with retinoblastoma. The normal red reflex to light, which may be red, orange, or yellow, is replaced by a white reflex in 60% of patients with retinoblastoma. The normal red reflex should be symmetric between both eyes. Leukocoria may be unilateral or bilateral and may occur with conditions other than retinoblastoma including congenital cataracts, Coats disease, persistent hyperplastic primary vitreous (PHPV), and toxocariasis. (From Augsburger JJ, Bornfeld N, Giblin ME. Retinoblastoma. In Yanoff M, Duker JS. *Ophthalmology,* 2nd ed. St. Louis, Mosby, 2004.)

ANATOMY

The Eye

The eyeball is formed as an outgrowth of the optic vesicle and consists of several layers:

- External fibrous region: sclera, cornea
- Middle vascular region: choroid, ciliary body, iris
- Internal region: retina

The internal region includes both the neural retina (optic disk, macula, fovea centralis, rods, and cones) and the pigmented retina. Retinal detachment occurs when the neural retina becomes separated from the pigmented retina.

An apparent paradox regarding tumor suppressor genes is voiced by the question: How can cancer due to tumor suppressor genes be autosomal dominant when both copies of the gene must be inactivated to permit tumor formation? In fact, the inherited or constitutional deleterious allele is transmitted in an autosomal dominant manner and most heterozygotes do manifest the disease. So, while the predisposition for cancer is inherited in a dominant fashion, pathology at the cellular level requires the loss of both alleles—a decidedly recessive mechanism. This explains why penetrance is incomplete in Rb, since only about 90% of heterozygotes ever undergo the second, somatic "hit" to their normal *RB1* allele.

Loss of Heterozygosity

Intensive molecular genetic analysis of the Rb locus revealed that, in a significant proportion of cases, individuals who were otherwise heterozygous in normal tissues contained tumors that harbored only a single *RB1* allele. In other words, one allele seemingly vanished. The tumor cells underwent a *loss of heterozygosity* (LOH) for part of chromosome 13q, including the RB1 locus. In familial Rb, the remaining *RB1* allele was the inherited and deleterious gene, and the loss of the nonmutated allele equaled a second "hit" and precipitated tumor formation. Several mechanisms may account for LOH, including interstitial deletion in chromosome 13q14, mitotic nondisjunction resulting in the loss of one chromosome 13, or mitotic recombination. In any case, *LOH represents the most common genetic mechanism for loss of the normal RB1 allele in patients.* If LOH is not found, the most likely explanation is a point mutation inactivation of the second *RB1* allele. LOH is considered an important genetic phenomenon in cancer and has been observed in a number of cancers that are perpetuated by the loss of tumor suppressor genes (Table 5-3).

Spontaneous Retinoblastoma

Spontaneous retinoblastoma accounts for roughly 60% of cases and results from the concerted action of two independent somatic *RB1* mutations in a single retinal cell (Table 5-4). Hence, these tumors are unifocal and unilateral,

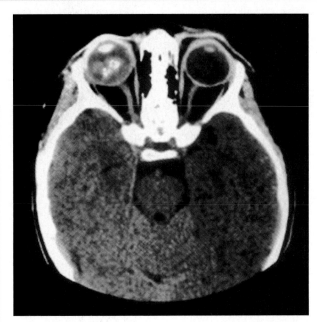
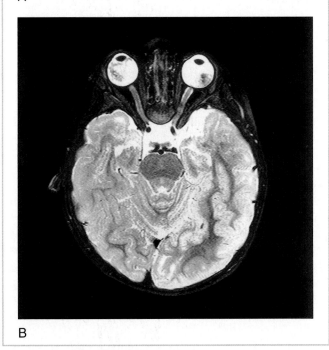

Figure 5-12. CT scan (**A**) and MRI (**B**) of retinoblastoma in a child with leukocoria showing a calcified mass in the globe of the eye. (Courtesy of Simin Dadparvar, MD)

extremely rare event, but the one million or so retinoblasts are mitotically active, giving ample opportunity for genetic error. Hence, Rb clinical expression is quite common in families with a germline *RB1* mutation, although penetrance is not complete owing to the random nature of the second, somatic mutation (see Fig. 5-13). It is proper then, to suggest that the predisposition for Rb is high in families carrying the mutation although some individuals heterozygous for an *RB1* mutation may not develop retinal tumors.

PATHOLOGY

Retinoblastoma

Tumors may contain both differentiated and undifferentiated cells. Differentiated cells may contain Flexner-Wintersteiner rosettes and fleurettes, whereas undifferentiated cells have hyperchromatic nuclei and appear as collections of small, round cells.

Calcification is characteristic of retinoblastoma and differentiates retinoblastoma from other tumors or lesions that mimic retinoblastoma in children under age 3 years. In older children, calcification may occur in other lesions, such as retinopathy of prematurity and *Toxocara* infections from pets.

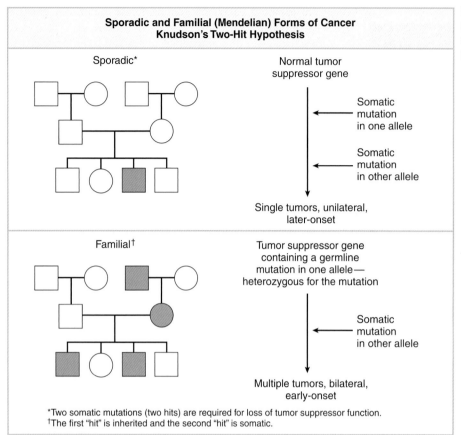

Sporadic and Familial (Mendelian) Forms of Cancer
Knudson's Two-Hit Hypothesis

Sporadic*

Normal tumor
suppressor gene

Somatic
mutation
in one allele

Somatic
mutation
in other allele

Single tumors, unilateral,
later-onset

Familial†

Tumor suppressor gene
containing a germline
mutation in one allele—
heterozygous for the mutation

Somatic
mutation
in other allele

Multiple tumors, bilateral,
early-onset

*Two somatic mutations (two hits) are required for loss of tumor suppressor function.
†The first "hit" is inherited and the second "hit" is somatic.

Figure 5-13. Comparison between sporadic and inherited forms of cancers, as seen with retinoblastoma and other cancers.

since they are truly monoclonal in origin. This can be contrasted to familial Rb in which tumors can be multifocal and are often bilateral—reflecting the need for only a single additional somatic mutational event within the normal *RB1* allele in a retinal cell.

Using Rb as a model, the key differences between the heritable cancer predisposing syndromes and sporadic cancer can be examined. Typically, the inherited cancer predisposition is passed through a family by autosomal dominant transmission. Because offspring of a carrier have a 50% chance to inherit the predisposing allele, the risk is high within families. There is a much lower risk for sporadic cases of a certain cancer in the general population. Individuals harboring a cancer predisposition allele tend to have an earlier onset, develop second tumors that tend to be bilateral

TABLE 5-3. Examples of LOH and Associated Tumor Suppressor Gene Cancers

Chromosome	Tumor Suppressor Gene	Gene Associated Cancer
1q	Unknown	Breast carcinoma
	HPC1	Prostate cancer
3p	Unknown	Small-cell lung carcinoma, renal cell carcinoma
	VHL	CNS hemangioblastoma
5q	APC	Familial polyposis coli, colorectal carcinoma
8p	MSR1	Prostate carcinoma, breast carcinoma
9p	INK4A	Non-small-cell carcinoma of the lung, melanoma
13q	RB1	Retinoblastoma, osteosarcoma
17p	TP53	Colorectal carcinoma, breast carcinoma
18q	DCC	Colorectal carcinoma

TABLE 5-4. Comparison Between Heritable and Nonheritable Retinoblastoma

Feature	Heritable Rb	Nonheritable Rb
Tumor	Usually bilateral	Unilateral
Family history	20% of cases	None
Average age at diagnosis	<1 year	About 2 years or later
Increased risk of second primary tumors	Osteosarcoma, other sarcomas, melanoma, others	None

as opposed to unilateral, and/or exhibit cancers in other organ systems more frequently than do sporadic cases. Although the sporadic form is much more common than the familial form for any particular cancer, there is still great value in forging a deep understanding of the molecular pathophysiologic mechanisms of heritable cancers. Advances in diagnosis, prognosis, presymptomatic detection and surveillance, and treatment will not only help those patients with the heritable form but also may lead to mechanistic insights into the sporadic forms.

Neurofibromatosis Type 1

Neurofibromatosis type 1 (NF1) is an autosomal dominant disease of the nervous system that features the cardinal signs of multiple benign neurofibroma tumors in the skin (Fig. 5-14), irregularly pigmented patches of the skin (café-au-lait spots), and small benign tumors on the iris known as Lisch nodules (Box 5-2). Occasionally, NF patients will develop cancer related to the nervous system, including neurofibrosarcoma, cancer of Schwann cell, or astrocytoma. The NF1 gene is located at chromosome 17q11.2 and its nucleotide and protein sequence analyses showed it has extensive similarity with a GTPase-activating protein (GAP). This, in turn, is significant to carcinogenesis because one of the GAP functions is to accelerate the hydrolysis of GTP bound to the RAS protein. Thus, the NF1 protein, neurofibromin, can be envisioned as a GAP specific to neural related cells that regulates RAS activity in neuronal tissues. Normally, neurofibromin interacts with RAS in the signal transduction pathway by down-regulating the activity of RAS. As the neurofibromatosis gene product is diminished or lost by mutation, RAS activity may increase in such a way to promote cell growth and inhibit cellular differentiation. In this case, the loss of NF1 serves as the "trigger" for increasing the activity of the *RAS* oncogene.

Box 5-2. DIAGNOSTIC FEATURES OF NEUROFIBROMATOSIS TYPE 1

Café-au-lait spots
  Prepubertal—6 or more >5 mm
  Postpubertal—diameter >15 mm
Neurofibroma
  Two or more of any type of neurofibroma *or*
  One plexiform neurofibroma
Freckling in the axillary or inguinal regions
Optic glioma
Two or more Lisch nodules (iris hamartomas)
A distinctive osseous lesion such as sphenoid dysplasia or thinning of the long bone cortex with or without pseudoarthrosis
A first-degree relative with NF1

When a deleterious *NF1* mutation occurs, the heterozygote exhibits typical neurofibromatosis. If the second *NF1* allele is inactivated, however, *RAS* activity may increase further and the chance for malignancy increases. This scenario suggests that the *NF1* gene is a tumor suppressor gene. Indeed, LOH for the normal (noninherited) *NF1* allele has been observed in a number of NF1-related malignancies.

●●● DNA REPAIR GENES

Colorectal Cancer and the Genetic Paradigm for Cancer Revisited

Nearly 2% of individuals in Europe and North America develop colorectal cancers, making it one of the most common cancers in the Western world. In 2006, it is estimated that 148,000 new cases will diagnosed and more than 56,000

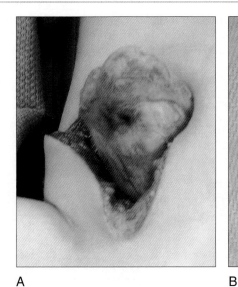
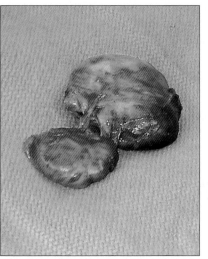

A   B

Figure 5-14. Neurofibroma removed from a child. Most neurofibromas present as active stage 2 tumors (G0, T0, M0) in the skin or associated with nerves. Occasionally they can be seen as stage 3 (M0, T1–2, M2) aggressive infiltrative forms. (Courtesy of Dr. Rahul Nath, Texas Nerve and Paralysis Institute, Houston, Texas.)

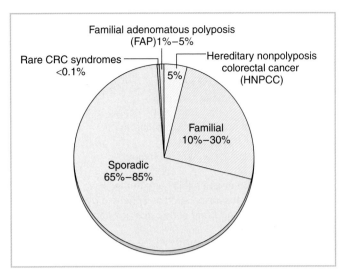

Figure 5-15. Causes of hereditary susceptibility to colorectal cancer. Single-gene mutations have been identified for HNPCC and FAP.

Likewise, p53 mutations and LOH for regions of chromosomes 5q and 18q seem to accumulate or increase in frequency as benign adenomas progress to malignant carcinomas. Molecular genetic dissection of colorectal cancer has demonstrated that the inactivation of the *APC* ("adenomatous polyposis coli") gene on chromosome 5q and the *DCC* ("deleted in colon cancer") gene on chromosome 18q is common in colorectal cancer. This, in turn, explains the increased frequency of LOH on chromosomes 5q and 18q in this form of malignancy—the *APC* and/or the *DCC* gene have been lost via LOH. The general genetic model for cancer evolution to colorectal cancer can now be applied (Fig. 5-16). It is important to remember that it is the accumulation of mutations that is key in this model—not necessarily the order. Empirically, for example, it has been reported that greater than 90% of carcinomas contain at least two of these genetic changes and roughly 40% show at least three accumulated mutations.

This genetic paradigm can be applied to the two forms of familial colorectal cancer syndromes, familial adenomatous polyposis (FAP) and hereditary nonpolyposis of the colon cancer (HNPCC). Like many of the autosomal dominant cancer syndromes, the familial form of colorectal cancer is recognized by an increased incidence of cancer in people with a family history of colorectal cancer and families exhibiting a number of affected individuals consistent with autosomal dominant transmission.

deaths from colorectal cancer will occur in the United States. Most of these will be sporadic cases, but up to 30% will be familial cases (Fig. 5-15). Two subclasses of familial colorectal cancers have been identified that are associated with the loss of tumor suppressor genes: familial adenomatous polyposis (FAP) and hereditary nonpolyposis colon cancer (HNPCC). Although the primary genes associated with these colorectal cancers have radically differing functions, the overall mechanism for carcinogenesis is quite similar.

Applying the Genetic Paradigm for Cancer Evolution

Most colorectal cancers proceed from benign adenomatous polyps to malignant tumors. This transition is associated with increasing polyp size and an accumulation of genetic alterations. For example, polyps less than 1 cm in diameter rarely appear cancerous histologically and harbor *RAS* mutations in only a few percent of examined cases. As polyps increase in size to 2 cm, however, *RAS* mutations appear in 40% of cases.

Familial Adenomatous Polyposis (FAP)

Approximately 1% to 5% of colorectal cancers are caused by FAP, an autosomal dominant disorder. FAP is a serious disorder in which penetrance is greater than 90% by age 35, reflecting the near 100% risk in untreated individuals. There is also an increased risk for extracolonic tumors in FAP, including upper GI tumors, osteomas, thyroid tumors, and brain tumors. The gene responsible for FAP is the *APC* gene. The *APC* gene product is a cytoplasmic protein that regulates the activity of β-catenin, one of three ubiquitously expressed cytoplasmic catenins. β-Catenin has two functions within the cell. First, it permits cell-cell interactions by anchoring cadherins, which are extracellular glycoproteins that form intercellular complexes necessary for cell adhesion. Second, β-catenin is also a transcription factor that promotes the

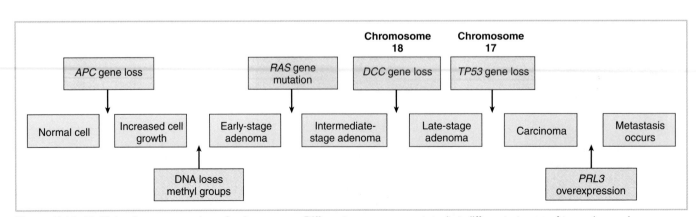

Figure 5-16. Multiple step progression of colon cancer. Different genes are mutated at different stages of tumorigenesis.

BIOCHEMISTRY

B-Catenin

Most β-catenins are bound to cadherins, a class of calcium-dependent proteins important in cell adhesion, at the cell membrane. The remaining β-catenins occur either in a free form and enter the nucleus or are part of a complex associated with APC (adenomatous polyposis coli) and GSK (glycogen synthase kinase) proteins. Nuclear β-catenins recruit transcription factors to regulate gene expression. In resting cells, however, cytoplasmic β-catenins turn over rapidly and few enter the nucleus. The APC/GSK complex controls degradation. GSK phosphorylates β-catenins, leading to ubiquination and degradation by proteosomes.

WNT proteins control β-catenin expression. WNTs bind to a seven-helix receptor at the cell membrane, leading to the inactivation of GSK. In the absence of GSK and β-catenin phosphorylation, β-catenin is not degraded. The increased concentration of free β-catenin can then enter the cell and affect transcription.

expression of MYC and cyclin D1 proteins. Under normal conditions, APC regulates β-catenin levels by binding to it and marking it for proteolytic degradation, thus preventing excessive levels of β-catenin. The loss of *APC* permits accumulation of β-catenin in the nucleus, where it facilitates cellular proliferation by activating cyclin D1 and MYC.

Individuals inheriting a deleterious *APC* allele develop numerous (hundreds or thousands of) adenomatous polyps at an early age. In some polyps, a second, somatic genetic "hit" occurs, thus effectively knocking out the *APC* gene product. This is possibly an early event in the pathway to malignancy; the association between colorectal cancer and FAP is strong, and LOH for the *APC* region is found in 70% of adenomatous polyps in non-FAP patients. More than 700 different *APC* mutations, which are mostly nonsense and frameshift mutations, have been found. However, molecular genetic diagnostics can identify carriers at an early age, permitting appropriate monitoring and treatment.

Hereditary Nonpolyposis Colon Cancer (HNPCC)

A small percentage of colorectal cancer is described by the autosomal dominant HNPCC, which is characterized by the presence of only one or a few adenomas in the proximal colon. Cancer is usually diagnosed by age 45, and the lifetime penetrance risk for cancer is 80%. Extracolonic tumors are not rare and include cancers of the endometrium, biliary and urinary tracts, ovary, and stomach.

HNPCC is due to mutations in one of the five genes (*MLH1, MSH2, PMSL1, PMSL2,* and *MSH6*) involved in DNA mismatch repair (MMR)—a class of genes that is highly evolutionarily conserved, supporting their importance in maintaining genome viability (Fig. 5-17). *MLH1* and *MSH2* mutations are most common and found in 60% to 80% of individuals developing HNPCC. Typical of the tumor suppressor gene model of carcinogenesis, in individuals heterozygous for mutations in these genes, only a second somatic mutation in the other allele via an LOH mechanism or point mutation is needed in order to promote cancer. Specifically, the loss of MLH1 or MSH2 proteins renders DNA mismatch repair inefficient and thus promotes genetic instability and an increased mutation rate. Indeed, much somatic variation in DNA microsatellite regions is observed in these patients owing to errors in DNA replication accompanied by decreased repair. Obviously an increased mutation rate could facilitate the second genetic hit in other tumor suppressor genes, or the initial activating mutation in an oncogene, again promoting malignancy.

Breast Cancer

Breast cancer is a malignancy that originates in the glandular tissue of the breast, primarily the milk-producing lobules and the milk ducts. It is, like colorectal cancer, one of the most common malignancies in humans. Roughly 10% of North American women will develop cancer in their lifetime. This translates to greater than 220,000 newly diagnosed cases per year—and greater than 40,000 deaths per year—in women living in North America. Overall, this form of cancer is the

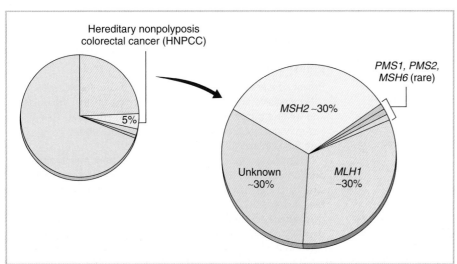

Figure 5-17. Five mismatch repair genes have been identified in HNPCC. Two of these are responsible for a majority of cases, and genetics laboratories that offer HNPCC testing examine only these two genes: *MLH1* and *MSH2*.

most commonly diagnosed malignancy in this group of women, and it is second only to lung cancer for cancer-related mortality.

Although most breast cancer is sporadic, the disease has been noted to cluster within families. In addition, a woman's risk for developing this cancer is three-fold higher if a first-degree relative has had breast cancer; the risk is ten-fold higher if more than one first-degree relative has developed breast cancer. This suggests a strong heritable genetic component in a subset of families. In fact, 15% to 20% of cases have been labeled as "familial clustering" and another 5% to 10% have been classified as heritable. Although the familial clustering cohort likely has a genetic etiologic component, there is no clear evidence of mendelian transmission within such families and no specific mutations have been associated with this group. Thus, any genetic component must be considered a polygenic or multifactorial genetic mechanism in which the gene or genes involved impart a predisposition to develop breast cancer, but other factors such as environment, socioeconomic status, diet, and more, also influence disease expression.

In the heritable form, the propensity for developing breast cancer appears to be transmitted among families in an autosomal dominant fashion. Besides multiple affected individuals in the pedigree, such families share certain clinical features including early onset (5 to 15 years before the average age of sporadic case onset), bilateral involvement, and the occurrence of other cancers, primarily ovarian. The availability of such families greatly facilitated genetic linkage analysis that led to the identification of several susceptibility genes including *BRCA1*, *BRCA2*, *TP53*, and *PTEN/MMAC1*. Because *BRCA1* and *BRCA2* mutations are much more commonly associated with breast cancer, these genes are featured in the subsequent discussion.

BRCA1 and BRCA2

The *BRCA1* gene maps to chromosome 17q21 and encodes a 1863-amino-acid polypeptide. Mutations in this gene are responsible for 40% to 50% of the autosomal dominant breast cancer families. For patients harboring a mutation, the risk for developing a breast cancer is 80% by age 70. Hence, penetrance in these families is not 100%. A second primary breast tumor forms in roughly 50% of the cases. As for other tumor suppressor genes, one deleterious *BRCA1* allele is inherited and the loss of both alleles is required for neoplasia. Here, greater than 600 mutations have been identified, mostly nonsense or frameshift mutations, predicting a truncated or nonfunctional gene product. Again in keeping with the tumor suppressor gene motif in cancer, the normal *BRCA1* allele is frequently absent in tumor tissue but is present in adjacent normal breast tissue, signaling LOH (Fig. 5-18).

BRCA2 localizes to chromosome 13q12 and produces a large protein of 3418 amino acids. Greater than 100 *BRCA2* variants have been characterized, and these account for roughly 30% of families with breast cancer. The risk for breast cancer associated with this gene is 50% to 85% in females and 6% for the rare male breast cancer. This gene is also associated with an increased risk for prostate, pancreatic, and laryngeal cancer. Just like *BRCA1*, this gene is a tumor suppressor gene and shares a similar profile of mutations (protein termination mutations and LOH resulting in no protein production) in tumor tissues. Hence, they share pathogenic characteristics with the *RB1* and *APC* tumor suppressor genes already discussed. However, unlike these genes, *BRCA1* and *BRCA2* mutations are not generally found in sporadic breast cancer cases.

Recent data suggest that *BRCA1* and *BRCA2* may be involved in more sporadic cancers than previously thought. Many of these are not due to mutations in the coding region of *BRCA1*, for example, but rather are promoter mutations that increase promoter methylation and lead to transcriptional silencing of the gene. As expected, the prognosis for disease with these mutations is poor. The mean survival of women with ovarian cancer with *BRCA1* promoter hypermethylation was 36.1 months compared with 63.3 months for women with ovarian cancer but with a normal *BRCA1* gene.

The BRCA1 and BRCA2 proteins do not share significant DNA or amino acid homology, but they do participate in the

---

ANATOMY

Breast Cancer

Sixty percent of breast cancer cases occur in the upper lateral quadrant. The cancer attaches to suspensory ligaments as progression occurs, shortening them and causing dimpling. The cancer may also attach to lactiferous ducts, causing inverted nipples, or invade the deep fascia of the pectoralis major muscle. Mastectomy may be performed to varying degrees:

- Radical: removal of breast and related structures— pectoralis major and minor muscles, axillary lymph nodes/fascia, part of thoracic wall
- Modified radical: removal of breast and axillary lymph nodes
- Lumpectomy: removal of palpable mass

PATHOLOGY

Breast Cancer Classification

Breast cancer is classified by histologic presentation.

Noninvasive (in situ) cancer growth occurs within the ducts and without penetration of the basement membrane. This includes ductal carcinoma in situ (DCIS) and lobular carcinoma in situ (LCIS).

Invasive carcinoma penetrates the basement membrane of a duct containing ductal carcinoma in situ and extends into the stroma. Ductal carcinoma accounts for 75% of all invasive breast cancer. Other examples include invasive lobular carcinoma, mucinous carcinoma, medullary carcinoma, papillary carcinoma, tubular carcinoma, apocrine carcinoma, squamous cell carcinoma, and spindle-cell type carcinoma.

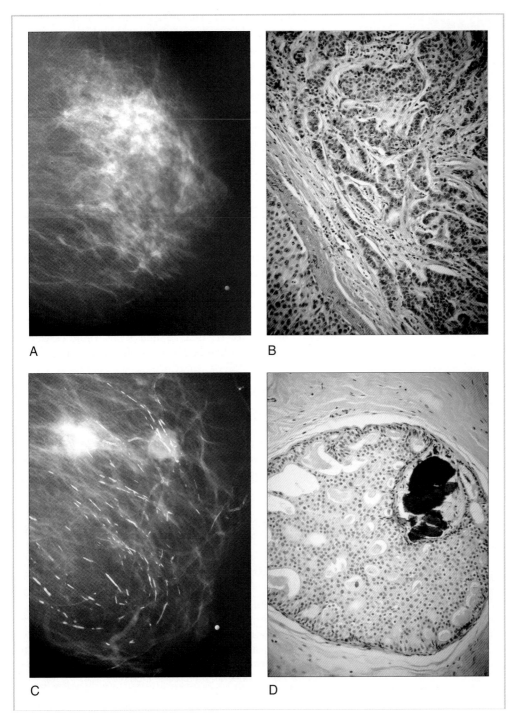

Figure 5-18. Invasive and noninvasive ductal carcinomas. **A**, Carcinoma has poorly defined edges that have begun to extend into surrounding tissue. Fibrous, or scar-like, tissue may form. Depending on the location, symptoms may include dimpling, retraction of the nipple, and nipple discharge. **B**, Histology of sample from patient in part A shows a random configuration of cells extending through the periductal connective tissue. **C**, Noninvasive ductal carcinoma (also known as interductal carcinoma or ductal carcinoma in situ) contains breast duct cells that have malignant characteristics but have not invaded surrounding tissue. **D**, Histology of sample from patient in part C shows proliferating malignant ductal cells limited to existing ductal units without invasion through the basement membrane. (Courtesy of Dr. Juan Lee, Mercer University School of Medicine, Georgia, and Dr. Emil Goergi, Dodge County Hospital, Georgia.)

same molecular complex. BRCA1 is a phosphorylated nuclear protein that has two functional motifs: a BRCT domain at the N-terminus and a ring-finger domain at the C-terminus. It is expressed in a variety of tissues, particularly in G_1 through S phase of the cell cycle. BRCA1 and also BRCA2 apparently interact with the RAD51 protein, a gene product involved in the repair of double-stranded breaks in the DNA. BRCA1 may also activate the p21 CDK inhibitor, which, as discussed for p53, is involved in suppressing growth at the G_1 to S cell cycle transition, presumably to repair DNA damage. *BRCA1* and *BRCA2* are therefore "caretaker" tumor suppressor

genes, since the homozygous loss of these alleles predicts genome instability that promotes the accumulation of mutations, consistent with the genetic model of cancer progression.

Worldwide, approximately 1 in 800 persons are likely to carry a deleterious *BRCA1* allele (Box 5-3). This carrier frequency for breast cancer predisposition varies from population to population. Affected families also rarely share the same pathogenic mutation; *BRCA1* mutations are therefore "private" to a family. In certain cases, however, seemingly unrelated breast cancer families have been found to have a deleterious allele in common. This phenomenon has been

Box 5-3. RISK FACTORS FOR BREAST CANCER

Nationality
  Most common in white women
  Least common in Hispanic, Asian, and black women
Age
  Uncommon before menopause
Positive family history
Early menarche—before age 12 years
Late menopause—after age 55 years
Atypical epithelial hyperplasia of breast on biopsy
Dense breast parenchyma on mammography
Hormone replacement therapy
Radiation exposure to breasts—before age 30 years
Life style
  Physical activity and weight management reduce risk
Alcohol use

observed, for example, in the Ashkenazi Jewish population, where two *BRCA1* alleles, 185delAG and 5382insC, and the 6174delT *BRCA2* alleles are common among families (Fig. 5-19). These three variants are found in 1%, 0.13%, and 1.5% of Ashkenazi Jews, respectively. Taken together, these three mutations result in an overall carrier frequency of one in 40 and account for 25% of early onset breast cancer and 90% of familial breast and ovarian cancer in this population. The unexpected high frequency of certain mutations within a subpopulation is consistent with a genetic *founder effect* whereby a modern population has derived recently from a small group of founders. For *BRCA1* and *BRCA2*, additional founder mutations have been characterized in northern European and Icelandic populations. The presence of certain disease-causing alleles in particular population subgroups can streamline DNA-based testing for the *BRCA1* and *BRCA2* mutations.

Ovarian Cancer

Ovarian cancer is the fifth leading cause of death from cancer among women and is the deadliest of all gynecologic cancers,

with a 5-year survival rate of less than 50%. In 2006, the diagnosis of 20,180 new cases is expected, coupled with 15,310 deaths due to this type of malignancy. Like breast cancer and most other cancers, the majority of ovarian cancers appear to be sporadic, and only 5% to 10% can be called hereditary on the basis of multiple affected family members and an age of onset 10 to 15 years before sporadic cases (Fig. 5-20). *BRCA1* (70%) and *BRCA2* (20%) mutations account for 90% of inherited ovarian cancer. In these families, both breast and ovarian cancer segregate among affected individuals. Mutations in *BRCA1* are associated with an earlier age of onset than is seen with *BRCA2* mutations: 54.6 years versus 64 years, respectively. A lifetime risk of developing ovarian cancer by age 75 years for heterozygous carriers of either mutated gene is 63% even though women with *BRCA1* mutations will develop ovarian cancer earlier.

Ovarian cancer is also not uncommon in the previously discussed HNPCC due to mutations in the *MLH1* and *MSH2* tumor suppressor genes involved in DNA mismatch repair. Up to 8% of familial ovarian cancer families do not have *BRCA1, BRCA2,* or *HNPCC*-related genes. These cases may be caused by an unidentified site-specific major allele.

●●● APOPTOTIC GENES
p53 Protein and Li-Fraumeni Syndrome

The *TP53* gene, producing the p53 protein involved in the cell cycle, holds a special place in cancer genetics; somatic mutations in this gene have been found in roughly half of all

ANATOMY

Ovaries

The ovaries lie on the posterior side of the broad ligament projecting into the ovarian fossae. They are supported by:

- Mesovarium: attaches ovary to the broad ligament
- Suspensory (infundibulopelvic) ligament of the ovary: attaches ovary to the pelvic brim
- Ovarian ligament: remnant of the gubernaculum lying within the mesovarium that attaches the ovary to the lateral surface of the uterus beneath the uterine tube

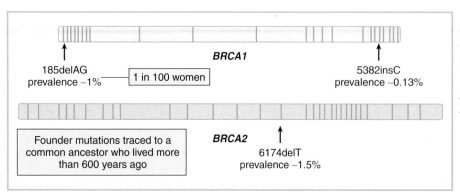

Figure 5-19. One in 40 Ashkenazi Jews carries a *BRCA1* or *BRCA2* mutation, demonstrating a founder effect. Since the prevalence of these specific mutations is high, population screening can be done in this population with a three-mutation test. Frequencies carriers of this allele in the population.

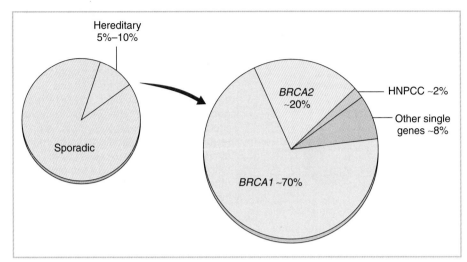

Figure 5-20. Causes of ovarian cancer. Most genetic causes of ovarian cancer are associated with *BRCA1* mutations. Unlike breast cancer, familial clustering does not appear to occur in ovarian cancer families.

human cancers, easily making it the most frequently altered gene in cancer. Over 50% of colorectal, lung, and bladder tumors have p53 mutations, as do roughly 40% of breast cancers. The extremely high frequency of p53 variants in various tumor types obviously suggests an important role in cell growth and differentiation.

The *TP53* gene maps to chromosome 17p and encodes a transcription factor that is expressed when the cell is stressed or damaged by such factors as ionizing radiation, environmental mutagens that damage the DNA, or ultraviolet light. Because p53 levels rise when DNA is damaged, this protein is often called the "guardian of the genome." One of the targets for p53 is the promoter for the *CDKN1A* gene encoding p21 (Fig. 5-21). p21 is a cyclin-dependent kinase inhibitor (CDI) in the Cip/Kip family of CDIs. It inhibits the activity of the cyclin/CDK complex, thereby disallowing inactivation of the pRB protein by phosphorylation. pRB therefore remains active in its hypophosphorylated state, resulting in halting the cell cycle prior to the S phase, as discussed previously. This, in turn, gives the cell time to repair any DNA damage prior to DNA replication. p53 also increases the expression of GADD45 (for growth arrest and DNA damage), a DNA repair enzyme. If the genome is successfully repaired and ready for subsequent replication, p53 down-regulates itself. In this way, p53 acts to preserve the integrity of the genome, inhibiting tumor formation. However, if the cell is unable to respond appropriately to excessive damage, p53 triggers apoptosis by inducing the pro-apoptotic *BAX* and *IGFBP3* genes. So, in a sense, if p53 cannot safeguard the cell by permitting DNA repair, it provokes death rather than allow continued genetic damage that would promote cancer.

Because somatic *TP53* mutations are clearly a key etiologic event in many cancers, the presence of germline *TP53* mutations would predict dire consequences. In fact, this condition is seen in Li-Fraumeni syndrome, a familial cancer disorder in which a deleterious *TP53* allele is transmitted in an autosomal dominant manner (Fig. 5-22). Li-Fraumeni families have a higher risk for early-onset cancer, predicting the multiple affected family members commonly found in

pedigrees. By age 30, roughly 50% of individuals harboring such a mutation will develop one of a variety of malignancies, including soft-tissue sarcomas, osteosarcomas, brain tumors, breast or colon carcinomas, adrenal carcinomas, and leukemia (see Fig. 5-22). Development of multiple primary tumors, however, is not uncommon, and 15% of individuals develop a second cancer. Bone and soft-tissue sarcomas are more commonly found in affected children, while breast cancer is most common in adult females.

The *TP53* gene product is a tumor suppressor, and both alleles need inactivating for cancer promotion. Following the

BIOCHEMISTRY & PATHOLOGY

Apoptosis

Apoptosis is a cascade of events leading to the activation of caspases and ending with cell death. There are three phases to apoptosis: initiation, intrinsic, and extrinsic. In the initiation phase, the caspases become active.

In the intrinsic pathway, BCL2 and BCLX antiapoptotic proteins are located on mitochondrial membranes and recognize internal damage to the cell such as that caused by reactive oxygen species. The balance of BCL2 and BCLX with the proapoptotic proteins BAK, BAX, and BIM changes, and the increase in the proapoptotic proteins causes an increase in mitochondria permeability. Cytochrome *c* then leaves the mitochondria and forms a complex with apoptotic protease-activating factor 1 (APAF1). These cytochrome *c* molecules and APAF1 molecules form apoptosomes that activate caspase-9. This leads to activation of caspases 3, 6, and 7 and to cell death through cleavage of cell substrates.

The extrinsic pathway involves signals from receptors that are members of the tumor necrosis factor (TNF) family, containing a "death domain." When bound to ligands, caspases are activated. For example, the type 1 TNF receptor and FAS located on the cell surface can bind TNF and FAS ligands and activate caspase-8. The proteolytic cascade is thus activated, as is caspase-9, leading to cell death followed by phagocytosis of debris.

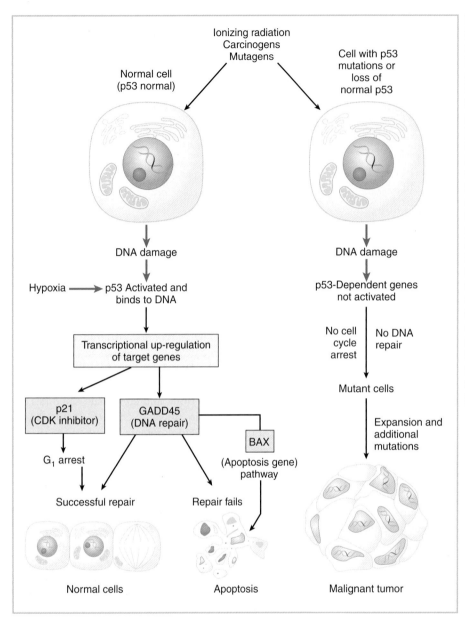

Figure 5-21. The role of p53 is pivotal to the integrity of DNA in each cell. In normal cells, p53 is present in low levels; however, DNA damage increases *TP53* gene transcription, leading to increased transcription of genes for p21 and GADD45, a CDK inhibitor and DNA repair gene, respectively. The *BAX* gene, which produces a proapoptotic protein, is up-regulated by p53 binding to its promoter and is subsequently expressed on mitochondrial surfaces. BAX interacts with other proteins to form pores that release cytochrome *c* from the mitochondria into the cytosol, leading to activation of caspases and cell death. (Not shown: *BCL2* inhibits p53-mediated cell death, but increased expression of *TP53* represses *BCL2* expression.) Shown at right are the consequences of inactivation of p53 through mutation or deletion. DNA repair does not occur in the presence of damage, and abnormal cells continue to expand unchecked. (Redrawn from Kumar V, Abbas A, Fausto N. *Robbins & Cotran Pathologic Basis of Disease,* 7th ed. Philadelphia, WB Saunders, 2004, p 303.)

model previously discussed for retinoblastoma, the mechanism of cancer in Li-Fraumeni syndrome is clear. Family members transmit the constitutional *TP53* mutation in an autosomal dominant fashion. Those who inherit the deleterious allele need only one additional mutational "hit" in the other *TP53* allele. This second hit may occur in any somatic cell, thus accounting for the wide variety of tumor types found in Li-Fraumeni syndrome.

Prostate Cancer

Prostate cancer is the most common malignancy in men and the second leading cause of death due to cancer in men. In 2006, it is estimated that 234,460 new cases will be diagnosed and that 27,300 deaths will occur due to prostate cancer (Box 5-4). The lifetime risk is 10% to 14%, although the diagnosis, surveillance, and prognostication efficiency of

Box 5-4. RISK FACTORS FOR PROSTATE CANCER

Age
    Risk increases over age 55
    75% of cases are diagnosed after age 65
Positive family history
Diet—risk increases with high saturated fat intake
Nationality/race
    Most common in North America and northwestern Europe
    Highest risk for blacks
    70% more common in blacks than in whites
    Lowest risk for Asians
Exposure to heavy metals
Life style
    Physical activity and weight management reduce risk
Smoking

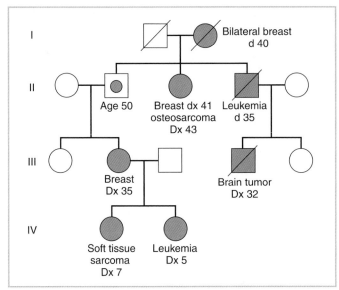

Figure 5-22. Pedigree of a Li-Fraumeni family demonstrating multiple types of cancers within a family. As shown here, male cancer may have a later onset (II-2) and multiple primary tumors can be seen in one person (II-3). d, died; Dx, diagnosis.

ANATOMY

Prostate

The prostate is located between the base of the urinary bladder and the sphincter urethrae muscle, and it consists of five lobes:

- Anterior
- Median—prone to benign hypertrophy causing obstruction of urethral orifice
- Posterior—prone to cancer transformation
- Right lateral
- Left lateral

It secretes PSA, prostaglandins, citric acid, acid phosphatase, and proteolytic enzymes.

PATHOLOGY

Prostate-specific Antigen

Prostate-specific antigen (PSA) is an enzyme produced by the prostate and normally secreted in semen from prostatic epithelium. It functions as a serine protease to cleave and liquefy seminal fluid. PSA is not specific to cancer; it is found in an increased amount in the blood during

- Prostate cancer
- Benign prostatic hyperplasia
- Infections or inflammations of the prostate

Serum levels below normal (4.0 ng/mL) may occur in 20% to 40% of patients with cancer.

prostate cancer has been greatly facilitated by laboratory testing for the prostate-specific antigen (PSA).

Typical of cancers, most cases of prostate cancer are sporadic. However, up to 20% of cases may be considered "familial" on the basis of at least one of the following criteria: (1) family history is positive for three or more first-degree relatives with the disease, (2) three or more generations exhibit the disease on the same side of the family, or (3) two or more close relatives have early-onset prostate cancer. Among the familial forms, 5% to 9% may be hereditary and these seem to follow an autosomal dominant mode of transmission within families (Fig. 5-23). Examination of tumors from such families indicates LOH at several loci, consistent with the tumor suppressor model of cancer.

Molecular genetic investigation of hereditary prostate cancer indicates two loci linked with the disease. The hereditary prostate cancer alleles 1 and 2, *HPC1* and *HPC2*, are linked

to chromosomes 1q24 and 17p11, respectively. Originally, it was believed that these two loci represented major susceptibility genes for this form of cancer. Subsequent detailed analysis of heritable prostate cancer, however, revealed that only *HPC1* represented a strong association with prostate cancer. Another gene, *MSR1*, also demonstrates a strong association with prostate cancer risk. The HPC1 protein participates in apoptosis and mutations in the gene result in apoptotic inhibition. MSR is a macrophage scavenger receptor localized to chromosome 8p22 and within an area frequently

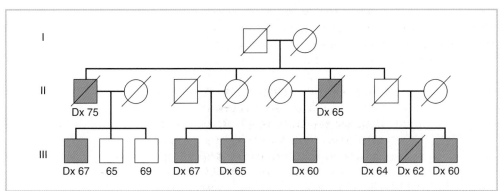

Figure 5-23. Family with prostate cancer linked to HNPC1 mutations. Hereditary prostate cancer accounts for about 10% of all prostate cancer. About 34% of cases are linked to mutations in this gene. The ages of two unaffected brothers (III-2 and III-3) are shown. Dx, diagnosis.

recognized for LOH, chromosome 8p21-25. The association of prostate cancer with LOH is greater for chromosome 8 than for any other chromosome.

●●● TELOMERES AND TELOMERASE

Telomerase is a ribonucleoprotein enzyme that acts as a cellular reverse transcriptase to maintain the length and integrity of chromosomal ends, or telomeres. In humans, telomeres are represented by hexameric DNA repeats of TTAGGG that are present in thousands of copies at the ends of chromosomes. Telomeres, in partnership with telomerase, serve to protect the ends of chromosomes from degradation due to incomplete double-strand DNA synthesis during DNA replication. Because DNA replication in mammals is bidirectional and DNA polymerase can process only in a 5′ to 3′ direction, the lagging strand of DNA must be replicated in a discontinuous fashion. This means that for DNA polymerase to initiate lagging strand discontinuous replication, an RNA primer must be utilized well 5′ of the replication fork. Replicating this strand at the terminus of the chromosome, however, is not possible using this mechanism because there is no DNA template for an RNA primer to pair with. Therefore, the lagging strand at the end of chromosomes cannot be replicated in the normal fashion, and this has been termed the "end replication problem." The telomeric ends of

chromosomes would get progressively shorter at each DNA replication, ultimately damaging coding sequences on chromosomal tips. Telomerase evolved as a solution to this problem. It uses its internal RNA moiety that is complementary to the single-stranded telomeric overhang as a template to synthesize telomeric DNA on the ends of the lagging strand (Fig. 5-24). This mechanism corrects for the continued erosion of chromosomal ends that occur in its absence.

Telomerase is composed of two major components: the catalytic subunit (hTERT) and the template RNA (hTER). The hTERT component is a reverse transcriptase that is involved in synthesizing DNA from the RNA template. Other proteins and kinases are additional components of the holoenzyme. Activation of the holoenzyme requires transcriptional and posttranscriptional levels of the hTERT. A number of transcriptional factors, including c-MYC, BCL2, and RAS, and acetylating and methylating changes in the chromatin structure may also play a role in the control of hTERT. To illustrate their role, the overexpression of c-MYC is correlated with increased hTERT expression in several cancers including prostate, neuroblastoma, and cervical. In studies using cells with down-regulated c-MYC expression, cell proliferation decreased; subsequently increasing hTERT resulted in increased proliferation through restored telomerase activity. A few approaches to directly target either telomerase and telomeres or the telomerase-associated regulatory mecha-

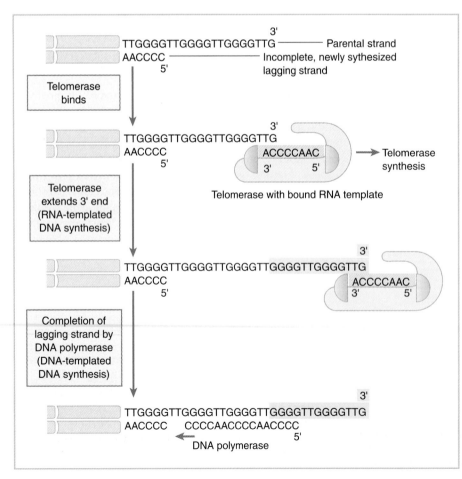

Figure 5-24. Telomere replication and the role of telomerase. Telomerase binds to the 3′ end of a parental strand—the terminal sequences of the chromosome—and provides a template (ACCCCAAC) for synthesis in the 5′→3′ direction. The newly extended sequence serves as the template for synthesis on the opposite strand.

TABLE 5-5. Examples of Several Therapeutic Approaches Targeting Components of the Telomerase Core

Target	Approach	Molecular Effect	Biological Effect	Application
hTER	2′-5′ Oliogoadenylate antisense	Inhibit telomerase	Apoptosis; increased sensitivity to cisplatin	Prostate, ovarian, bladder, cervical cancers
	N3′-P5′ thiophosphoramidate oligonucleotides		Apoptosis, senescence	Prostate cancer
hTERT	Ribozyme		Inhibition of proliferation; sensitivity to topoisomerase inhibitors	Breast and ovarian cancer
	Peptide nucleic acids		Decreased survival	Prostate cancer

Data from Birrocio A, Leonetti C. Telomerase as a new target for the treatment of hormone-refractory prostate cancer. *Endocr Relat Cancer.* 2004;11:407-421.

nisms are shown in Table 5-5. Additionally, it is worth noting that an increase in hTERT activity is regulated by androgens and so removing androgens is reflected in decreased expression of hTERT.

In normal cells, telomerase activity decreases with age and the number of cell divisions, yielding progressively shorter telomeres over time. Normal cells also have a limited potential for cell division, and it is believed that the shortening of the telomeres is associated with the limited proliferative capacity of the typical somatic cell. Indeed, after hundreds of cell divisions, certain telomeres may be dangerously short such that terminal genes are threatened. Such damage may signal p53 and pRB expression that halts the cell cycle and places the cell into a G_0 state. At this point, the cell is said to be in "senescence."

In many cancer cells, telomerase activity is reactivated, allowing tumor cells to proliferate indefinitely. Experimentally, two lines of data underscore the potential importance of telomerase to cancer. First, tumor cells show no telomeric shortening over repeated cell divisions, strongly suggesting that this enzyme is required for indefinite proliferation. Second, 90% of tumors show telomerase activity but adjacent normal tissues do not. Hence, in sharp contrast with normal cells, a reactivation of telomerase activity is a common finding in highly proliferative and immortal tumor cells. Telomerase expression, and thereby availability, may be enhanced in tumor cells due to mutations that enhance activity or by an oncogenic transcription factor. Telomerase activity has been correlated with aggressiveness in several cancers including prostate. In any case, the observation that telomerase is active in tumor cells and may facilitate proliferation provides a diagnostic substrate as well as a potential new target for anticancer drugs (Fig. 5-25).

●●● CYTOGENETIC ALTERATIONS IN CANCER AND TUMOR HETEROGENEITY

Cytogenetic changes such as translocations, deletions, inversions, and aneuploidy are common in tumor cells and decidedly uncommon in normal cells. Certain of these play a strong causal role in certain cancers such as Burkitt lymphoma, chronic myeloid leukemia, and neuroblastoma— all of which result from earlier discussed chromosomal abnormalities that transform proto-oncogenes into oncogenes. Some chromosomal numerical defects such as aneuploidy appear later in the more malignant stages of cancer. Such changes suggest either that the loss of genetic control of chromosomal stability and number is key to late-stage cancer or that chromosomal instability is secondary to the cellular deregulation found late in tumor progression.

Human tumors are clonal and derived from a single progenitor cell. However, as the tumor grows, the constituent cells become extremely heterogeneous, as sublineages of variant types are generated. Because a hallmark of tumor growth is genetic instability, each sublineage differs in the accumulation of genetic alterations ranging from an accumulation of point mutations to karyotypic differences. In turn, these genetic changes provoke variation in invasiveness,

PHARMACOLOGY

Antitelomerase Therapy

Telomeric DNA and the core telomerase components, hTR and hTERT, are good targets for antitelomerase pharmacologic strategies.

- Approaches to targeting hTR
  - Antisense 2′-5′ oligoadenylate inhibits telomerase and increases apoptosis
  - N3′-P5′ thiophosphoramidate oligonucleotides (GRN163) increase apoptosis and senescence
  - Ribozymes
  - Peptide nucleic acids to stop growth and initiate apoptosis
- Approaches to targeting hTERT
  - Ribozyme inhibits telomerase
  - Peptide nucleic acids
  - Small molecules such as BIBR1532 induce senescence-like growth arrest
- Approach to targeting the telomeric G-quadruplex
  - Acridine compounds bind the G-quadruplex and induce growth arrest and increase sensitivity to paclitaxel

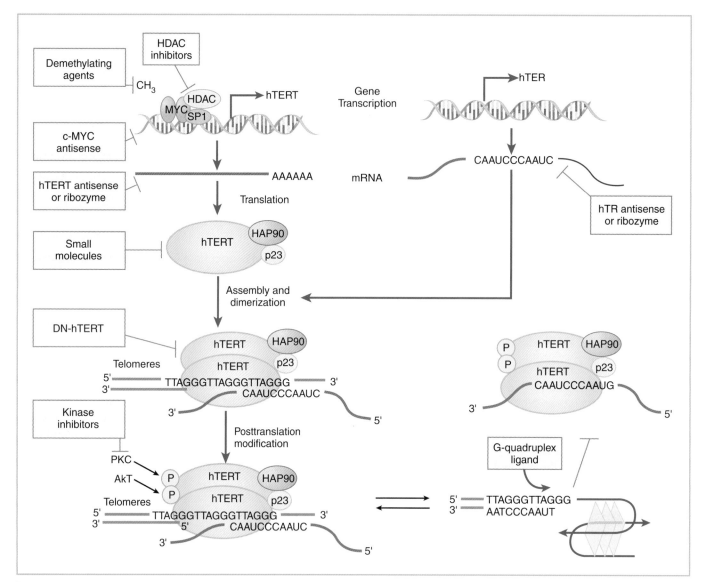

Figure 5-25. Some of the most promising approaches that directly target either telomerase and telomeres or the telomerase-associated regulatory mechanisms are reported in the boxes at the targeting sites. HDAC, histone deacetylase; DN-hTERT, dominant-negative hTERT; PKC, protein kinase C. (Reproduced by permission from Biroccio A, Leonetti C. Telomerase as a new target for treatment of hormone-refractory prostate cancer. *Endoc-Relat Cancer.* 2004;11:407–421 (Fig. 1). © Society for Endocrinology, 2004.)

growth rate, hormonal responsiveness, and metastatic abilities. From a genome point of view, the most frequent chromosomal alteration in solid tumors, such as colon cancers, is a change in chromosome number. Colon cancers are frequently hyperdiploid, i.e., possessing chromosomes in excess of the diploid number. However, not all chromosomes are fully intact, and it can be speculated that tumors exhibiting LOH not only suffer from the functional loss of suppressor genes but have also lost growth-promoting genes. The unintended deletion of growth-promoting genes might restrict the cell's growth potential. The cancer cell would thus be expected to obtain a selective advantage from an endomitosis, or chromosomal replication within a cell nucleus that does not divide, leading to hyperdiploidy; this would restore copies of the growth-promoting genes necessary to maintain tumor progression. This extreme chromosomal heterogeneity may or

may not facilitate certain features, such as metastasis, of a tumor, but at the very least, it demonstrates the dysfunctional biology of the cancer cell while serving as a cancer biomarker.

●●● DNA-BASED CANCER SCREENING

As the number of cancer-related genes increases, attention is turning to the role of DNA testing for early detection and prevention of cancer. This method is primarily applicable to familial cancers with a known mutational association, since sporadic cancer implies unknown molecular etiology. Until recently, cancer surveillance in families predisposed to the disease relied on phenotypic or symptomatic monitoring with or without indirect diagnostic tests. As familial cancer genes and mutations are identified, however, cancer screening can

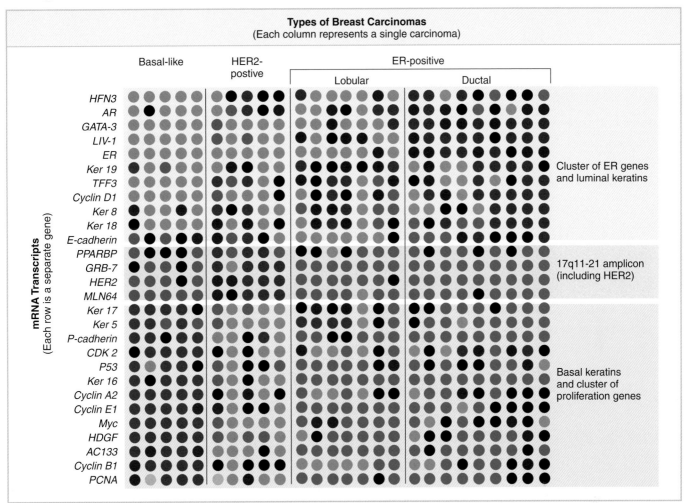

Figure 5-26. Selected data from mRNA expression profiling of 26 breast carcinomas. Each vertical column represents one carcinoma, and each horizontal row represents the data for a gene identified at the left. Red circle, increase in expression; green circle, decrease in expression; black circle, no difference in expression between normal and carcinoma cells. (Redrawn from Kumar V, Abbas A, Faust N. *Robbins & Cotran Pathologic Basis of Disease*, 7th ed. Philadelphia, WB Saunders, 2004, p 1137.)

be performed noninvasively and well before the onset of early symptoms. The identification of a cancer-predisposing mutation therefore permits an aggressive surveillance or treatment plan for at-risk individuals as well as reproductive planning. In certain cases, such as FAP (colectomy), familial ovarian cancer (oophorectomy), and familial breast cancer (bilateral mastectomy), prophylactic surgery is considered a viable option to eliminate the genetically identified and verified malignancy risk.

A new technique, called microarray analysis, which compares patterns of gene expression in normal and abnormal tissues, is demonstrating great promise for diagnostic use (see Chapter 13). This gene expression profiling has proved most useful in cancer diagnosis and surveillance (Fig. 5-26). Here, cDNA probes are used that are derived from tumor and adjacent normal tissues. Gene chip expression studies have, for example, permitted the classification of new subtypes of breast cancers and have produced a rapid diagnostic tool for the distinction between acute lymphoblastic leukemia and acute myeloid leukemia. Prior to such tests, it was often difficult and time consuming to classify tumor subtypes. Overall, gene expression analysis can be applied to neoplasia classification, diagnosis of malignant versus benign tumors, prognosis including metastatic potential, and the development of a cell-based surveillance platform to monitor the response to therapy.

Hematologic Disorders 6

The heritable blood disorders are a heterogeneous group of diseases that historically account for significant morbidity and mortality around the world. The advent of transfusion techniques and appropriate surgical and pharmacologic approaches and the emergence of DNA-based carrier and prenatal testing have rendered most of these disorders manageable through early detection and diagnosis. In this chapter, a number of the more common inherited hematologic disorders that are genetically well characterized and therefore serve as paradigms for the genetic basis of blood disease are discussed. Disorders of white blood cells are more appropriately addressed in other chapters.

●●● RED BLOOD CELL MEMBRANE

The red blood cell (RBC) membrane consists of a lipid bilayer (primarily phospholipids and unesterified cholesterol), integral membrane proteins, and structural proteins that form the membrane infrastructure. Membrane proteins are often glycoproteins that confer either *functional* or *antigenic* properties, illustrated by anion exchange band 3 protein and glycophorins, respectively. The structural proteins define an inner membrane coating lattice that forms the typical biconcave shape and promotes the deformability of normal RBCs. Such proteins include spectrin, ankyrin, actin, and protein 4.1. Spectrin is composed of two chains, α and β, that

form heterodimers by wrapping around each other. These heterodimers associate in a head-to-tail manner, resulting in heterotetramers. Spectrin heterotetramers interact with two other structural proteins, actin and protein 4.1, at the spectrin "tail" end. At the "head" end, the spectrin heterotetramer is attached to ankyrin, and this complex is stabilized by protein 4.2. This proteinaceous "membrane skeleton" is connected to the lipid bilayer by an association between ankyrin and band 3 protein. Mutations in these structural proteins affect the ability of RBCs to appropriately change shapes when circulating through narrow and tortuous vessels. Decreasing the flexibility of RBCs can lead to an increased opportunity for abnormal pathology.

●●● HEMOLYTIC ANEMIAS

Anemia can result from many causes, some congenital and some acquired. Among the most serious are the hemolytic

BIOCHEMISTRY

Membranes

Lipids that consist predominantly of aliphatic or aromatic hydrocarbons form the framework of cell membranes. The major lipid components are phosphoglycerides (sometimes just referred to as phospholipids), sphingolipids, and sterols. Cholesterol is the major sterol. There are hundreds of minor lipids, and differences in specific composition cause different cell membrane fluidity; in some situations, differences are reflected by disease.

Lipids in membranes usually contain C16 saturated fatty acids and longer fatty acids with the presence of double bonds. The presence of double bonds is critical, since C18 fatty acids are solid at physiologic temperatures without double bonds. Double bonds create specific conformational changes that affect membrane fluidity. Fluidity is particularly influenced by the amount of cholesterol in membranes because the rigid steroid ring binds and immobilizes other fatty acids. Thus, modest changes in cholesterol concentrations have great impact on membranes. Spur cell anemia illustrates the impact of an increased ratio of cholesterol to phospholipids. This condition is usually seen in alcoholic cirrhosis, in which cholesterol content increases from 25% to 65%. The increased cholesterol leads to a progressive increase in RBC deformation and ultimately hemolysis and anemia.

anemias resulting from increased RBC destruction. In general, hemolytic anemias share two characteristics: the life span of the red cell is reduced and iron is retained after hemolysis. Congenital hemolytic anemias in this chapter are classified into three general etiologic categories: erythrocyte membrane defects, metabolic defects, and hemoglobin defects.

Red Blood Cell Membrane Defects

Hereditary Spherocytosis and Hereditary Elliptocytosis

Hereditary spherocytosis (HS) and hereditary elliptocytosis (HE) are the most common hemolytic anemias caused by RBC membrane defects. HS is the most common hereditary hemolytic anemia found in individuals of Northern European descent and results from structural defects linking the underlying membrane skeleton with the lipid bilayer. Mutations causing HS have been found in the genes encoding ankyrin, spectrin, band 3, and protein 4.2 (Fig. 6-1). Such defects cause a loss of membrane and an associated decreased surface area to volume ratio. These changes account for the spheroidal shape of the HS erythrocytes and the decreased ability of RBCs to change shape as they circulate through small vessels and capillaries. The deformed erythrocytes, called spherocytes, become trapped in the splenic microcirculation and undergo hemolysis (Fig. 6-2).

The mutational spectrum in ankyrin, α-spectrin, β-spectrin, band 3 protein, and protein 4.2 includes missense, nonsense, frameshift, splicing and promoter variants. The majority of patients have unique (or "private") mutations. This indicates an absence of a mutational "hot spot." Unique mutations are more difficult to identify and are not well suited for screening tests; however, once a mutation is identified within a family, other members may be screened. HS is most commonly an autosomal dominant disease with variable expressivity (Table 6-1). α-Spectrin, however, is a notable exception. Roughly four times more α-spectrin than β-spectrin is expressed within

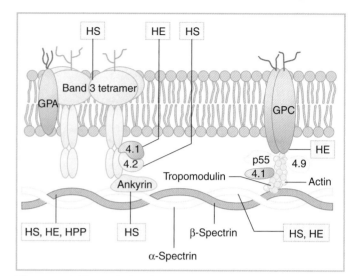

Figure 6-1. The red blood cell membrane has several proteins that affect the structure of the cell. Mutations in proteins leading to hereditary spherocytosis (HS), hereditary elliptocytosis (HE), and hereditary pyropoikilocytosis (HPP) are shown.

an RBC. This seeming excess of α-spectrin is reflected in heterozygotes for α-spectrin mutations. In these individuals, enough α-spectrin protein is usually produced without serious consequence. However, homozygous or compound heterozygous α-spectrin mutations can precipitate a severe HS presentation.

HE is similar to HS in that both may have mutations in α-spectrin and β-spectrin genes. These disorders differ in the effect the mutations have on the membrane and its resulting shape. Typically in HE, spectrin heterodimers cannot self-associate into heterotetramers. This is consistent with the fact that most HE mutations are found in the protein domains that directly participate in the self-association process. HE is also typically an autosomal dominant disease (Table 6-2).

Patients with the most common form of HE are usually asymptomatic. Only 5% to 20% develop hemolysis with anemia, splenomegaly, scleral icterus, pallor, gallstones, or occasional leg ulcers. In many cases, splenectomy eliminates

---

PATHOLOGY

Hemolytic Disorders

Hemolytic disorders are characterized by premature destruction of red cells. Hemolysis can occur either intravascularly or extravascularly. During intravascular hemolysis, hemoglobin is released and bound to haptoglobin. The hemoglobin-haptoglobin complex is removed by hepatic RES cells; thus, the haptoglobin levels generally fall; the resulting excess hemoglobin is converted to ferritin and hemosiderin. With rapid intravascular hemolysis, hemoglobinuria can be seen.

Most hemolytic disorders demonstrate extracellular hemolysis. Red cells are sequestered in the spleen and/or liver and phagocytized with the hemoglobin escaping into plasma and thus causing the haptoglobin to decrease. In this case, hemosiderinuria and hemoglobinuria generally do not occur.

TABLE 6-1. Mutation Frequency in Hereditary Spherocytosis (HS)

Gene Product	Transmission	Frequency in HS Patients (%)
Ankyrin	AD, some AR	40–50
Band 3	AD	20–30
Spectrin	α-Spectrin, AR	10
	β-Spectrin, AD	10
Protein 4.2	AR	Rare

AD, autosomal dominant; AR, autosomal recessive.

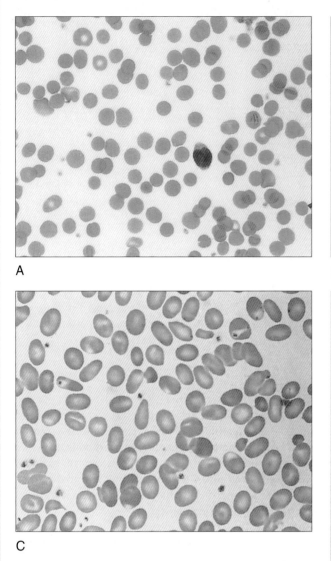

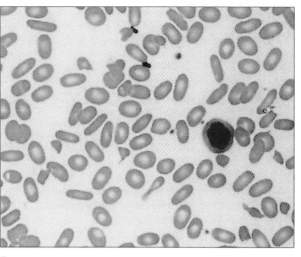

Figure 6-2. A, Hereditary spherocytosis. Spherocytes lack central pallor, stain more darkly and are smaller in diameter than nonspherocytic RBCs. **B**, Hereditary elliptocytosis. Many cells are elliptical rather than oval. The marker ellipsoidal cell has an axial ratio of >2:1. Cell fragments and microelliptocytes are present. Note that they maintain an area of central pallor. **C**, Hereditary pyropoikilocytosis. Almost all cells are misshapen. Fragmented spheroidal cells and elliptical forms predominate. (Courtesy of Dr. Anna Walker, Mercer University School of Medicine, Georgia.)

symptoms by decreasing the number of ruptured RBCs. This defect is common in individuals of African and Mediterranean descent, and many of these individuals harbor similar genetic backgrounds, or *haplotypes*. This indicates a genetic founder effect and persistence within the population. Such persistence can be explained by selection, since elliptocytosis appears to confer some resistance to malaria. This contrasts with the situation for HS, which is much more common in European-derived individuals than African-derived individuals and does not exhibit a founder effect or allele persistence due to selection.

Hereditary Pyropoikilocytosis

Hereditary pyropoikilocytosis (HPP) has been called a subtype of homozygous elliptocytosis as well as an "aggravated" form of elliptocytosis. Both HPP and HE result from mutations in α-spectrin, but the clinical presentations differ in severity. Hereditary elliptocytosis has a wide spectrum of clinical manifestations ranging from no symptoms to severe. Pyropoikilocytosis is a severe form of hemolytic anemia with thermal instability of red cells. The consequences of this severe anemia are evident in children who exhibit growth retardation, frontal bossing, and gallbladder disease.

HPP is rare; however, it is worth considering along with HE because it illustrates that some mutations affect the *rate of expression* rather than the structure or function of the protein produced. The differences between HPP and HE in disease severity are explained by allele specificity resulting from mutations in the same gene. Specific mutations in α-spectrin associated with HPP are called "low expression" alleles. There are at least four of these alleles that produce fewer α-spectrin chains. When any of these alleles combine with other α-spectrin alleles that are more commonly associated with HE, fewer α-spectrin chains are produced from one allele and defective α-spectrin chains produced from the other allele fail to form spectrin tetramers.

TABLE 6-2. Red Blood Cell Membrane Defects Leading to Hemolysis

Feature	Elliptocytosis	Spherocytosis	Pyropoikilocytosis
Inheritance	Dominant	Dominant	Recessive
Incidence	1 in 2000–4000	1 in 5000	Rare
Ethnicity	In all racial and ethnic groups; more common in blacks	Common in people of Northern European descent, but found in all people	Predominantly in blacks
Mutation	Spectrin, glycophorin C, protein 4.1	Spectrin, ankyrin, band 3, protein 4.2	Compound heterozygous α-spectrin functional mutation, reduced synthesis mutation
Clinical presentation	Most asymptomatic or with minimal (15%) compensated anemia	Asymptomatic (80%) to moderate anemia (20%); jaundice, pallor, splenomegaly	Splenomegaly, intermittent jaundice, aplastic crises
Laboratory findings	Elliptocytosis, few or no poikilocytes, no anemia, little or no hemolysis, reticulocytes 1%–3%, normal osmotic fragility	Reticulocytosis, spherocytosis, elevated MCHC, increased osmotic fragility, normal Coombs' test	Severe hemolysis; microspherocytes, poikilocytes, reticulocytosis, decreased MCV, increased osmotic fragility, decreased red cell heat stability

MCHC, mean corpuscular hemoglobin concentration; MCV, mean corpuscular volume.

Erythrocyte Metabolic Defects

Glucose-6-Phosphate Dehydrogenase Deficiency

Glucose-6-phosphate dehydrogenase (G6PD) deficiency reigns as the most prevalent enzyme disorder in the world. It occurs in an estimated 400 million people in the world population. As an X-linked disorder, it affects mostly males. The highest frequencies occur in Mediterranean countries, Africa, and China. The worldwide distribution of G6PD deficiency parallels that of malaria, which suggests a genetic state of balanced polymorphism associated with resistance to falciparum malaria. It has been observed that female heterozygotes for G6PD deficiency, who have both normal and G6PD-deficient RBCs, have lower parasite counts in G6PD-deficient red cells and are relatively resistant to malaria. This selective advantage has been observed for other diseases such as sickle cell disease and β-thalassemia.

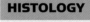

BIOCHEMISTRY

Hexose Monophosphate Shunt

The hexose monophosphate shunt (HMP) is also called the pentose phosphate pathway. It occurs in the cytoplasm and is a major source of NADPH. The HMP consists of two irreversible oxidative reactions and a series of reversible sugar-phosphate conversions. No ATP is consumed or produced directly. Carbon 1 is released from glucose 6-phosphate (G6P) as CO_2, and 2 NADPH are produced for each G6P entering the pathway. The HMP also produces ribose-phosphate for nucleotide synthesis.

G6PD activity is essential to normal functioning of the hexose monophosphate (HMP) shunt. This pathway generates reduced nicotinamide adenine dinucleotide phosphate (NADPH), a cofactor in glutathione metabolism in human RBCs. The HMP shunt is tightly coupled to glutathione metabolism, which serves to protect RBCs from oxidant injury. Accordingly, a marked deficiency of G6PD leaves the red cell vulnerable to oxidant damage.

There are two normal alleles of *G6PD*—the B allele (*G6PD^B^*), which is widespread in the Mediterranean, Middle East, and Orient, and the A allele (*G6PD^A^*), which is largely confined to sub-Saharan Africans and their descendants. The normal enzyme products of these alleles are designated G6PD^B+^ and G6PD^A+^, respectively, where the "+" denotes normal enzyme activity. Both enzymes are slowly degraded normally over the life span of a normal red cell, but G6PD activity is still sufficient in the oldest normal RBCs to withstand oxidant stresses (Fig. 6-3). The mutations causing *G6PD^A−^* and *GGPD^B−^* differentially affect the rate of degradation of the enzyme. The G6PD^A−^ enzyme is more rapidly degraded than the normal enzyme, but young *G6PD^A−^* cells are capable of withstanding oxidant stresses. In stark contrast,

HISTOLOGY

Heinz Bodies

Heinz bodies are intracellular inclusions composed of denatured hemoglobin. Found at the cell membranes of erythrocytes, they are seen in thalassemias, enzymopathies, hemoglobinopathies, and after splenectomy.

both the catalytic ability and stability of the variant G6PD^{B-} enzyme are reduced so drastically that virtually the entire G6PD^{B-} RBC population, young and old cells, is susceptible

MICROBIOLOGY

Sickle Cell Trait and Malaria Resistance

Erythrocytes in a person with sickle cell trait (heterozygote) confer protection from infection with falciparum malaria. RBCs develop "knobs" on the cell membrane surfaces that cause the cells to stick to the endothelium of small vessels. This sticking occurs because of low oxygen concentration, presumably caused by the parasite.

The parasite requires a high K$^+$ environment, and when the RBC membrane is damaged potassium is lost from the RBC as well as the parasite. Infected RBCs are more acidic and hypoxic. These conditions increase sickling, leading to the sequestration of infected cells (but not uninfected cells) and elimination of the sickled cells by phagocytes.

Neonates have an increased resistance to malaria because Hb F is very stable and resistant to malaria hemoglobinases. Hb F cells are infected preferentially to Hb A cells.

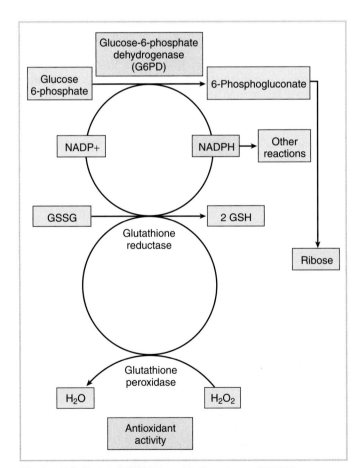

Figure 6-3. Role of G6PD in oxidative stress. G6PD is required to generate NADPH and break down H$_2$O$_2$. GSH, reduced glutathione; GSSG, oxidized glutathione; NADP+, nicotinamide adenine dinucleotide phosphate; NADPH, reduced nicotinamide adenine dinucleotide phosphate.

to oxidant-induced hemolysis. The A form of G6PD deficiency is contrasted with the B form in Table 6-3.

There are more than 400 variant (mutant) alleles of G6PD. The allelic changes result in varied forms of enzyme deficiency: decreased enzyme synthesis, the presence of an enzyme with abnormal kinetics, or the presence of an unstable enzyme whose catalytic activities become diminished as cells age. Two prominent hemolytic conditions, primaquine sensitivity and favism, illustrate effects of the mutated alleles.

Primaquine Sensitivity

In the mid-1900s, a strain of vivax malaria with a long latent period was common in Korea. During the Korean War (1950–1953), American soldiers were prophylactically administered an antimalarial drug, primaquine (a 6-methoxy-8-amino-quinoline). It was observed that about 10% of black soldiers experienced an intravascular hemolytic reaction following administration of primaquine. Intravascular hemolytic reactions had long been known to occur in some individuals from Mediterranean areas after eating broad beans (*Vicia fava*); however, soldiers of Mediterranean ancestry in Korea were largely spared the hemolytic reaction to primaquine that befell certain black soldiers. An important clinical observation was that this primaquine-induced hemolytic anemia was

TABLE 6-3. Comparison between G6PD^{A-} and G6PD^{B-}

Feature	G6PD^{A-}	G6PD^{B-}
Frequency	Common in African populations	Common in Mediterranean populations
Enzymatic activity		
G6PD^{A+}	100%	—
G6PD^{B+}	—	100%
G6PD^{A-}	10%–20%	—
G6PD^{B-}	—	0–5%
Degree of acute hemolysis	Moderate	Severe
Abnormal G6PD activity	Old RBCs	All RBCs
Hemolysis with		
Fava beans	Unusual	Common
Primaquine	Common	Rare
Other drugs	Moderately common	Very common
Infection	Common	Common
Need for transfusion	Rare	Sometimes

self-limited and not life threatening. It was discovered that the differential sensitivity to primaquine was a function of RBC age. Young RBCs were resistant to the hemolytic effect of primaquine while older RBCs were sensitive. Hence, in an affected individual, once older cells are destroyed, hemolysis stops despite continuation of drug treatment.

Primaquine sensitivity among sub-Saharan Africans and their descendants is associated with a mutation of the normal $G6PD^A$ allele. The frequency of the normal $G6PD^A$ allele is about 10% to 15% in American black males and over 20% among males in many parts of Africa.

Favism

Fava beans are a staple of the diet in many Mediterranean countries. A severe hemolytic anemia is associated with the ingestion of fava beans and can even be induced by inhalation of fava bean pollen. The culpable mutant allele is $G6PD^{B-}$ (sometimes written $G6PD^{Mediterranean}$). This allele is responsible for severe hemolytic episodes when G6PD-deficient individuals acquire infections such as pneumonia, salmonellosis, and hepatitis. During acute infections, phagocytic activity of macrophages liberates oxidants that RBCs cannot adequately degrade because of inadequate G6PD, and hemolysis occurs. A dire consequence of G6PD deficiency in Mediterranean and Asian neonates is hyperbilirubinemia. Severe hyperbilirubinemia can result in kernicterus and severe neurologic sequelae. The affected neonates manifest jaundice at 1 to 4 days of age.

Severe hemolysis following exposure to fava beans occurs in G6PD-deficient whites and Asians; it is rarely seen in black Africans. Acute infections, however, do trigger hemolytic

---

NEUROSCIENCE

Kernicterus

Kernicterus results from bilirubin deposition in the basal ganglia and causes diffuse neuronal damage. Elevated bilirubin moves out of blood and into brain tissue, causing lethargy, hypotonia, and poor sucking reflex in the first few days of life, followed by marked hypertonia—especially of extensor muscles. Children are hypotonic for years before hypertonicity returns and have marked developmental and motor delays in the form of choreoathetoid cerebral palsy. Mental retardation may be present. Other sequelae include extrapyramidal disturbances, auditory abnormalities, gaze palsies, and dental dysplasias.

---

episodes in black Africans. The physiologic properties of $G6PD^{Canton}$, the variant common in Asians, are very similar to those of $G6PD^{Mediterranean}$.

The experience of the black soldiers during the Korean War and of favism among Mediterranean and Asian individuals clearly established differences in the expression of G6PD deficiency between Mediterranean and black males. In the RBCs of blacks with primaquine-induced G6PD deficiency, a residual enzyme activity of 10% to 20% is regularly found, whereas affected Mediterranean males show only minimal, often barely detectable, activity below 5%. The young red cells of primaquine-induced G6PD deficiency have a sufficient level of catalytic activity to provide protection against oxidative damage and hemolysis. In fava-induced hemolysis in Mediterranean males, virtually all RBCs are susceptible to destruction, and the acute hemolytic episodes are thus life threatening.

Sex-linked Inheritance

The $G6PD$ gene is located on the X chromosome. As a result, males are typically more severely affected than females, who have two X chromosomes and demonstrate lyonization. A G6PD-deficient cell in a female is as vulnerable to hemolysis as an enzyme-deficient cell in a male. However, the presentation of G6PD deficiency in female heterozygotes may be mild, moderate, or even severe, depending on the proportion of RBCs in which the abnormal G6PD enzyme is expressed. A female may even have two different $G6PD$ alleles and, accordingly, produce two different biochemical types of enzyme.

●●● ERYTHROCYTE HEMOGLOBIN DEFECTS

Hemoglobinopathies

The primary function of an RBC is its role in delivering O_2 to cells and tissues. As seen with HS, HE, and HPP, compromising the integrity of the cell membrane can lead to hemolysis and thus affect oxygen delivery. The role of hemoglobin molecules is equally or more critical. Globin is the protein that surrounds a heme molecule that mediates

---

BIOCHEMISTRY

G6PD and Oxidative Stress

The metabolism in erythrocytes is almost entirely anaerobic, and the major source of energy is derived from the glucose that is metabolized by the glycolytic pathway and the pentose phosphate pathway. These cells are very sensitive to oxidative stress.

Glucose-6-phosphate dehydrogenase is the only RBC enzyme that produces NADPH through glutathione reductase, and therefore any variation in the function of G6PD can decrease the amount of NADPH available to the cell. A deficiency in G6PD diminishes the amount of NADP available for glutathione reductase. This is not an issue in other cells, because they have several enzymes. A reduction in glutathione allows reactive oxygen products to damage cell proteins, lipids, and DNA.

Individuals deficient in G6PD should not be given oxidative drugs such as antimalarial drugs (primaquine), certain analgesics/antipyretics, cardiovascular drugs (procainamide, quinidine), sulfonamides, and cytotoxics/antimicrobials. These oxidant drugs can induce immediate acute hemolytic episodes characterized by progressive anemia, hemoglobinuria, and reticulocytosis caused by hemolysis of cells with low G6PD activity.

oxygen binding. Several types of hemoglobins are produced, beginning in the fetus, before the "adult" form appears. Two distinct globin chains combine with each heme. The fetus and embryo have hemoglobins that differ from the mature "adult" form. Adult hemoglobin, Hb A, is composed of α- and β-chains. Generally speaking, mutations causing a structural change in the β-globin gene result in sickle cell anemia, whereas mutations causing an absence or reduced amount of hemoglobin, from either the α- or the β-globin allele, result in thalassemias.

Nomenclature

It is important to clarify certain terminologies that can be confusing. Greek letters have been used historically by biochemists to designate protein chains with complex molecules. Geneticists have used Greek letters to name genes within a family that produce related proteins. For example, "α" and "β" have been used to designate two different spectrins in RBC membranes. The gene symbols for spectrins are in the *SPT* gene family. Globin genes are another family of closely related genes using Greek symbols to indicate loci. Several letters, some less commonly used than others, designate the gene, but these designations are not the gene name or symbol. The α-globin locus and protein may be shown as α or α-globin, but the genes are designated as *HBA1* and *HBA2*.

It is also important to recognize that *types* of hemoglobin have a single letter designation or a combination of two letters. This is demonstrated by normal adult hemoglobin, which is Hb A, or sickle cell hemoglobin, which is Hb S. All hemoglobins consist of four polypeptide chains—two of one type and two of another type. For Hb A, these chains are two α chains and two β chains. For Hb S, mutations have occurred and the hemoglobin is composed of two normal α-chains and two mutated β-chains. These are discussed in greater detail below.

Hemoglobin

Different hemoglobins exist at various phases of human development (Fig. 6-4). Two hemoglobins, Gower 1 and Gower 2, are found in embryos of up to 8 weeks of gestation. Hemoglobin Portland, which was first characterized in an infant with a chromosome abnormality, is a third normal embryonic hemoglobin. The predominant hemoglobin from the eighth week to term is fetal hemoglobin, Hb F, and is composed of $\alpha_2\gamma_2$. There are two distinct γ-chains, one with glycine and the other with alanine at position 136. These two γ-chains are expressed at distinct loci. The rate of production of β-chains increases coincidentally with a decline in γ-chain synthesis. In adult life, Hb A ($\alpha_2\beta_2$) makes up about 97% of the total hemoglobin, the remaining 2% to 3% being represented by Hb A_2 and a small amount of Hb F.

Genetic studies have established that the α-globin gene and the β-globin gene reside on different chromosomes. Indeed, a cluster of α-like genes has evolved from a single ancestral α-gene by a series of duplications on one chromosome, and a comparable family of β-genes has emerged on another chromosome. As shown in Figure 6-4, the linked group of α-like genes on human chromosome 16 contains an active embryonic ζ-gene and two active α-genes. The β-like cluster on human chromosome 11 comprises five active genes—one ε (epsilon), two γ, one δ (delta), and one β.

The β and δ genes are nearly identical in composition, which reflects their recent duplication during evolution. Indeed, the δ gene arose only 40 million years ago and is found only in higher primates. The divergence of the δ gene occurred prior to the separation of the phylogenetic lineage leading to the Old World monkey assemblage and the line represented by the great apes and humans.

Both families of hemoglobin genes contain loci called pseudogenes, depicted as psi (ψ), which do not encode functional polypeptides. Although each pseudogene shares many base sequences with its corresponding normal gene, the presence of frameshift mutations has shifted the triplet of bases so that polypeptide synthesis is prematurely halted. Thus, pseudogenes are products of gene duplication that have accumulated debilitating base changes during sequence divergence.

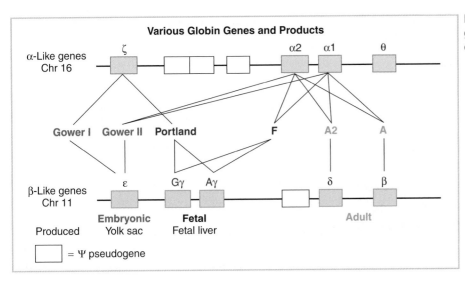

Figure 6-4. Genetic control of various globin genes and products in the embryo, fetus, and adult.

PATHOLOGY

Hematologic Indices

Red blood cell indices are part of the complete blood count (CBC).

- Mean corpuscular volume (MCV): average RBC size
- Mean corpuscular hemoglobin (MCH): amount of hemoglobin per RBC
- Mean corpuscular hemoglobin concentration (MCHC): amount of hemoglobin relative to the size of the cell

Sickle Cell Anemia

Sickle cell anemia afflicts one in every 500 black children born in the United States. This is an inherited disorder in which the RBCs, normally discoidal, are contorted into rigid crescents ("sickled") (Fig. 6-5). Sickle cell disease is characterized by chronic hemolytic anemia, recurrent vaso-occlusive painful "crises" of variable duration and severity, and infarctions of tissues and organs. Pain is the most frequent cause of recurrent morbidity. Life expectancy has increased in recent years owing to pharmacologic advances; however, the mean survival age remains at less than 50 years (Table 6-4). A disproportionate number of deaths occur in infancy or early

TABLE 6-4. Median Survival Age of Individuals with Sickle Cell Disease

Genotype	Mean Survival
Male HbSS	42 years
Female HbSS	48 years
Male HbSC	60 years
Male HbSC	68 years

Data from Office of Genomics and Disease Prevention, Centers for Disease Control and Prevention (CDC), May 5, 2005.

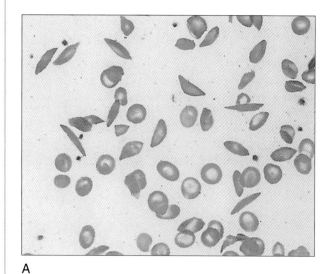

A

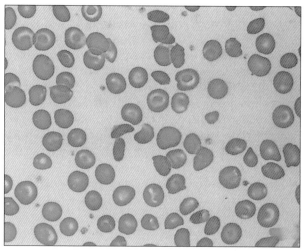

B

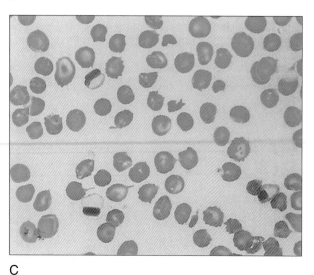

C

Figure 6-5. **A**, Sickle cell disease. Crescent- and cigar-shaped cells are present along with target cells and teardrop cells. **B**, Hemoglobin sickle cell disease. The striking sickle forms of sickle cell are not evident, but densely staining, elongated RBCs with rather blunt ends are present. (It has been said these are trying to "sickle like S, and crystallize like C.") Cells appear dense on the smear, with many target cells. **C**, Hemoglobin C disease. Target cells are present as are some spherocytic cells. Hemoglobin crystals can be seen within intact cell membranes. These are pathognomonic. (Courtesy of Dr. Anna Walker, Mercer University School of Medicine, Georgia.)

childhood, usually resulting from overwhelming bacterial infections, a sudden severe splenic crisis, or acute cerebrovascular occlusion.

Genetic Aspects of Sickle Cell Anemia

Sickle cell anemia results from the single substitution of valine for glutamic acid at amino acid 6 in the 146-amino-acid chain of the β-hemoglobin chain. This abnormal hemoglobin is known as hemoglobin S (Hb S), and its cause is an alteration of a single base of the triplet of DNA that specifies an amino acid, as depicted in Figure 6-6. Another abnormal hemoglobin molecule, hemoglobin C, results from a mutation at the same DNA triplet; however, whereas the glutamine residue is replaced by valine in hemoglobin S, it is replaced by lysine via a different missense mutation in hemoglobin C. Hemoglobin S and hemoglobin C are *allelic*; two independent mutations occurred in the same sequence of bases in the DNA that make up alleles of a single gene (Table 6-5). This example demonstrates that there may be more than one mutation site within a single allelic locus, which can lead to different alterations in the function of the gene. Hemoglobin C disease is usually a benign hemolytic anemia, whereas sickle cell anemia can have severe consequences. Because Hb S and Hb C are allelic, an allele could be inherited from each parent, resulting in HbSC disease (see Fig. 6-6). The severity of this condition is between that of sickle cell disease and Hb C except that visual damage due to retinal vascular lesions is worse.

Sickle cell anemia is an autosomal recessive disease. Individuals with one normal and one defective allele are

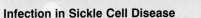

MICROBIOLOGY

Infection in Sickle Cell Disease

Splenic dysfunction can occur in sickle cell disease by age 3 months. These infants have a high risk for septicemia and meningitis, pneumococci, and infections by other encapsulated bacteria. The most common cause of death in children with sickle cell disease is *Streptococcus pneumoniae* sepsis. There is also an increased risk of osteomyelitis caused by *Staphylococcus aureus*, *Salmonella* species, and others.

PHARMACOLOGY

Penicillin Prophylaxis in Infants with Sickle Cell Anemia

Prophylactic penicillin therapy prevents 80% of life-threatening *Streptococcus pneumoniae* sepsis. Infants should receive 125 mg of penicillin V PO_4 prophylaxis orally twice a day. Children aged 3 to 5 years should receive 250 mg of penicillin V PO_4 prophylaxis orally twice a day. Erythromycin prophylaxis is an alternative for individuals allergic to penicillin. Folic acid supplementation may also be considered.

PHYSIOLOGY

Hemoglobin and O_2 Binding

Hemoglobin is a tetramer with each monomer composed of a heme and a globin. Heme is a general term for a metal ion chelated to a porphyrin ring. Central to the pyrrole rings of porphyrin is Fe^{++}. Oxygen binds to hemoglobin only when iron is in the ferrous state (Fe^{++}), and therefore hemoglobin in the Fe^{+++} state (methemoglobin) does not bind oxygen. However, O_2 interaction can bind reversibly to Fe^{++} because of the interaction of heme with specific amino acids in hemoglobin. The interaction of histidine with Fe^{++} stabilizes the Fe-O_2 complex. When O_2 binds to Fe^{++}, the shape of the hemoglobin molecule is changed to a planar conformation. This change in the shape of hemoglobin corresponds to a change from the tense (T) form to the relaxed (R) form. Oxygen binding is sterically inhibited in the T form. In the R form, the affinity for O_2 is approximately 150-fold greater than in the T form. The binding of the first O_2 is energy dependent, but affinity for binding increases after the first O_2 is bound. These affinity changes account for the S shape of the initial slope of the oxyhemoglobin dissociation curve. The capacity to bind O_2 is dependent on the availability of Fe^{+++}. Pao_2 determines the binding of hemoglobin with O_2, or the hemoglobin saturation level, and this oxyhemoglobin saturation level can be influenced by alterations in $Paco_2$, pH, and temperature.

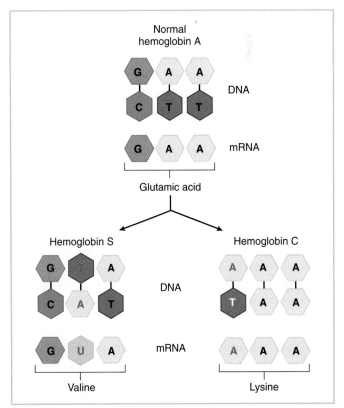

Figure 6-6. Hemoglobin A mutations. Two different missense mutations at the same codon result in two different proteins. The mutations are allelic.

TABLE 6-5. Mutations in β-Globin Gene Producing Sickle Cell Anemia, Hemoglobin C Disease, and HbSC Disease

Hemoglobin	Composition	Genotype	Clinical Status
Hb A	$\alpha_2^A\beta_2^A$	$\alpha\alpha/\alpha\alpha$ β/β	Normal
HbAS	$\alpha_2^A\beta_2^A$ $\alpha_2^A\beta_2^S$	$\alpha\alpha/\alpha\alpha$ β/β^S	Sickle cell trait
HbCC	$\alpha_2^A\beta_2^C$	$\alpha\alpha/\alpha\alpha$ β^C/β^C	Hemoglobin C disease
HbSC	$\alpha_2^A\beta^S\beta^C$	$\alpha\alpha/\alpha\alpha$ β^S/β^C	HbSC disease
HbSS	$\alpha_2^A\beta_2^S$	$\alpha\alpha/\alpha\alpha$ β^S/β^S	Sickle cell disease

generally healthy carriers. Such heterozygous individuals are said to have a sickle cell trait. Two million blacks (8% to 9% of African Americans) have sickle cell trait. Although heterozygous individuals are typically asymptomatic, even RBCs of heterozygotes can undergo sickling under certain circumstances, such as low oxygen tension, and produce clinical manifestations. Since the detrimental allele can occasionally express itself in the heterozygous state, the gene should be considered dominant. Thus, dominance and recessiveness are somewhat arbitrary concepts that depend on the point of view. From a molecular standpoint, the relation between the normal and the defective allele in this instance may best be described as *codominant*, since the heterozygote produces both normal and abnormal hemoglobin. As with many heterozygous conditions, both normal and abnormal proteins are produced with possible consequences due to reduced amounts of normal protein and increased amounts of abnormal protein.

Hemoglobin and Pathophysiology of Sickle Cell Anemia

Sickle cell anemia does not manifest itself in the first few months of neonatal life. There is a protective action of Hb F to the very low levels of the disease-causing abnormal hemoglobin (Hb S) during early life. The percentage of Hb F at birth is high, often as high as 85%, but the quantity drops precipitously as the synthesis of the adult form of hemoglobin accelerates. In sickle-cell anemic infants, the proportion of abnormal hemoglobin rises to near adult levels by 6 months of age. After 6 months of age, the sickling of RBCs is a constant finding.

In individuals with the sickle cell trait, the proportion of Hb S is between 35% and 45%. Of course, two types of hemoglobin would be expected to be synthesized in equal amounts. However, it appears that Hb S is synthesized at a lower rate than Hb A. It has been suggested that this difference is the result of a specific delay in translation of mRNA on the polyribosome.

The substitution of valine for glutamic acid causes the abnormal hemoglobin S molecules to aggregate, or polymerize, into strands that are laid down to form cable-like fibers. As greater numbers of fibers accumulate, the large aggregates, or polymers, of linearly arranged fibers attain sufficient length and rigidity to distort the cell membrane into a crescent shape. Polymerization of Hb S occurs at low oxygen tensions. In the fully oxygenated state, Hb S behaves like normal hemoglobin (Hb A) and remains in solution. The sickling phenomenon is reversible with reoxygenation of Hb S; the aggregated molecule dissociates and the distended cell returns to its normal shape. The continual dual process, however, of polymerization and depolymerization ultimately takes its toll, and many RBCs become irreversibly sickled—even in the fully oxygenated state.

The sickling of RBCs leads to the obstruction of microvasculature that can result in vaso-occlusion, blocking of blood flow, and perhaps infections in postoccluded areas. In lungs, gas exchange becomes difficult and individuals may suffer breathing difficulties (dyspnea). Increased pressure from fluid seeping into the lung parenchyma from capillaries will also activate cough receptors. These physiologic alterations induce intensely acute problems, such as acute chest syndrome, and may require intervention with oxygen either through inhalation or extracorporal administration. Transfusions may also be necessary. If microemboli are trapped in bone marrow, infections may develop and fat emboli may be released into the blood. These emboli may then also be trapped in the lung and exacerbate the crisis.

DNA Analysis of Sickle Cell Anemia

DNA technology has made it feasible to examine DNA directly and to identify sickle cell anemia with a high degree of precision during early development. A variety of polymerase chain reaction (PCR)–based techniques is used yielding 99% to 100% detection of specific mutations in the β-hemoglobin gene.

As noted previously, an A to T substitution in the sixth triplet of the globin gene causes the substitution of valine for

PATHOLOGY & PHYSIOLOGY

Acute Chest Syndrome (ACS)

ACS is a common complication of sickling disorders such as Hb SS, Hb SC, Hb S β^+-thalassemia, and Hb S β^0-thalassemia. It is responsible for considerable morbidity and mortality in these patients owing to the altered hemoglobin that causes erythrocytes to accumulate on endothelial microvasculature surfaces. Because of these accumulations, ACS presents with a pulmonary infiltrate (infection or infarction) on radiography that may have been induced by or associated with cough, fever, sputum, dyspnea, or hypoxia.

Major clinical problems are distinguishing between infection and infarction and establishing the clinical significance of fat embolism.

BIOCHEMISTRY

Techniques to Demonstrate Hemoglobin Variation

Various techniques are used to differentiate between different hemoglobins. High-performance liquid chromatography (HPLC) resolves protein bands that are not separated by other tests. It can achieve accurate quantitation even at low concentrations but does not enable the identification of HbS-β° thalassemia, which requires hemoglobin electrophoresis.

Isoelectric focusing (IEF) has better resolution and quantitation than does electrophoresis.

Electrophoresis is used for quick screening. Bands may overlap, and quantitation is inaccurate at low concentrations. It is being replaced by HPLC.

---

glutamine. This results in the subsequent production of sickle cell hemoglobin. The sequence CCTGAGG in the region coding for amino acids 5–7 in the normal globin sequence is recognized by the restriction enzyme *Mst*II. A PCR test can be designed to utilize this ability to cleave a normal DNA fragment containing this site. Failure of the restriction enzyme to cleave the DNA demonstrates an amplified fragment containing the altered site (Fig. 6-7).

Thalassemias

Thalassemia is a potentially fatal blood disorder that is associated with a marked suppression or absence of hemoglobin production. This differs from sickle cell and hemoglobin C diseases, which result from a structural alteration of hemoglobin.

α-Thalassemia

The α-thalassemias are characterized by reduced synthesis of α-chains. Anemia stems both from the lack of adequate hemoglobin and from the effects of excess unpaired non-α chains. Since different non-α chains are synthesized at different times of development, different conditions prevail. In the newborn with α-thalassemia, the excess unpaired γ-chains form γ tetramers called Hb Barts. In the adult, the excess β-chains aggregate to form tetramers called Hb H (Fig. 6-8).

The α-thalassemias most often result from deletions of one or more of the α genes (Fig. 6-9). These deletions occur by unequal crossing-over between homologous sequences in the α-goblin gene cluster. When this occurs, one chromosome will have only one α-gene (α-) and the other chromosome will have three (ααα). Since there are normally four α-globin genes, the severity of α-thalassemia depends on the number of available and normally functioning α-globin genes (see Fig. 6-9). Each α-gene normally is responsible for 25% of the α-chains, and each may be deleted independently of the other α-genes. If only one of these genes is lost, there is no detectable clinical abnormality. Such a "silent" carrier of α-thalassemia is asymptomatic, with a hematologic profile that is within normal limits. The silent carrier can transmit the deletion to offspring, who could manifest a symptomatic form of α-thalassemia if the other parent also transmits a chromosome with one or more α-deleted genes.

The loss of two of the four genes is referred to as α-*thalassemia trait*. The pair of deleted genes may be from the same chromosome, or one α-globin gene may be deleted from each of the two chromosomes. The former situation is more common in Asian populations, whereas the latter is witnessed more often in those of African origin. Although both of these

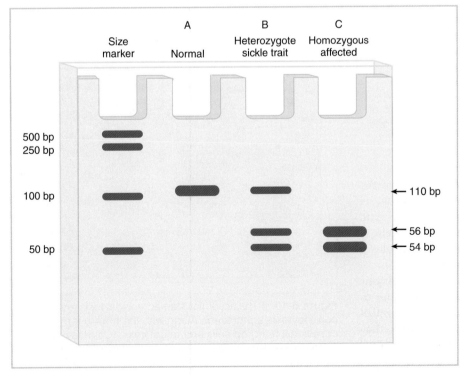

Figure 6-7. The region of the β-globin gene corresponding to codon 6 was amplified by polymerase chain reaction (PCR). Using primers, 20 bases in length, to flank the region, DNA from individuals being tested, free nucleotides in buffer, and DNA *Taq* polymerase, the region can be copied millions of times in a short period of time. For sickle cell, the knowledge that the mutation changes a restriction enzyme recognition site is used to identify the mutation. As shown here, a 110-base-pair fragment of the normal β-globin gene was amplified in lane A; in lane B, a normal fragment and one fragment that was cleaved by the restriction enzyme *Mst*II. Amplified and digested products are visualized after separation on a 3% agarose gel by electrophoresis. This pattern (B) represents the heterozygote Hb AS. If both alleles are cleaved by *Mst*II, sickle cell disease occurs, Hb S, as shown in lane C.

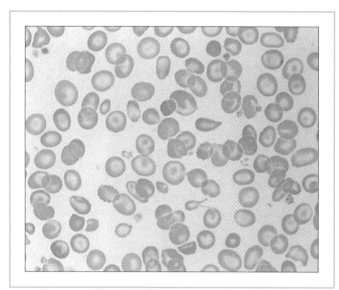

Figure 6-8. α-Thalassemia. RBCs are hypochromic and microcytic and vary considerably in shape. Target cells are present. (Courtesy of Dr. Anna Walker, Mercer University School of Medicine, Macon, Georgia.)

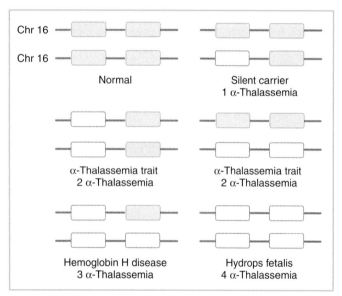

Figure 6-9. α-Thalassemia results from reduced synthesis of α-globin chains. This occurs most often from deletion of one to all four genes found on chromosome 16. Open boxes represent deleted genes.

genetic patterns are identical clinically, the position of the deleted genes is important in terms of the likelihood of severe α-thalassemia in the offspring. Accordingly, progeny with *hydrops fetalis*, who have no α-globin chains, rarely occur in black African populations because each parent contributes a chromosome containing one functional α-gene.

Hemoglobin H disease, most commonly found in Asiatic populations, is associated with the loss of three of the four α-genes. The outcome is a significant imbalance in globin synthesis. Although β-chains are produced in normal amounts, they are actually present in relative excess owing to the marked suppression of α-chain production. The excess β-chains form

unstable β_4 tetramers (Hb H). These tetramers form insoluble inclusions in mature red cells (see Fig. 6-8). The spleen removes the older red cells with precipitates of Hb H.

The most severe form of α-thalassemia, hydrops fetalis, results from the deletion of all four α-genes. In the fetus, excess γ-chains form tetramers (Hb Barts) that have extremely high oxygen affinity but are unable to deliver oxygen to tissues. Severe tissue anoxia invariably leads to intrauterine fetal death. Presently there is no effective therapy for the hydropic fetus. Exchange transfusions will fail because the fetus has no capacity for endogenous production of functional hemoglobin.

β-*Thalassemia*

β-Thalassemia is the second most common cause of hypochromic, microcytic anemia; iron deficiency anemia is the most common. Homozygous β-thalassemia, in which the patient has inherited two defective β-alleles, results in impaired β-chain synthesis. The production of α-chains continues at normal, or elevated, levels in β-thalassemia, but the unmatched α-chains accumulate and precipitate as inclusion bodies in the RBC precursors (Fig. 6-10). Most damaged RBC precursors do not leave the marrow; those which are released to the circulation are disadvantaged and rapidly destroyed by the spleen. The suppressed synthesis of β-chains is compensated by overproduction of fetal hemoglobin. The compensation, however, is incomplete, since the blood cells are still deficient in hemoglobin.

Clinically, β-thalassemias are classified as thalassemia major, thalassemia intermediate, or thalassemia minor. The three differ in severity of disease and types of interventions. As suggested, thalassemia major is the most severe and requires transfusions. Thalassemia minor is often asymptomatic. Each

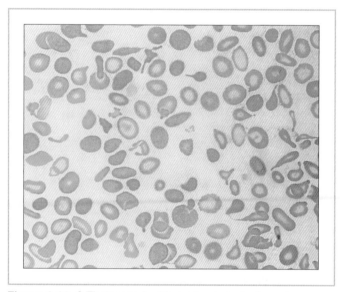

Figure 6-10. β-Thalassemia. Marked anisocytosis and poikilocytosis are present. Along with the bizarre forms are occasional teardrop cells and target cells. (Courtesy of Dr. Anna Walker, Mercer University School of Medicine, Macon, Georgia.)

of these disease classes is caused by a particular molecular defect in the α- or β-globin genes that prevents normal expression of these genes. Because the α-globin gene is essential both to fetal life and to postpartum life, α-thalassemia generally is either *fatal in utero* or compatible with a normal life style. On the other hand, the β-globin gene is not imperative in fetal life and is not even fully expressed until after birth. Hence, β-thalassemia in its full expression is the crippling disease of childhood. α- and β-thalassemias are compared in Table 6-6.

To reiterate the role of Hb F in the etiology of the disease, as Hb F ($\alpha_2\gamma_2$) γ-chain production switches off postpartum, the deficit of β-chains in β-thalassemia becomes a significant problem. Anemia is compounded by the death of RBC precursors, which leads to compensatory erythropoietin-induced marrow hypertrophy. This, in turn, leads to a hypermetabolic state, skeletal changes, and increased intestinal absorption of iron and iron overload. Iron overload is compounded by administration of transfusions to treat the anemia.

The majority of individuals with minor and intermediate thalassemia do not need regular transfusions although some individuals do require either occasional or regular transfusions. The most effective therapy, if needed, is the use of transfusions with prophylactic antibiotics. Unfortunately, just as with thalassemia major, repeated transfusions, especially in children, can create a state of iron overload, which damages the tissues in which it is deposited, such as the heart and liver. Chelation with an iron-binding resin is administered to prevent this overload. The intensive use of transfusions and chelation can extend the life expectancy of a patient for 20 to 30 years. Bone marrow transplantation is available but has been successful in only a small percentage of patients.

β-Thalassemia is a heterogeneous disorder. Some patients with homozygous β-thalassemia are unable to synthesize any β-chains; this is known as β^0-thalassemia. The production of *some* β-chains is known as β^+-thalassemia. In either event, the lack of or marked reduction in β-chain synthesis is accompanied by the unimpaired synthesis of α-chains. The clinical severity of β-thalassemia reflects the extreme insolubility of α-chains, which are present in relative excess because of the deficiency of β-chain synthesis. Therefore, the fewer functional β-chains present, the more insoluble α-chain aggregates occur and the more severe is the disease.

PATHOLOGY

Erythropoietin-induced Marrow Hypertrophy

Erythropoietin (EPO) secretion from the kidney is stimulated by hemolysis and a decrease in hemoglobin. Tissue anoxia also leads to EPO production. EPO causes excessive iron absorption and iron overload and increases erythroid hyperplasia in bone marrow and extramedullary sites.

Marrow expansion leads to skeletal deformities by invading bone and impairing proper growth. It also affects extramedullary sites—the liver and spleen. Extreme cases involve extra-osseous masses in the thorax, abdomen, and pelvis.

TABLE 6-6. Comparison Between α- and β-Thalassemias

Clinical Condition	Genotype	Disease	Molecular Genetics
α-Thalassemias			
Silent carrier	-α/αα	Asymptomatic; no RBC abnormality	
α-Thalassemia trait	--/αα (Asian) -α/-α (Black African)	Asymptomatic, like β-thalassemia minor; microcytosis	
HbH disease	--/-α	Severe, resembles β-thalassemia; intermediate, moderately severe hemolytic anemia	Gene deletions usually
Hydrops fetalis	--/--	Lethal in utero, Hb Barts	
β-Thalassemias			
Thalassemia major	Homozygous β^0-thalassemia (β^0/β^0)	Severe, requires blood transfusion regularly	
Thalassemia intermediate	β^0/β	Severe, but does not require regular blood transfusions	Rare gene deletions in β^0/β^0. Defects in transcription, processing, or translation of β-globin mRNA
Thalassemia minor	β^0/β β^+/β	Asymptomatic with mild or absent anemia; RBC abnormalities seen	

Deleted genes are indicated by hyphens (-) in α-thalassemias. The absence of chain production in β-thalassemia is indicated by (°), whereas mutations resulting in decreased β globin chains are indicated by ($^+$).

The loss of β-chain gene function results from a variety of different structural mutations within or surrounding the β-gene. The level of β-chain synthesis is determined by the specific manner in which gene expression is altered. Unlike α-thalassemia in which α-globin genes are deleted, the β-globin gene is present in most cases, and defects in gene expression have been identified that alter gene transcription, mRNA processing, and translation. The varying clinical severity observed in β-thalassemia is directly correlated with the degree to which such mutations decrease β-globin gene expression.

●●● BLEEDING DISORDERS

The most common hereditary deficiencies of coagulation, resulting in excessive bleeding, are hemophilia A, hemophilia B, and von Willebrand disease. Among these, the hemophilias affect one in 10,000 individuals per year and are best known because of their historic association with European royal families. However, von Willebrand disease is the most common coagulation disorder, affecting 1% to 2% of the U.S. population (Table 6-7).

Hemophilia A and B are characterized by defects in key components of the clotting cascade—factors VIII and IX, respectively—which render the patient incapable of normal coagulation processes. Clinical expression can range from mild to excessive bleeding due to major insult to frequent spontaneous internal bleeding without insult. As exhibited by a number of recessive disorders, the degree of clinical manifestation depends on the amount of clotting factor available. Accordingly, the amount of available clotting factor is determined by the severity of the genetic mutation. Finally, both hemophilias are sex-linked diseases and serve as a paradigm for X-linked recessive disorders. Females only exhibit bleeding problems via unfortunate lyonization, or the co-occurrence of two independent allelic mutations.

In von Willebrand disease, both platelet aggregation and clot formation fail to occur properly. The von Willebrand protein, also known as the von Willebrand factor or vWF, normally promotes platelet adhesion to endothelium and is a carrier for factor VIII in the clotting cascade. Therefore, von Willebrand disease has an association with hemophilia A that is caused by a mutation in the factor VIII gene.

Hemophilia A

Hemophilia A occurs with an incidence of approximately 1 in 5000 live male births. A deficiency or absence of clotting factor VIII ultimately results in impaired thrombin production. The gene for factor VIII is large, encoding 26 exons that span 186 kb on the tip of the long arm (Xp28) of the X chromosome. Base pair changes, deletions, frameshift mutations, and protein-truncating mutations have been found in the factor VIII gene, and clinical severity is proportional to the loss of factor VIII activity conferred by the mutation. Hence, it is possible for a female to exhibit a modest reduction in factor VIII due to X inactivation. About 45% of the most severe cases of hemophilia A are caused by the so-

TABLE 6-7. Comparison between Hemophilia A, Hemophilia B, and von Willebrand Disease

Feature	Hemophilia A	Hemophilia B	Von Willebrand Disease
Inheritance	X-linked	X-linked	Dominant with variable expressivity; chromosome 12
Mutations	Flip inversion, deletions, rearrangements, frameshift mutations, splicing errors, and nonsense mutations; mild form—missense mutations	Severe form—frameshifts, splicing errors, nonsense and missense mutations; mild-to-moderate form—missense mutations	Missense, deletion
Primary sites of hemorrhage	Muscle, joints; posttrauma, postoperative	Muscle, joints; posttrauma, postoperative	Mucous membranes; skin cuts; posttrauma, postoperative
Platelet count	Normal	Normal	Normal
Bleeding time	Normal	Normal	Prolonged
Prothrombin time	Normal	Normal	Normal
Partial thromboplastin time	Prolonged	Prolonged	Prolonged or normal
Factor VIII	Low	Normal	Normal
Factor IX	Normal	Low	Normal
VWF	Normal	Normal	Low
Ristocetin-induced platelet aggregation	Normal	Normal	Impaired

Data from Hoffbrand AV, Pettit JE, Moss PAH, *Essential Haematology*, 4th ed. Oxford, Blackwell, 2001, p 265.

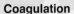

PHYSIOLOGY

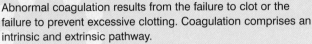

Coagulation

Abnormal coagulation results from the failure to clot or the failure to prevent excessive clotting. Coagulation comprises an intrinsic and extrinsic pathway.

The intrinsic pathway is initiated by a negatively charged surface, which may occur with damaged endothelium or by surface contact with certain foreign substances. Partial thromboplastin time (PTT) detects intrinsic factor abnormalities reflected by increased PTT.

The extrinsic pathway is activated by tissue thromboplastin (factor III), which is released after *cell injury* of endothelium or other cells. Prothrombin time (PT) mainly detects abnormalities in extrinsic factors (prothrombin; factors V, VII, and X) although prothrombin is commonly considered the major factor measured by PT. Most factors adversely affecting the extrinsic coagulation pathway, including clotting factors, result in an increased PT. However, a few situations such as vitamin K supplementation, thrombophlebitis, and use of certain drugs will decrease PT.

called "flip" inversion in intron 22. Here, recombination with nearly homologous X chromosome sequences located near the chromosome-terminating telomere disrupts the normal reading frame. Approximately 50% of remaining cases of severe hemophilia have deletions, rearrangements, frameshift mutations, splicing errors, or nonsense mutations. Mild-to-moderate cases typically harbor missense mutations. For both forms of hemophilia, nearly one third of cases are due to new, spontaneous mutations.

In severe cases, the diagnosis of hemophilia may be made during the first year of life. If the diagnosis is not made, an affected child may have large bruises from minor injuries, which may even suggest a "battered" child. The child or adult with severe forms of the disease may have five or more spontaneous bleedings per month. Often, these are in joints and deep muscles and can be painful. This is in contrast to individuals with mild disease who may not have spontaneous bleeding and may experience abnormal bleeding once a year to once every 10 years.

Hemophilia B

Hemophilia B, sometimes referred to as Christmas disease, results from a reduction in the amount of factor IX, a serine protease, available for thrombin generation by the clotting cascade. The incidence of hemophilia B is roughly one seventh that of hemophilia A. This is in part attributable to the much smaller size of the factor IX gene—8 exons comprising 34 kb—at the tip of the X chromosome (Xp27) and very close to the factor VIII gene. Still, hundreds of different missense, nonsense, frameshift, and deletion mutations have been found with hemophilia B. The most common cause of mild-to-moderate hemophilia B results from missense mutations. There have been occasional reports of large deletions associ-

ated with severe disease, but usually cases are associated with frameshifts, splicing errors, nonsense, and missense mutations.

The presentation of hemophilia B is quite similar to hemophilia A. For both disorders, there may be prolonged bleeding, spontaneous bleeding, hemarthrosis, deep muscle bruising, intracranial bleeding at birth, unexplained GI bleeding, and excessive bruising. Both hemophilias have mild to severe forms. Only by determining the deficient factor can a proper diagnosis be made.

Von Willebrand Disease

Von Willebrand disease differs from the hemophilias in its mode of inheritance. It is transmitted in an autosomal dominant manner with variable expression. In hemophilia, bleeding is generally in joints and muscles; whereas in von Willebrand disease, bleeding is more common in mucous membranes and after routine operations. As with hemophilia, there are mild to severe forms. Missense mutations or large deletions cause either a reduced amount of vWF or an abnormal function of the protein. The most common is the mild form, type I, in which vWF and perhaps factor VIII are reduced. Type II results from a structural defect in vWF, and the presentation reflects the severity of the defect. In type III, there may be a complete absence of vWF and factor VIII levels are often less than 10%.

●●● THROMBOPHILIA

A final group of disorders to be considered are those abnormalities which cause excessive clotting; in other words, this group could be considered the antithesis of those coagulation disorders discussed above that result in excessive bleeding. Their occurrence is sometimes not recognized as a coagulation disorder. Eighty percent of all strokes result from ischemic events—blood clots blocking a vessel. One in 1000 individuals in the United States is at risk for venous thrombosis, most commonly occurring in the lower extremities.

BIOCHEMISTRY

Serine Proteases

Serine proteases are a family of enzymes that cleave between specific amino acids. They are grouped according to structural homology and play important roles in coagulation, inflammation and immunity, and digestion. Generally, there is an enzyme-specific preference for cleaving adjacent to a specific type of amino acid. For example, trypsin cleaves after the basic amino acids arginine and lysine. The coagulation factors, except for factors VIII and V, which are glycoproteins, are all serine proteases. Serine proteases are synthesized in an inactive form (zymogen) and require proteolysis for activation. Those participating in the coagulation cascade are synthesized in the liver, secreted as zymogens, and activated following vascular injury. The zymogen, or proenzyme, form generally has an -ogen suffix.

There are 2 million cases per year in the United States, with mortality estimated at 60,000 from pulmonary emboli. Several genetic conditions contribute to these clotting disorders. Antithrombin III (AT3) deficiency, protein C deficiency, and protein S deficiency account for 5% to 15% of these inherited thrombophilias.

Activated Protein C Resistance and Factor V Leiden

In families suspected of having a familial thrombotic disorder, 20% to 65% of these disorders have been attributed to activated protein C resistance. Known as factor V Leiden, this defect is present in 2% to 5% of the asymptomatic white population and 1.2% of the black population. The factor V Leiden mutation is relatively uncommon in the native populations of Asia, Africa, and North America. In contrast, in Greece and southern Sweden, rates above 10% have been reported.

Risk of venous thrombosis is increased 3- to 8-fold for heterozygous individuals and 30- to 140-fold for homozygous individuals (Table 6-8). It accounts for about 40% of idiopathic venous thromboembolic disease. It has been associated with recurrent venous thromboembolism and thrombosis following pregnancy and the use of oral contraceptives.

The primary factor V Leiden mutation is an A to G missense mutation in the factor V coagulation factor, leading to an arginine to glutamine substitution at position 506 of the protein, which represents the proteolytic site of the protein.

TABLE 6-8. Risk of Deep Vein Thrombosis with Factor V Leiden Mutation

Risk (age)	Average Population	Factor V Leiden Mutation
<40 years	1 in 10,000	1 in 1750
40–50 years	1 in 1250	1 in 1100
50–60 years	1 in 1100	1 in 476
60–70 years	1 in 833	1 in 250
70–80 years	1 in 625	1 in 120

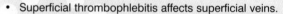

PATHOLOGY

Venous Thrombosis

- Superficial thrombophlebitis affects superficial veins.
- Deep vein thrombosis affects deep veins.
- Prolonged thrombosis can lead to chronic venous insufficiency with edema, pain, stasis pigmentation, dermatitis, and ulceration.
- Almost always associated with phlebitis, "thrombosis" and "thrombophlebitis" are used interchangeably.
- It may occur as a result of a coagulation disorder or related to an underlying malignancy.

This mutation occurs in over 95% of cases and is the most common genetic risk factor for venous thrombosis.

The function of protein C in the clotting cascade is to inactivate factor V and factor VIII. The arginine to glutamine substitution prevents factor V from being cleaved by activated protein C and thus it remains active. The reality is that factor V Leiden is inactivated by activated protein C but at a much slower rate. The factor V Leiden mutation has been associated with venous thrombotic clots, pulmonary emboli, and arterial clots. The probability of thrombosis before age 33 is 44% and 20% in homozygous and heterozygous individuals, respectively. In addition, it may play a role in stillbirths or recurrent miscarriages, preeclampsia, and eclampsia.

ANATOMY

Thrombosis of the Leg

Three major veins drain the lower leg, so thrombosis in one does not obstruct venous return. Deep vein thrombosis involving the popliteal, femoral, and iliac may be tender and palpable over the involved vein. With iliofemoral venous thrombosis, dilated superficial collateral veins may appear over the leg, hip, and lower abdomen.

Musculoskeletal Disorders 7

CONTENTS

In this chapter, the most common forms of a heterogeneous group of inherited musculoskeletal diseases are highlighted. Musculoskeletal disorders have many etiologic origins, including connective tissue/extracellular matrix deficiencies such as osteogenesis imperfecta, Ehlers-Danlos syndrome, and Marfan syndrome; faulty growth factor biology as seen in achondroplasia; and both structural and metabolic muscle cell abnormalities represented by Becker and Duchenne muscular dystrophies and mitochondrial myopathies, respectively. Although individually these may be somewhat rare, collectively the musculoskeletal diseases constitute a significant proportion of human disease.

●●● CONNECTIVE TISSUE AND BONE DISEASES

Extracellular Matrix and Connective Tissue

The extracellular matrix is found in the spaces between cells, forming a large proportion of tissue volume. It is also found between organs and as such contributes to the body's shape, plasticity, and partitioning. The extracellular matrix (ECM) is composed of three associated macromolecules: (1) fibrous structural proteins such as collagen and elastin, (2) glycoproteins, and (3) proteoglycans and hyaluronic acid. Typically, the ECM forms either basement membrane or interstitial matrix and, in doing so, performs several functions including retaining water, minerals, and nutrients as well as acting as substrate for cell-cell contact, migration, and adherence.

Connective tissues have an extensive extracellular matrix that serves to bridge, interconnect, and support a variety of cellular and organ structures. These structures are typically made up of cells, blood vessels, and a particular type of ECM. For example, in skin, fibroblasts and blood vessels are interwoven within an extracellular matrix that is an amalgam of structural proteins, proteoglycans, and adhesion molecules. Other types of connective tissue include tendon and cartilage. Here, the discussion of connective tissues focuses on skin connective tissue, since much is known about the structure and function of this anatomic element and many well-characterized connective tissue diseases are localized to the skin. Central to any discussion of skin connective tissue is collagen.

BIOCHEMISTRY

Extracellular Matrix (ECM)

The extracellular matrix occupies the intercellular spaces. It is most abundant in connective tissues such as the basement membrane, bone, tendon, and cartilage, where definition is given to the ECM by the proportions and organization of various components. The elastin of skin and blood cells provides resiliency, collagen provides strength to tendons, and the calcified collagen matrix of bone provides strength and incompressibility.

Integrins are a family of heterodimeric proteins composed of α- and β-subunits that are the main cellular receptors for the ECM. Integrins have several distinctive features from other adhesion proteins. They interact with an arginine-glycine aspartic acid (RGD) motif of ECM proteins. Integrins link the intracellular cytoskeleton with the ECM through this RGD motif. Without this attachment, cells normally undergo apoptosis. Integrins can bind to more than one ligand and many ligands can bind to more than one integrin. Examples of integrins include fibronectin receptors and laminin receptors.

Types of Connective Tissue

Connective tissues are classified by the cells and fibers present in the tissue as well as the characteristics of the ground substance.

Connective tissue (CT) proper consists of loose connective tissue (areolar tissue) and dense connective tissue, which has more and larger fibers than loose CT. Dense connective tissue can be either irregular, in which the fibers are usually arranged more or less haphazardly, or regular, in which the fibers are arranged in parallel sheets or bundles. Specialized CT is distinct in either structure or function from CT proper. Examples are adipose tissue, blood, bone, cartilage, hemopoietic tissues, and lymphatic tissues.

Embryonic CT encompasses mesenchymal and mucoid CT.

HISTOLOGY

Skin

Skin is composed of the epidermis and the dermis. The epidermis is composed of two main zones of cells:

- Stratum corneum: outer layer of cells without nuclei
- Stratum germinativum: composed of three strata (basal, spinous, granular)

The dermis consists of a three-dimensional matrix of loose connective tissue including fibrous proteins such as collagen and elastin as well as proteins embedded in ground substance (glycosaminoglycans). Skin collagen (type I) is rich in glycine, proline, and hydroxyproline. Hydroxyproline is unique to collagens, and synthesis requires vitamin C.

Collagen

A major component of skin connective tissue is the fibrous structural protein collagen. The collagens form a family of insoluble, extracellular proteins that are produced by a number of cell types but primarily by fibroblasts. Collagen is the most abundant protein found in the human body and is a key structural component of bone, cartilage, tendons, ligaments, and fascia in addition to skin. Nineteen types of collagen have been characterized and each localizes to a specific part of the body. The major collagens are type I of skin, tendons, bone and ligaments; type II found in cartilage; type III found in skin and hollow tubular structures such as arteries, intestines, and uterus; and type IV represented in all basal laminae (Table 7-1). Types I through III form strong fibers and thus are called fibrillar collagens, while type IV is associated with a multibranched network. Fifteen additional types of collagen perform essential functions but are less abundant.

Collagens have a distinctive primary amino acid sequence featuring a repeated motif of (glycine-X-Y)$_n$, where Y is often proline or hydroxyproline and X can be any amino acid. Typically, a fibrillar collagen is synthesized in the endoplasmic reticulum as a precursor molecule—procollagen—which is composed of a short signal peptide, an amino- and carboxyter-

minal propeptide, and a central α-chain segment (Fig. 7-1). The α-chain segment includes the repeated motif in which glycine represents every third amino acid, and it is this chain that constitutes the biochemical core of collagen. Three separate chains coalesce in the Golgi to form a triple helix, or tropocollagen, that is characterized by numerous disulfide bonds. The formation of a stable triple helix requires the presence of glycine in the restricted space where the three chains come together. Collagen triple helices are either heterotrimers or homotrimers, depending on the collagen type. The heterotrimeric type I collagen molecule has two identical polypeptide chains called α$_1$ (I) and one slightly different chain called α$_2$ (I). The homotrimeric type II and type III collagen molecules are composed of three identical α$_1$ (II) chains and three identical α$_1$ (III) chains, respectively. Upon secretion from the originating cell, tropocollagen is processed into individual fibrils that, in turn, assemble into large, linear, insoluble fibers that are strengthened by lysine-mediated covalent cross-links between individual fibrils.

Collagen Genes

Collagen genes are named starting with the prefix COL, followed by an Arabic numeral indicating the collagen type, the letter "A," and finally a second Arabic number denoting

TABLE 7-1. Characteristics of the Major Collagens

Collagen Type	Chain	Gene	Location	Disorder
I	α$_1$(I)	COL1A1	17q21-22	Osteogenesis
	α$_2$(I)	COL1A2	7q21-22	Ehlers-Danlos syndrome
II	α$_1$(II)	COL2A1	12q13-q14	Chondrodysplasias
III	α$_1$(III)	COL3A1	2q31-q32	Ehlers-Danlos syndrome
IV	α$_3$(IV)	COL4A3	2q35-q36	Alport syndrome
	α$_4$(IV)	COL4A4	2q36-q37	
	α$_5$(IV)	COL4A5	Xq22.3	

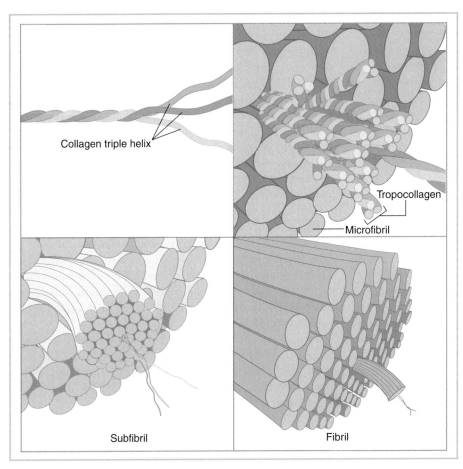

Figure 7-1. Structure of collagen. The triple helical structure of collagen—tropocollagen—is the basic unit of microfibrils. Many microfibrils bundled together form a macrofibril. (Redrawn with permission from Dr. J. P. Cartailler at Symmation LLC [www.symmation.com].)

Collagen triple helix

Tropocollagen

Microfibril

Subfibril

Fibril

the particular α-chain. Four distinct genetic loci (*COL1A1, COL1A2, COL2A1,* and *COL3A1*) collectively encode the unique chains of the three classic fibrillar collagens—types I, II, and III—and these genes are dispersed throughout the genome. *COL1A1* is found on chromosome 17, *COL1A2* on chromosome 7, *COL2A1* on chromosome 12, and *COL3A1* on chromosome 2. Type IV collagen is a nonfibrillar, or amorphous, form coded for by the *COL4A3* gene on chromosome 2. Overall, there are more than 34 different collagen genes dispersed on at least 15 chromosomes.

Collagen genes have several interesting features. Genes encoding fibrillar collagen are quite similar in structure; the triple helical domain regions consist of greater than 40 exons all of which are multiples of nine nucleotides. Exons are typically 54 nucleotides in length, but multiples of 54 or combinations of 45 and 54 base exons are not uncommon. Consistent with the (Gly-X-Y)$_n$ primary amino acid sequence motif, each exon begins with a glycine codon. The gene *COL1A1* that encodes α$_1$ (I) will serve as an example. The gene is large, spanning 18 kb of genomic DNA and encoding 52 exons that are 45, 54, 99, 108, or 162 base pairs in length. Hydroxyproline occupies the Y position in about a third of the triplets and is often preceded by proline.

The model exon in all collagen loci is a 54-bp unit that codes for 18 amino acid residues, or six triplets of Gly-X-Y repeats. This has led to the hypothesis that the varied collagen genes, although now widely scattered in the human genome, were derived from a single ancestral gene more than 50 million years ago. It is surmised that the numerous genes evolved by successive duplications of a primitive procollagen gene consisting of 54 bp with six Gly-X-Y repeats that underwent subsequent chromosomal rearrangements and sequence divergence. These genes have remained highly conserved during evolution.

Disorders of Connective Tissues

The large number of collagen genes, the widespread distribution of collagen within the body, and the high degree

BIOCHEMISTRY

Glycine

Glycine is the smallest amino acid and is a nonessential amino acid. Its size is convenient for "small places" in proteins such as the turns of helices. These are evolutionarily very stable. Substituting the glycine with a larger amino acid can dramatically change the shape of the protein.

Glycine can also function as an inhibitory neurotransmitter and serve as a coagonist with glutamate to activate NMDA (*N*-methyl-D-aspartate) receptors.

of evolutionarily conserved primary amino acid sequence all strongly suggest that functional collagen is critical for health. Accordingly, it follows that defects in collagen synthesis, processing and maturation, and structure would result in tissue dysfunction and human disease. This is the case, as more than 1000 mutations have been described in the collagen genes. Here, we discuss three such diseases: osteogenesis imperfecta and Ehlers-Danlos syndrome as paradigms of collagen disorders and Marfan syndrome as an important noncollagen disorder.

Osteogenesis Imperfecta

Osteogenesis imperfecta (OI) represents a collection of type I collagen disorders due to mutations in the COL1A1 or COL1A2 genes that are generally characterized by weak bones, dentinogenesis imperfecta, short stature, and adult-onset hearing loss. Classically, four types of OI have been recognized (Table 7-2). However, with the availability of DNA-based diagnostics, there are now seven subtypes of OI that stand as distinct clinical entities. Considering all forms of OI, the overall prevalence is roughly 7 per 100,000, and the disease crosses all racial and ethnic boundaries. Types I to IV illustrate the more common forms of OI.

Type I OI is the most common form of OI. It is relatively mild and exhibits autosomal dominant inheritance with variable expressivity. Clinically, type I individuals exhibit skeletal osteopenia and fractures, dentinogenesis imperfecta (Fig. 7-2), joint hypermobility, and blue-colored sclerae. Stature is usually within the normal range, but conductive hearing loss that progresses to sensorineural loss occurs in roughly 50% of adult patients. Type I OI is most often associated with protein-shortening nonsense, frameshift, or splice site mutations in the COL1A1 gene leading to decreased α_1 chains. Because type I collagen is a heterotrimer consisting of two α_1 chains and one α_2 chain, triple helix formation is greatly reduced.

Mutations in either COL1A1 or COL1A2 can cause OI types II to IV. Each of these forms of OI is transmitted in an autosomal dominant fashion and most often results from missense mutations that alter the important glycine codon in the triple helical domain. Interestingly, the phenotypical consequence depends on the nature and position of the glycine amino acid substitution. For example, substitutions with large side-chain amino acids or in the C-terminal two thirds of the gene usually predict a severe clinical outcome. Some splice site mutations have also been found. There is a rare form of OI III that has autosomal recessive transmission. This form is associated with consanguinity and is the most common form of OI observed in Africa.

Types II and III are severe forms of OI. Type II is characterized by multiple fractures and perinatal lethality. The mean birth weight and length is below the 50th percentile. Twenty percent of these infants are stillborn and 90% die within 4 weeks after birth.

Type III features progressive skeletal abnormalities including frequent early-onset fractures and progressive kyphoscoliosis. Fractures are frequently present at birth. Generalized

TABLE 7-2. Summary of Osteogenesis Imperfecta (OI) Types

OI Type	Clinical Features	Inheritance	Biochemical Abnormality
I	Normal stature, little or no deformity, blue sclerae, hearing loss	AD	50% reduction in type I collagen synthesis
II	Lethal in perinatal period, very few survive to 1 year; minimal calvarial mineralization, beaded ribs, compressed femurs, long bone deformity, platyspondyly	AD	Structural alteration in type I collagen chains—overmodification
III	Progressively deforming bones, moderate deformity at birth, sclerae hue varies, dentinogenesis imperfecta, hearing loss, very short stature	AD/AR (rare) Structural alteration in type I collagen chains—overmodification	Increased collagen turnover
IV	Normal to gray sclerae, mild-to-moderate deformity, variable short stature, dentinogenesis imperfecta, some hearing loss	AD	Excessive posttranslational modification to one type I collagen chain
V	Similar to OI type IV plus calcification of interosseous membrane of forearm, anterior radial head dislocation, hyperplastic callus formation, normal sclerae	AD	None identified
VI	Similar to OI type IV with early-onset vertebral compression fractures, mineralization defect	Unknown	None identified
VII	Mild symptoms, short stature, shortened limbs, normal sclerae	AR	

Data from Sillence DO, Senn A, Danks DM. Genetic heterogeneity in osteogenesis imperfecta. *J Med Genet.*1979;16:101–116.
AD, autosomal dominant; AR, autosomal recessive.

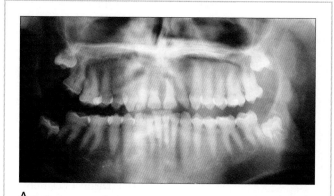

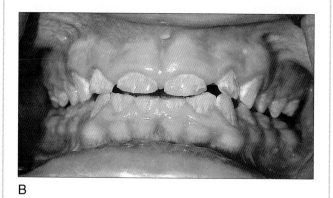

Figure 7-2. Dentinogenesis imperfecta is characterized by translucent gray to yellow-brown teeth and involves both deciduous (baby) and permanent teeth. The enamel fractures easily. This condition occurs in osteogenesis imperfecta, or it can be caused by a separate inherited autosomal dominant trait. **A**, Panoramic radiographic view of permanent dentition with bulb-shaped crowns and large pulpal chambers. **B**, Frontal view showing irregularly formed, opalescent teeth. (Courtesy of Rebecca Slayton, DDS, PhD, University of Washington School of Dentistry.)

NEUROSCIENCE

Hearing Loss

Hearing loss is classified as conductive, sensorineural, central hearing disorder, and presbycusis. Lesions involving the external or middle ear characterize conductive hearing loss. It is most commonly caused by cerumen impaction, although otitis media is the most common serious cause.

A lesion of the cochlea or auditory parts of cranial nerve VIII indicate sensorineural hearing loss, which includes hereditary deafness. Intrauterine factors causing sensorineural hearing loss include infection, metabolic and endocrine disorders, and anoxia. When hearing loss is unilateral, there is usually a cochlear basis, whereas bilateral loss is often due to drug use. Aminoglycoside antibiotics are toxic; salicylates, furosemide, and ethacrynic acid can cause transient loss.

Central hearing disorders occur with lesions of the central auditory pathways. The loss is unilateral if there is unilateral pontine cochlear nuclei damage in the brainstem owing to ischemic infarction of the lateral brainstem, multiple sclerosis plaque, neoplasia, or hematoma. Bilateral degeneration of nuclei is seen in rare childhood disorders.

Presbycusis is gradual age-related loss, which may be conductive or central.

ANATOMY

Dentinogenesis Imperfecta

Dentinogenesis imperfecta results from a failure of odontoblasts to differentiate normally. Odontoblasts produce dentin; ameloblasts produce enamel. Dentinogenesis imperfecta affects deciduous and permanent teeth, giving them a brown to grayish-blue appearance with an opalescent sheen. The enamel wears down quickly, exposing the dentin. It occurs because of autosomal recessive inheritance, drug toxicity (tetracycline), and syndromic association.

osteopenia leads to poor longitudinal growth that is well below the third percentile in height. Blue sclerae are another frequent clinical sign. Infants that survive the first months of life generally live reasonably long lives, and approximately one third survive long-term. In one example, a child was born with 132 fractures at birth and missing bones of the skull. This person attained a maximum height of 36 inches and weight of 50 pounds by adulthood. This young woman was above average in intelligence, completing college and mastering five languages before her death at age 32.

Type IV OI is the most clinically variable of the four paradigm types. Presentation may be severe to mild. Clinical signs may include somewhat reduced stature, dentinogenesis imperfecta, adult-onset hearing loss, and variable degrees of skeletal osteopenia.

A particularly interesting skeletal anomaly found in osteogenesis imperfecta is the presence of wormian bones. These are irregularly shaped bones within the sutures of the skull; they are found most often within the lambdoid suture and arranged in a mosaic pattern (Fig. 7-3). These intrasutural

bones have been associated with several congenital disorders but most commonly with OI. Other disorders associated with wormian bones include cleidocranial dysplasia, hypophosphatasia, hypothyroidism, and pycnodysostosis. They may also occur with no anomaly. In this last case, these extra bones tend to be smaller and fewer in number. Wormian bones tend to represent a pathologic condition when greater than 4 to 6 mm and when more than 10 are present. Interestingly, the name wormian has nothing to do with the appearance of the bone but honors Olaus Worm, the Danish anatomist who first described them in 1643.

It is important to emphasize that children with undiagnosed osteogenesis imperfecta or another type of bone disease may have the same symptoms as an abused child. Bruising, unexplained fractures, and evidence of old fractures in various stages of healing on radiography can lead a physician to consider abuse when a genetic defect has not been eliminated. A thorough family history may reveal other minor or variable phenotypes not previously recognized in family members.

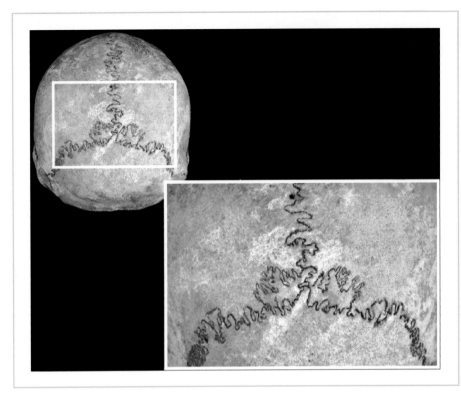

Figure 7-3. Wormian bones are intrasutural cranial bones. They are often associated with the lambdoid suture and are generally only considered pathologically significant when greater than 6 × 4 mm in size and 10 or more are arranged in a mosaic pattern. Pathologic associations of wormian bones include osteogenesis imperfecta, cleidocranial dysplasia, pycnodysostosis, hypophosphatasia, hypothyroidism, and acro-osteolysis. The majority of observations represent normal variants. (Courtesy of Owen Lovejoy, PhD, Kent State University, and Melanie McCollum, PhD, University of Virginia School of Medicine.)

A careful physical examination of the child may reveal additional features associated with OI such as blue sclerae, opalescent and undermineralized teeth, bruising, a triangular face, a barrel-shaped chest, and scoliosis.

Ehlers-Danlos Syndrome

Ehlers-Danlos syndrome (EDS) is a group of connective tissue disorders featuring joint hypermobility, hyperelasticity of the skin, and abnormal wound healing (Fig. 7-4). Historically, EDS was classified into two subtypes, EDS type I and type II, the discriminator being clinical severity. However, it is now recognized that EDS represents a continuum of clinical manifestations. Today, most of EDS types I and II have been reclassified as classical EDS on the basis of diagnostic criteria. Three of four major criteria must be met for diagnosis of EDS: skin

hyperextensibility; wide, atrophic scars; joint hypermobility; and a positive family history for EDS. There are six major types of EDS (Table 7-3). Newer terminology has replaced the use of Roman numerals to designate types.

Classic EDS is an autosomal dominant disease caused by mutations in genes encoding the α-chains of type V collagen. Specifically, approximately 50% of patients presenting with classical EDS have mutations in either *COL5A1* or *COL5A2*. The genetic defects responsible for the remaining half of the patients have not been identified. Of patients with *COL5A* mutations, one half have inherited the mutation from a parent and the other half harbor a new mutation that occurred in a parental gamete or during their own early embryonic development. Both protein-truncating mutations and glycine substitution mutations have been found in *COL5A*-associated EDS.

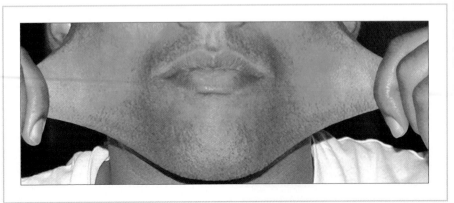

Figure 7-4. Ehlers-Danlos syndrome, characterized by hyperelastic skin and hypermobile joints, may also be characterized by easy bruising, poor healing, and "cigarette paper" scarring. (Courtesy of Joshua Lane, MD, Mercer University School of Medicine.)

TABLE 7-3. Summary of Ehlers-Danlos Syndrome Types

Type	Former Type	Clinical Features	Prevalence
Classical	I and II	Skin hyperextensibility, velvety skin Fragile skin—bruises and tears easily Poor wound healing leading to widened, atrophic scarring Molluscoid pseudotumors on elbows and knees; spheroid bodies on shins and forearms Hypermobile joints Mitral valve prolapse	1 in 20,000 to 40,000
Hypermobility	III	Hypermobile, unstable joints Chronic joint pain Mitral valve prolapse Fragile blood vessels and organs—at risk for rupture, aneurysm, dissection Thin, fragile skin—bruises easily	Most common form: 1 in 10,000 to 15,000
Vascular	IV	Veins visible beneath skin Characteristic facies—protruding eyes, thin nose and lips, malar flattening, hypoplastic mandible	One of the most serious forms: 1 in 100,000 to 200,000
Kyphoscoliosis	VI	Progressive scoliosis Fragile eyes Progressive muscle weakness	Rare
Arthrochalasis	VIIA VIIB	Hypermobile joints prone to dislocations, especially hips Skin hyperextensibility—prone to bruising Early-onset arthritis Increased risk of bone loss and fracture	Rare
Dermatosparaxis	VIIC	Extremely fragile, sagging skin Hypermobile joints—may delay development of motor skills	Rare

Marfan Syndrome

Marfan syndrome is a systemic connective tissue disorder that typically manifests as skeletal, ocular, and cardiovascular defects. Individuals are typically tall with arachnodactyly (Fig. 7-5). Ectopia lentis, mitral valve prolapse, and dilation of the ascending aorta are also common.

Unlike osteogenesis imperfecta and Ehlers-Danlos syndrome, Marfan syndrome is caused by mutations in the *FBN1* gene that encodes fibrillin, a glycoprotein that is the major structural component of extracellular microfibrils. Microfibrils are part of the ECM and form a network for elastin deposition in the formation of elastic fibers. Microfibrils are widely distributed in the body, but they are most abundant in ligaments, the aorta, and the ciliary zonules of the lens—all tissues prominently affected in Marfan syndrome.

Several skeletal phenotypes are associated with Marfan syndrome. These individuals are noted for tall stature, where the mean height is greater than the 97th percentile, along with a decrease in the upper body segment to lower body segment ratio, designated as US:LS. Normally, US:LS is 0.93, but in individuals with Marfan syndrome it is 0.85 or at least 2 standard deviations below the mean for age, sex, and race.

Often the arm span exceeds height, an advantageous characteristic for some sports such as basketball. However, it is not unusual for normal males and females to also meet this criterion, but the greater the arm span exceeds height the less likely that normal individuals will be identified. Arm span exceeds height by more than 8 cm in only 5% to 6% of normal individuals. Other skeletal features frequently found in individuals with Marfan syndrome are dolichocephaly (Fig. 7-6), prominent brow, hypognathic or retrognathic mandible, and high-arched and narrow palate. Vertebral and pectus deformities are present in 30% to 60% of individuals.

Although the skeletal features may be the most readily recognized phenotype of Marfan syndrome, the earliest

ANATOMY

Ciliary Body of the Eye

The ciliary body lies behind the iris and is attached to the lens by ciliary zonules. It produces aqueous humor and controls accommodation—the changing of lens shape.

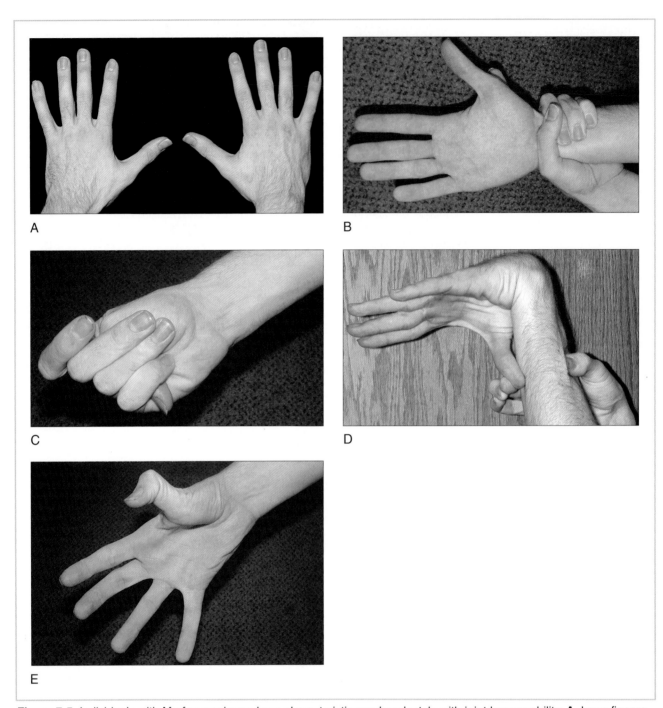

Figure 7-5. Individuals with Marfan syndrome have characteristic arachnodactyly with joint hypermobility. **A**, Long fingers. **B**, Positive wrist sign (Walker sign). **C**, Positive thumb sign (Steinberg sign). **D** and **E**, Hypermobile joints.

manifestation may be mitral valve disease. Eighty percent of individuals will show evidence of prolapse; in more than 25% of these individuals, prolapse will progress to regurgitation by adulthood. Aortic regurgitation is also common and progressive in 70% of individuals. Because of the altered fibrillin within the aorta, dilatation of the aortic root, where maximum stress occurs, is a serious concern (Fig. 7-7). Dilatation is seen in approximately 25% of children and 70% to 80% of adults. These individuals carry a significant risk of aortic dissection that may begin as a gradual dilatation at the aortic root that

progresses into the ascending aorta. Marfan syndrome does not preclude childbirth by females, but these women must be monitored regularly by echocardiography.

Marfan syndrome is an autosomal dominant disease; approximately 75% of the cases are inherited and 25% represent de novo mutations. Over 500 independent *FBN1* gene mutations have been associated with Marfan syndrome, nearly 70% of which are missense mutations. This suggests that the production of normal microfibrils is altered by the presence of mutant fibrillin. In the heterozygous state, this defines

Craniosynostosis

Craniosynostosis is the premature closure of sutures in the skull that leads to a change in the shape of the skull. Major sutures include coronal, sagittal, metopic, and lambdoid. There are several types of craniosynostosis:

- Brachycephaly: premature closure of coronal sutures
- Scaphocephaly, also called dolichocephaly: premature closure of the sagittal suture
- Trigonocephaly: premature fusion of the metopic suture
- Plagiocephaly: premature fusion of one of the coronal or lambdoid sutures
- Acrocephaly, oxycephaly, and turricephaly: premature closure of coronal and lambdoid sutures; creates pyramidal shape.

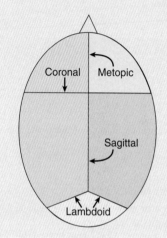

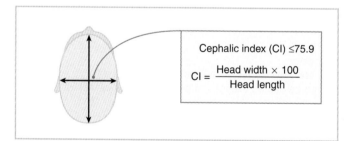

Cephalic index (CI) ≤ 75.9

$$CI = \frac{\text{Head width} \times 100}{\text{Head length}}$$

Figure 7-6. Dolichocephaly. The head is long and narrow. The cephalic index can be calculated to determine whether a shape is dolichocephalic or within normal limits.

autosomal dominant disorders—the interaction between mutant and normal fibrillin is sufficient for disease expression, suggestive of a dominant negative pathogenetic mechanism.

Allelic heterogeneity at the *FNB1* locus accounts for the overall symptom variability observed in individuals with Marfan syndrome and between different affected families. Some clinical variability can also be seen within a family sharing the same mutation, suggesting that other genetic or epigenetic factors play a role in disease expression.

Differential Considerations

Osteogenesis imperfecta, Ehlers-Danlos syndrome, and Marfan syndrome all share variably expressed phenotypic features. This is also true for other conditions discussed throughout this text as well as other conditions. Careful consideration of all physical and clinical findings is important in establishing a presumptive diagnosis. A definitive diagnosis is easily attainable with molecular analysis for each of these disorders with a specific known family mutation or in situations in which limited mutations are associated with a disorder, such as for achondroplasia (see next section). An equally definitive diagnosis is also possible with other tests such as muscle biopsy used for muscular dystrophies. Less secure diagnoses are described in Table 7-4.

●●● MUSCULOSKELETAL DISEASE DUE TO GROWTH FACTOR RECEPTOR DEFECT

Achondroplasia

Achondroplasia, also known as short limb dwarfism, is the *most common form of dwarfism* and occurs in roughly 1 in 20,000 live births. In short-limbed dwarfism, affected individuals have short stature and particularly short arms and legs; the average height of adult men is 132 cm and of adult women is 125 cm. Although all bones formed from cartilage are involved in achondroplasia, the proliferation of cartilage is greatly retarded in the metaphyses of long bones. In essence, the maturation of the chondrocytes in the growth plate of the cartilage is affected. Other skeletal abnormalities include macrocephaly with frontal bossing, mid-face hypoplasia, and genu varum (Fig. 7-8). The spine and ribs are also affected, as is the cartilaginous base of the skull. Life span and intelligence are typically normal, although 5% to 7% of infants with achondroplasia die within the first year of life from central or obstructive apnea due to brainstem compression or mid-face hypoplasia.

Achondroplasia results from mutations in the fibroblast growth factor receptor 3 (*FGFR3*) gene. Four *FGFR* genes

Appendicular Skeleton

The appendicular skeleton consists of the pectoral and pelvic girdles with the limbs. Ossification of long bones begins by the eighth week of development although all primary centers and most secondary centers of ossification are present at birth. For the diaphysis of long bones, bone is ossified from a primary center, whereas for the epiphysis, ossification occurs from a secondary center. The epiphyseal plate consists of cartilage formed between diaphysis and epiphysis, and it is eventually replaced by bone when bone growth ceases. Flat and irregular bones have no diaphysis or epiphysis.

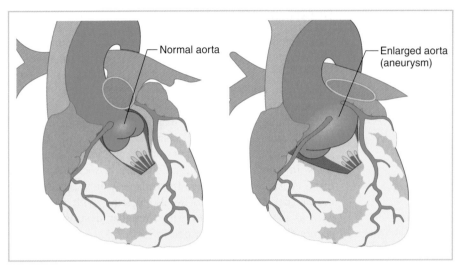

Figure 7-7. Aortic aneurysm. The aortic root is the site of greatest pressure. Mutations in fibrillin weaken the connective tissue of the aorta, causing bulging, tearing, and dissection.

Normal aorta

Enlarged aorta (aneurysm)

TABLE 7-4. Security of Diagnosis

Security	Level of Security	Explanation
Definite	100%	The diagnosis is absolutely not in question Full genetic counseling is appropriate relative to prognosis, treatment, and recurrence risk
Probable	80% to 99%	Absolute diagnosis is not able to be made A remote possibility of other diagnoses exists Reevaluation of diagnosis should occur with each follow-up visit. Full genetic counseling is given just as for "definite diagnosis"
Possible	50% to 79%	Diagnosis is considered likely, but the presence or absence of some historical, clinical, or laboratory findings leave some question about the diagnosis No specific genetic counseling can be offered, but the family should be informed of the diagnostic possibilities and of any opportunities for helping arrive at a diagnosis
Rule out	1% to 49%	The diagnosis being considered is among a list of possibilities, none being particularly likely Specific genetic counseling cannot be given Follow-up is very important to monitor growth and development and to check for new findings that may make the diagnosis more likely
Unknown	0%	There is no real clue to the diagnosis Continued follow-up is essential, and new diagnostic tests should be pursued No specific genetic counseling can be offered except that a 4% to 6% empiric risk of recurrence can be given

have been identified that interact with at least 23 different fibroblast growth factors; the receptors are all transmembrane tyrosine kinases involved in binding fibroblast growth factor and subsequent cell signaling. The FGFRs share a common protein structure, characterized by three extracellular immunoglobulin-like domains, an acidic box, a lipophilic transmembrane domain, and intracellular tyrosine kinase domains (Fig. 7-9). FGFR3 is expressed at high levels in the prebone cartilage rudiments of all bones and in the central nervous system. Defective FGFR proteins lead to altered interaction with fibroblast growth factor, which affects signal transduction. The most common mutations, G1138A and G1138C (discussed below), introduce a charged amino acid into the hydrophobic domain of the receptor and activate dimerization. This region of the receptor regulates the kinase

activity. The mutations, therefore, cause constitutive activation in a ligand-independent manner. Since FGFRs are widely expressed in bone, consequences of mutations are more profound in bone development.

Achondroplasia-associated *FGFR3* mutations exhibit autosomal dominant transmission with complete penetrance. Over 200 independent *FGFR3* mutations have been identified. Remarkably, 99% of individuals with achondroplasia have one of two missense mutations in the gene. Approximately 98% of individuals harbor a G-to-A mutation at nucleotide 1138 (G1138A) of the *FGFR3* gene that causes the replacement of a glycine with an arginine at amino acid residue 380. One percent of patients have a G1138C mutation that substitutes a cysteine for glycine at the same nucleotide. Hence, nearly all achondroplasia worldwide is due to the alteration

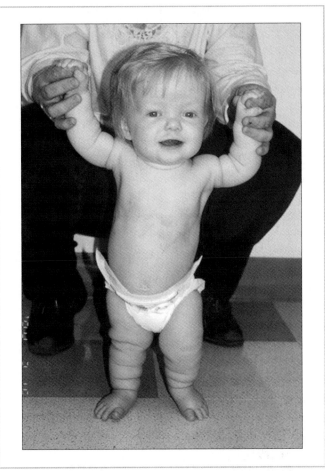

Figure 7-8. Achondroplasia. Note the short limbs relative to the length of the trunk. Also note the prominent forehead, low nasal root, and redundant skin folds in the arms and legs. (From Jorde LB, Carey JC, Bamshad MJ, White RL. *Medical Genetics,* 3rd ed. Philadelphia, Elsevier, 2006, p 67.)

BIOCHEMISTRY

Receptors

Transmembrane receptors have three parts: intracellular domain, transmembrane domain, and extracellular domain. Extracellular domain recognizes and responds to specific ligands such as hormones, neurotransmitters, and antigens. The transmembrane domain may form a channel or pore when the extracellular domain is activated. The intracellular domain interacts with the inside of the cell to relay a signal through effector proteins or enzymatic activity.

Receptor tyrosine kinases are single membrane-spanning receptors that can autophosphorylate as well as phosphorylate other proteins, such as EGF, PDGF, insulin, insulin-related growth factor type 1 (IGF1), FGF, and NGF. Binding of a ligand causes a conformational change that facilitates dimerization of two cytoplasmic domains and phosphorylation of tyrosines to activate the complex. The active complex then signals effectors downstream. Therefore, the phosphorylation of the intracellular domain is a regulatory mechanism for effector function.

of a single amino acid (glycine 380) in *FGFR3*, thus demonstrating once again the importance of glycine in protein function. A very rare mutation that substitutes lysine for methionine at position 650 results in severe achondroplasia with developmental delay and acanthosis nigricans (SADDAN).

Achondroplasia is a *congenital defect*, a defect present at birth. A significant number of achondroplastic infants are stillborn or die in infancy; those surviving to adulthood produce fewer offspring than normal. The mortality and low fecundity generate a strong force of selection against affected individuals. About 80% of the children born with this condition do not produce offspring. If this selective force were the only one operating, the frequency of the disorder would steadily decrease from one generation to the next. But this force is opposed by mutation. Greater than 80% of individuals with achondroplasia have normal parents, and thus de novo mutation occurs within a parental germ cell or very early in embryologic development. The former is strongly suspected, since *FGFR3* de novo mutations have been associated with advanced *paternal* age. The magnitude of recurrent mutations at *FGFR3* nucleotide 1138 represents one of the highest new mutation frequencies observed for autosomal dominant diseases. Obviously, the remaining 20% of patients have at least one parent with achondroplasia. Couples in whom both individuals are heterozygous for achondroplasia are not uncommon, and their offspring have a 25% risk of being homozygous for the achondroplasia mutation. The homozygous state of achondroplasia is not compatible with survival, and affected infants inevitably die of respiratory failure in the first or second year of life.

Prenatal diagnosis of homozygous achondroplasia can be accomplished by ultrasonography in the mid to late second trimester. However, women who are heterozygous for achondroplasia face maternal obstetric risks, several of which increase during gestation and may complicate a late pregnancy termination. Moreover, prenatal diagnosis in the second trimester creates anxiety for the couple and increases the emotional burden of terminating a homozygous fetus at a relatively late stage. Identification of the key mutations in the *FGFR3* gene enables first-trimester DNA-based prenatal diagnosis. In the simplest case, a disease mutation either creates or destroys a restriction endonuclease site. Thus, PCR-amplification of the relevant portion of the *FGFR3* gene, followed by mutation-specific restriction endonuclease digestion and gel electrophoresis, enables the visualization of the heterozygous

PATHOLOGY

Acanthosis Nigricans

Acanthosis nigrans are dark, thick, velvety skin in body folds and creases that are most commonly seen in individuals of African descent. They can occur with some drugs—particularly growth hormone and oral contraceptives—and with obesity and diabetes, GI or genitourinary cancers, lymphoma, and certain genetic conditions.

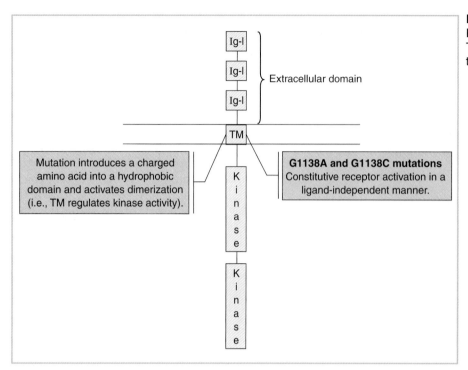

Figure 7-9. Typical FGFR structure. Ig, immunoglobulin domain; TM, transmembrane domain; kinase, tyrosine kinase domain.

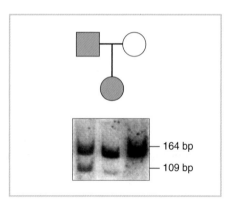

Figure 7-10. Prenatal analysis of *FGFR* mutation. Paternal DNA demonstrates the *Sfc*I restriction fragments created with the G1138A mutation. Maternal DNA does not have the mutation. Fetal DNA isolated from maternal serum has the G1138A mutation. The normal amplified fragment is 164 bp. Following digestion, one allele produces a 109-bp allele and a 55-bp allele that is not shown on the gel. Solid-colored symbols indicate affected individuals. (Gel from Li Y, Holzgreve W, Page-Christiaens GC, Gille JJ, Hahn S. Improved prenatal detection of a fetal point mutation for achondroplasia by the use of size-fractionated circulatory DNA in maternal plasma—case report. *Prenat Diagn.* 2004;24: 896–898. Copyright, John Wiley and Sons Ltd. Reproduced with permission.)

and homozygous states. Accordingly, both the G1138A transition and the G1138C transversion create new recognition sites for restriction enzymes, rendering it straightforward to test for the presence or absence of the mutation in genomic DNA. For example, the G-to-A transition produces a new restriction site for the enzyme *Sfc*I, which recognizes the sequence CTACAG (Fig. 7-10) (see Chapter 13). As a result,

prenatal diagnosis of heterozygous achondroplasia, homozygous achondroplasia, and the homozygous unaffected state is rapid, accurate, and unequivocal.

● ● ● MUSCLE CELL DISEASES

Muscular Dystrophies

The muscular dystrophies are a large and heterogeneous group of disorders distinguished by the progressive loss of muscular strength and morphologic integrity. Individual muscle fibers show variation in size, metabolic oxidative stress, sarcolemmal fragility, and ultimately, fiber loss due to necrosis and replacement by fat or connective tissue. As a group, the muscular dystrophies are represented by greater than 30 independent disorders with etiologic links to nearly 30 different genetic loci. Here, we focus on the most common and severe form of muscular dystrophy, Duchenne muscular dystrophy (DMD) and its associated milder form, Becker muscular dystrophy (BMD), as illustrative muscle diseases.

DMD is an X-linked disease of childhood. The incidence is approximately 1 in 3600 live male births. Unfortunately, for those males who inherit or harbor the DMD mutation, penetrance is essentially complete and their muscles rapidly deteriorate during early childhood. The earliest symptom is usually clumsiness in walking with a tendency to fall. At about age 3, the child experiences difficulty in climbing stairs and rising from the floor (Fig. 7-11). One of the most obvious physical features in the early stages of the disease is pseudohypertrophy of the calf muscles due to the replacement of muscle with adipose and fibrous connective tissue.

As the profound wasting of muscles progresses, the majority of affected individuals are unable to walk by

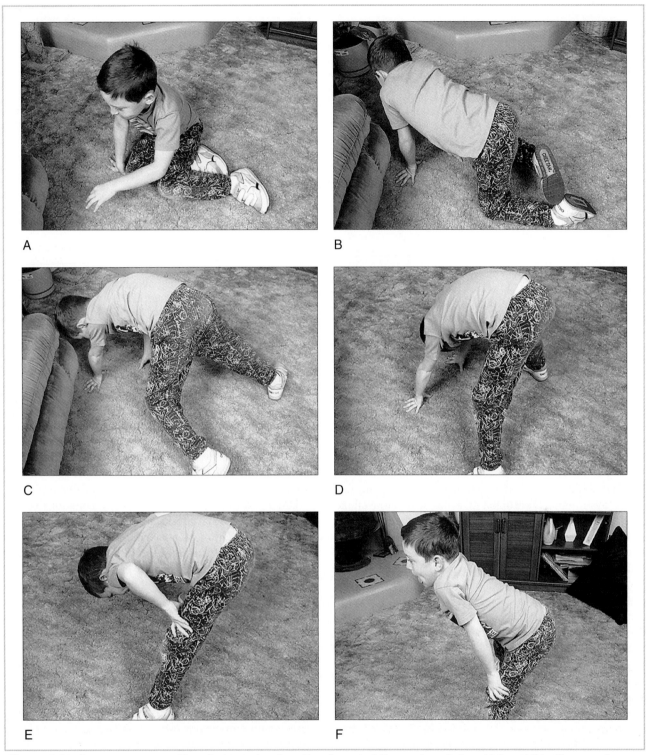

Figure 7-11. Gowers maneuver. The photographs show the characteristic movements by which a child with muscular dystrophy uses his hands to walk up his legs to a standing position. (Used with permission from the MDA Foundation.)

12 years of age (Fig. 7-12). As the disease progresses, loss of strength in shoulders and proximal arms is often noted and cognitive abilities decline. Respiratory muscles weaken, and cardiomyopathy is essentially ubiquitous in patients over 18 years. Most patients die before the age of 20 years of chronic respiratory insufficiency or pneumonia and, occasionally, of heart failure.

BMD is a milder variant of DMD and is distinguished from DMD by the later onset of skeletal muscle weakness and the ability to walk into the third decade of life. The disease

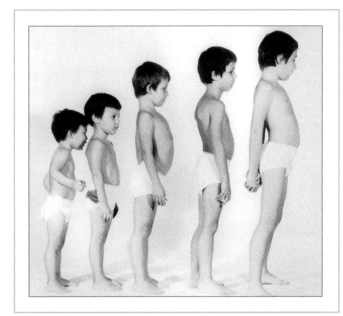

Figure 7-12. As muscle wasting progresses, postural changes occur in Duchenne muscular dystrophy (DMD). (Used with permission from the MDA Foundation.)

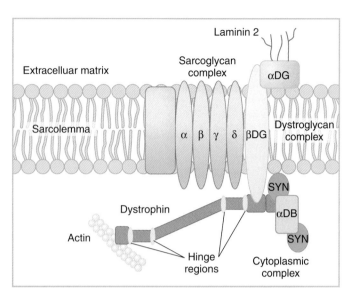

Figure 7-13. Skeletal muscle membrane organization. DB, dystrobrevin; DG, dystroglycan, SYN, syntrophin. (Used with permission and adapted from Blake DJ, Weir A, Newey SE, Davies KE. Function and genetics of dystrophin and dystrophin-related proteins in muscle. *Physiol Rev.* 2002; 82:291–329.)

usually progresses to death due to cardiomyopathy-related heart failure in mid to late adulthood.

Molecular Basis and Genetics of Duchenne and Becker Types of Muscular Dystrophy

DMD and BMD are caused by mutations in the gene that encodes dystrophin. Dystrophin is a 427-kDa intracellular protein, found predominantly in skeletal, smooth, and cardiac muscle. Low levels are also found in the central nervous system. Dystrophin has been localized to the sarcolemmal membrane, where it functions in a mechanical fashion by linking the ECM with actin components of the cytoskeleton, thereby helping to resist stresses associated with muscle contraction.

The N-terminal region of the dystrophin molecule (Fig. 7-13) is an actin-binding domain, homologous to the actin-binding portion of spectrin in the cytoskeleton of the red blood cell (see Chapter 6). This is followed by a rod-like domain consisting of 24 repeats of similar sequences of nearly 109 amino acids. The rod-like domain terminates at a cysteine-rich region of about 150 amino acids. The C terminus comprises a 420-amino acid region that is interactive with other membrane proteins.

There is tissue-specific expression of the 427-kDa protein that is controlled by different promoters. Brain dystrophin is expressed in the cortex and hippocampus; muscle dystrophin is expressed in skeletal muscle, cardiomyocytes, and some glial cells; and Purkinje dystrophin is expressed in cerebellar Purkinje cells and skeletal muscle. These three dystrophins have a unique first exon followed by 78 common exons. Four internal promoters give rise to shorter forms of dystrophin isoforms. Figure 7-14 shows the seven different promoters

within the dystrophin gene. In addition to the three 427-kDa proteins already mentioned, four other dystrophins are present in the retina (260 kDa); the brain and fetal kidney (140 kDa); Schwann cells and nodes of Ranvier (116 kDa); and the glia, kidney, liver, and lung (71 kDa). These findings are correlated with abnormal electroretinograms and electroencephalograms in individuals with abnormal dystrophins.

DMD and BMD are caused by many mutations within the dystrophin gene that are located in the middle of the short arm of the X chromosome (Xp21). It is the largest known human gene, spanning about 2000 kb and containing more than 70 exons. The gene is approximately 0.001% of the total human genome, representing about one third the amount of the entire *Escherichia coli* genome. Although the gene is 2 million base pairs in size, the mature dystrophin mRNA is 14 kb, which encodes a very large polypeptide of 3685 amino acids in muscle.

DMD is *allelic* with BMD in that both are caused by different mutations within the same gene locus. BMD affects about 1 in 30,000 male newborns. Both diseases usually result from deletions—65% of DMD cases and 85% of BMD cases—with duplications (6% of DMD cases) and point, small insertion, or deletion mutations (30% of DMD cases) accounting for the remainder of cases. The deletions are widely scattered over the length of the gene with two areas representing clusters of deletions (see Fig. 7-14). No clustering of deletions differentiates DMD from BMD. The deletions are not uniform in size, ranging from 6 to greater than 1000 kb. There is no apparent correlation between the size and location of the deletion and the severity and progression of the disorder. Large deletions have been found in some patients with the milder BMD, whereas some of the patients with severe DMD have small deletions.

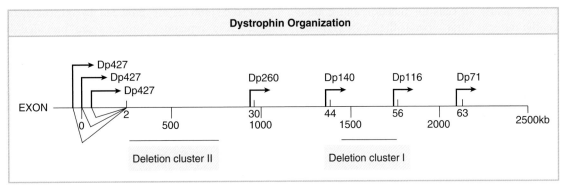

Figure 7-14. Exon of the dystrophin gene showing the seven different promoter sites for each of the isoforms: three full-length and four shortened forms. The 427-kDa forms differ only at the NH$_2$-terminal sequences. Two "hot spots" for deletions are shown: cluster I between exons 45 and 53 affects the rod domain of the protein, and cluster II between exons 2 and 20 affects the actin-binding domain. Dp, dystrophin protein. (Used with permission and adapted from Blake DJ, Weir A, Newey SE, Davies KE. Function and genetics of dystrophin and dystrophin-related proteins in muscle. *Physiol Rev.* 2002; 82:291–329.)

The enigma regarding deletion size and disease severity is resolved by the understanding of *reading frames.* The DNA deletions resulting in the clinically less severe BMD bring together exons that maintain the translational reading frame ("in-frame" deletions) of the messenger RNA. If two "compatible" exons (multiples of three bases) are juxtaposed in the sliced message, then the reading frame is preserved, and a functional, although shorter than normal, transcript is produced. Conversely, deletions associated with the more severe DMD bring together exons that disrupt the translational reading frame and inevitably lead to a stop codon. The outcome is the production of a severely truncated and nonfunctional protein. Likewise, duplications and point mutations associated with DMD typically render little or no dystrophin.

The integrity of the dystrophin protein is the key to distinguishing between the two diseases. Most DMD patients have between 0 and 5% detectable dystrophin while most BMD patients have between 20% and 80% of functional dystrophin. Based on dystrophin quantification, an intermediate or "outlier" form (IMD) can be recognized with a cognate intermediate phenotype. Thus, the presence or absence of dystrophin is of diagnostic and prognostic significance.

In its typical form, DMD is expressed in affected males with complete penetrance. Hence, affected males experience reduced reproductive fitness, since they cannot transmit the deleterious gene. Roughly one-third of the mutant alleles are "lost" each generation. Because the incidence of DMD is maintained at 1 in 3600 live male births, de novo mutations must occur in a significant number of cases either in parental gametes or very early in zygotic cleavage just as seen with achondroplasia. Indeed, the extremely large size of the dystrophin gene makes it an excellent target for mutation, and the DMD locus accordingly has a high new mutation frequency. As a result, the affected male is often the solitary member of the family to be afflicted.

Although heterozygous females generally are normal, about 8% have muscle weakness, fatigability, and mild respiratory and cardiac problems. The overt muscle weakness in female carriers is explicable by the chance predominance of mutant-expressing X chromosomes during lyonization. Indeed, monozygotic females have been identified with one normal twin and one DMD-affected twin resulting from skewed X chromosome inactivation.

Mitochondrial Myopathies

Mitochondrial myopathy (MM) is a muscle disease caused by mitochondrial dysfunction. Mitochondria provide several functions to the cell, but the primary function is producing cellular energy in the form of adenosine triphosphate (ATP). This is accomplished by the electron transport chain (ETC) and oxidative phosphorylation (OXPHOS). The ETC comprises four enzyme complexes (complexes I to IV) that systematically oxidize NADH and FADH$_2$ molecules and ultimately reduce molecular O$_2$ to form water. Concurrent with the flow of electrons down the ETC is the pumping of protons from the inner membrane space to the matrix, forming an electrochemical gradient across the mitochondrial inner membrane. This gradient, known as a membrane potential, is utilized by ATP synthase (complex V) to condense inorganic phosphate with ADP to form ATP, which

PATHOLOGY

Creatine Phosphokinase

Creatine phosphokinase (CK) is an important indicator of muscle damage. Both the muscle and the brain have high ATP demands, and CK functions to regenerate ATP rapidly. Muscle breakdown causes elevated serum CK (>10 times normal in DMD; >5 times normal in BMD) even before clinical symptoms appear. CK is also elevated in many muscle diseases and is a dimer of muscle-specific (M) or brain-specific (B) monomers.

- Muscle: MM form
- Brain: BB form
- Heart: MB form

is then utilized by nearly all cells for function and maintenance. Hence, the mitochondria serve as the "powerhouses" of the cell and are essential for aerobic respiration. However, mitochondria are also central players for two other relevant cellular metabolic processes: oxidative stress and programmed cell death, or apoptosis. In fact, mitochondrial myopathy, and mitochondrial diseases in general, can be envisioned as resulting from the interplay between bioenergetic deficiency, increased cellular oxidative stress, and the provocation of apoptosis.

Complexes I to V (Fig. 7-15) are generated from two different genetic systems. Eighty percent of the ETC and OXPHOS proteins are provided by nuclear-encoded (nDNA) genes. The remaining proteins are provided by the only extranuclear DNA found in cells, the mitochondrial DNA (mtDNA). mtDNA is a closed, circular molecule 16,569 bases in length that encodes 37 different gene products including 13 mRNAs that contribute polypeptides to complexes I to V (see Fig. 7-15). Specifically, the mtDNA provides seven subunits to complex I, one subunit to complex III, three subunits to complex IV, and two subunits to complex V. The remaining mtDNA genes code for 22 tRNAs and 2 rRNAs. Transcription and translation of mtDNA gene products take place within the mitochondrial matrix. Thus, the mtDNA-

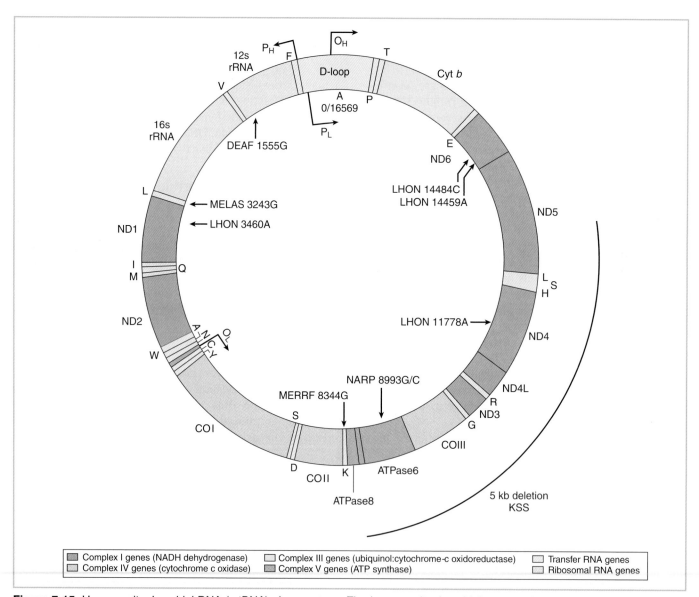

Figure 7-15. Human mitochondrial DNA (mtDNA) chromosome. The human mitochondrial genome is 16,569 bp in length and encodes 37 gene products, including 13 mRNAs, 22 tRNAs, and 2 rRNAs. The chromosome is present in multiple copies per cell. DNA replication is initiated at the origins of DNA replication (O_H and O_L), and polycistronic RNAs are produced by the two major promoters (P_H and P_L). The large RNAs are then processed to yield the mRNAs, tRNAs, and rRNAs. tRNA genes are identified by a single letter code that refers to the cognate amino acid in the charged tRNA. ND, NADH dehydrogenase genes; CO, cytochrome oxidase genes; Cyt b, cytochrome b gene; D-loop, noncoding displacement loop. (From MITOMAP: A human mitochondrial genome database. Available at: http://www.mitomap.org.)

encoded polypeptides are essential for aerobic respiration and, therefore, life. Because most of the well-characterized inherited mitochondrial diseases are due to mtDNA mutations, these will be discussed further. However, it should be noted that because most mitochondrial proteins are provided by the nucleus, the number of nDNA-based mitochondrial diseases will grow rapidly in the foreseeable future, thanks in large part to the recent elucidation of the complete *Homo sapiens* genome sequence.

mtDNA has a number of features distinguishing "mitochondrial genetics" from the better known nuclear genetic principles. First, mitochondria are present in multiple copies per organelle, and thus a cell harbors thousands of mtDNAs. Second, mitochondria are strictly maternally inherited in mammals. Defects in mtDNA that result in human disease show maternal (and no paternal) transmission. Third, the mtDNA has an extremely high mutation rate; perhaps in part due to lack of an efficient DNA repair mechanism. Fourth, when a new mutation occurs within a mitochondrion of a cell, a mixture of mutant and normal mtDNA is produced. This mixture is called *heteroplasmy* and, unlike the homozygous/heterozygous situation found for nDNA mutations, a heteroplasmic proportion can be anywhere from 0 to 100%. When heteroplasmic mitochondria divide, heteroplasmy can be propagated to an entire tissue, organ system, or organism, depending on when and where a mutation originated. Fifth, different organ systems and tissues rely on OXPHOS for energy to varying extents and thus display varying "threshold expression" of mitochondrial products. For example, the central nervous system and skeletal/cardiac muscle depend most strongly on mitochondrial ATP production. Thus, deleterious mtDNA mutations tend to feature neurologic and neuromuscular clinical signs, since these tissues are the least tolerant of perturbations in mitochondrial function.

As noted, mtDNA-encoded genes are essential for cellular energy in multiple cell types and these genes suffer a very high mutation rate. Therefore, it is reasonable that a number of mutations in mtDNA will be deleterious and result in mitochondrial dysfunction and human disease. In practice—again owing to the ubiquity of the mitochondrion—mitochondrial diseases that originate from both the mtDNA and the nDNA include a large spectrum of disorders ranging from lethal, perinatal disease to late-onset, progressive, aging-related disorders. Typically, mitochondrial diseases progress and involve more than one organ system. Exceptions to this generality demonstrate the tremendous clinical variability found in bioenergetic disease. For example, Leber hereditary optic neuropathy (LHON), a late-adolescence blindness, does not progress after rapid-onset degeneration of only the retinal ganglion cell and its axon, the optic nerve. Below, mtDNA-based mitochondrial myopathy is presented as the paradigm for mitochondrial muscle disease.

Mitochondrial myopathy is characterized by the degeneration of individual muscle fibers associated with an accumulation of abnormal mitochondria in the subsarcolemma of the fiber. The proliferation of abnormal mitochondria represents a compensatory response by the cell to bioenergetic deficiency and is perhaps the most reliable pathologic sign of a mitochondrial myopathy. Histochemical studies consistently demonstrate that such aggregates of abnormal mitochondria form red subsarcolemmal blotches, providing the pathognomonic name ragged red fibers (RRFs) (Fig. 7-16). Likewise, staining for mitochondrial electron transport chain enzymes (typically complex IV or cytochrome *c* oxidase [COX]) suggests COX-deficient fibers. Electron microscopic examination of RRF mitochondria reveal disordered cristae and often have paracrystalline inclusions ("parking lot" inclusion bodies), consisting of precipitated mitochondrial creatine phosphokinase. Thus, from a histochemical and ultrastructural point of view, mitochondrial myopathy is characterized by RRFs, an absence or diminution of mitochondrial respiratory chain enzyme signals, and morphologically abnormal mitochondria.

Clinically, mitochondrial myopathies encompass a fairly wide range of symptoms of varying severity. Most often, however, these are characterized by onset prior to age 20, muscle weakness, and exercise intolerance with lactic acidosis. Although mitochondrial myopathy can stand alone as the sole clinical presentation of mitochondrial disease, it frequently is part of a more complex clinical picture. Hence, vomiting, seizures, dementia, movement disorder, stroke-like episodes, ptosis, ophthalmoplegia, blindness, and cardiomyopathy/cardiac conduction abnormalities often occur in patients. Neurologic signs are common in mitochondrial myopathy, and when present, this group of disorders can be termed mitochondrial encephalomyopathies. Classic examples of mitochondrial myopathy include Kearns-Sayre syndrome (KSS); chronic progressive external ophthalmoplegia (CPEO); myoclonic epilepsy with ragged red fiber syndrome (MERRF); and mitochondrial encephalomyopathy, lactic acidosis and stroke-like symptoms (MELAS).

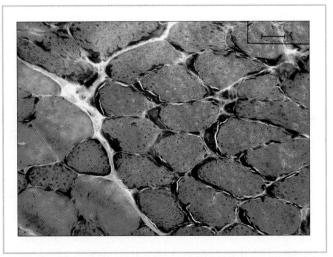

Figure 7-16. Ragged red fibers in skeletal muscle section. Muscle cells in mitochondrial myopathy contain a mitochondrial defect and exhibit a classical subsarcolemmal accumulation of abnormal mitochondria, which stain red with Gomori's trichrome stain.

Most cases of mitochondrial myopathy arise from either point mutations in mtDNA tRNA mutations (MERRF, MELAS) or deletions or rearrangements (KSS, CPEO). MERRF and KSS illustrate the general principles behind mitochondrial myopathy.

Myoclonic Epilepsy with Ragged Red Fiber Syndrome

MERFF typically presents with mitochondrial myopathy and myoclonic epilepsy—a periodic, uncontrolled jerking that often begins focally but progresses to generalized cyclic muscular contractions. Roughly 85% of the cases are due to an A to G mutation in the mtDNA tRNA^{Lys} gene at nucleotide position 8344, and many of the remaining cases result from a G to C mutation at position 8356 in the same tRNA gene (Fig. 7-17). Both of these mutations disrupt the TψC loop of tRNA^{Lys}. These mutations have consistently been found to be heteroplasmic in patients and have never been found in normal mtDNA.

As indicated above, clinical variability and age-related progression of symptoms are common in the mitochondrial disorders. Upon diagnosis of MERRF, examination of the clinical status of maternally related individuals within the proband's family often reveals affected individuals exhibiting a spectrum of clinical signs including mitochondrial myopathy, ataxia, cardiomyopathy, sensorineural hearing loss, diabetes, or dementia. The wide range of clinical signs and the variable expression found within families is in part due to the varying heteroplasmic proportioning found in affected individuals. MERRF pedigrees show a strong association between phenotype and genotype (heteroplasmic proportion) in relation to aging. For example, a young (15- to 25-year-old) patient with 95% mutant tRNA^{Lys} often will have a complex and severe clinical picture including mitochondrial myopathy, reduced muscle oxidative capacity, and diminished mitochondrial respiratory chain enzyme activities. In contrast, similarly aged individuals harboring 85% mutant tRNA^{Lys} can appear healthy and unaffected, exhibiting normal muscle bioenergetic capacity, OXPHOS enzyme activity, and phenotype. Interestingly, maternally related individuals aged 60 years and

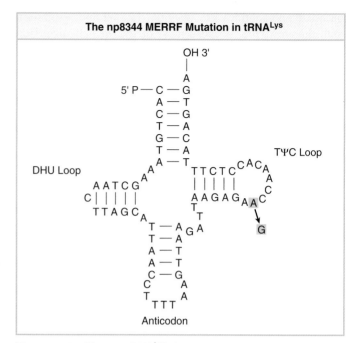

The np8344 MERRF Mutation in tRNA^{Lys}

Figure 7-17. Human tRNA^{Lys} showing the MERFF-associated A to G transition at mtDNA nucleotide position 8344.

greater, with the same 85% mutant tRNA^{Lys}, can be severely affected with mitochondrial myopathy, little muscle energy capacity, and dramatically reduced respiratory chain enzyme activities. Hence, for mitochondrial diseases due to tRNA mutations, age of onset often reflects the proportion of mutant mtDNA inherited and symptoms tend to progress with age in terms of the number and severity of clinical signs. This suggests that at least two factors—an inborn error mutation and an age-related factor—collaborate to precipitate many forms of mitochondrial disease.

Chronic Progressive External Ophthalmoplegia and Kearns-Sayre Syndrome

Frequently, a mild-to-moderate mitochondrial myopathy features ophthalmoplegia and ptosis in addition to frank mitochondrial myopathy. This combination of symptoms is termed chronic progressive external ophthalmoplegia (CPEO). Some patients manifest CPEO before age 20, with retinitis pigmentosa and at least one of the following: cardiac conduction abnormality, cerebellar ataxia, or cerebral spinal protein level above 100 mg/dL. These patients have the more severe Kearns-Sayre syndrome (KSS). Occasionally, other signs manifest with KSS or CPEO, including optic atrophy, sensorineural hearing loss, dementia, seizures, cardiomyopathy, diabetes, and lactic acidosis. Like the mtDNA tRNA mutations that result in MERRF and MELAS, KSS and CPEO patients typically feature RRFs and diminished histochemical staining of respiratory chain enzymes in skeletal muscle.

Nearly 85% of KSS patients harbor rearrangements of the mtDNA that take the form of a group of interrelated,

NEUROSCIENCE & ANATOMY

Ocular Mitochondrial Myopathies

Kearns-Sayre syndrome (KSS) and chronic progressive external ophthalmoplegia (CPEO) are known as ocular mitochondrial myopathies characterized by blepharoptosis and ophthalmoparesis. Extraocular muscles are affected preferentially because the fraction of mitochondrial volume is several times greater in these muscles than in other skeletal muscles. The levator palpebrae superioris (CN III), one of eight extraocular muscles, is weakened. As ptosis progresses, the individual may use the frontalis muscle to elevate the eyelids. Ophthalmoplegia occurs when a general weakness of extraocular muscles progresses to paralysis.

complex molecules including normal, duplicated, and deleted mtDNA. Occasionally, insertions are found. Such rearrangements are almost always heteroplasmic in patients, and the vast majority of patients are singleton cases representing a new mutational event that occurred either in the maternal oocyte or early in embryonic development.

In practice, deleted mtDNA is easiest to detect, characterize, and quantitate; hence, this form of mitochondrial myopathy has historically been erroneously associated strictly with deletions. Nevertheless, a consideration of mtDNA deletions associated with KSS and CPEO illustrates the magnitude and mechanism of the genomic rearrangements. Nearly all deletions, for example, are associated with direct repeats 4 to 16 nucleotides in length, suggesting that a specific DNA sequence motif is necessary for mtDNA rearrangement. Nearly 100 different rearrangement breakpoints and 200 different deletions have been characterized in KSS and CPEO patients, suggesting that this is a relatively common pathogenic mutational mechanism in mitochondrial diseases.

Currently there is no effective treatment for mitochondrial diseases. Administration of vitamins, O_2 radical scavengers, artificial electron acceptors (in an attempt to bypass a blockage in the electron transport chain), and the dimunition of harmful metabolites have been tried with anecdotal success. Frequently, a combination of the above is formulated as a "cocktail," indicating the dearth of knowledge regarding the underlying pathophysiologic basis of mitochondrial disorders.

Neurologic Diseases 8

●●● OVERVIEW

The advent of molecular techniques initiated a remarkable period of achievement in the understanding of inherited neurologic diseases. Linkage analysis, combined with molecular analysis, provided powerful tools for mapping genes for which no gene product was previously known. Investigators were then able to proceed with isolating, cloning, and sequencing mutant alleles. The determination of the normal and disease mutant allele products permitted an explanation for the molecular pathogenesis of disease. This isolation and characterization process of a gene before the gene product is known as *reverse genetics* and has been responsible for better understanding of many diseases.

The classification of genetic neurologic disorders is confusing because there are an immense number that may be classified in several different ways. For example, disorders classified by gene function may not represent the clinical manifestation of the disease. In some disorders, more than one gene may be involved, such as in neurofibromatosis—a disease that results from two different genes. In Duchenne and Becker muscular dystrophies, mutations in the same gene yield different clinical presentations.

The disorders discussed in this chapter represent two broad categories: single-gene disorders and complex disorders. Among the single-gene disorders, neurofibromatosis represents a disorder characterized by tumors, and Lesch-Nyhan syndrome is a metabolic disorder of purine and pyrimidine metabolism. Thus, the former could be discussed along with cancer disorders and the latter as an inborn error of metabolism. However, both have a significant neurologic impact. Lysosomal storage disorders are also single-gene disorders and underscore the importance of lysosomes and proper degradation of substrates. A discussion of two triplet repeat disorders—fragile X syndrome and Huntington disease—serves as a bridge between the easier to understand classical single-gene disorders and complex, multifactorial disorders. Triplet repeat amplification occurs at or near a specific gene and affects that specific gene. These amplifications are also inherited in the mendelian manner; however, expression of complex disorders is more intricate than noted in the earlier discussed examples. The amplifications in these disorders demonstrate effects in brain development and disease. The second group of disorders represents more complex diseases that have both a genetic and an environmental component affecting expression. The effects of Alzheimer disease, Parkinson disease, schizophrenia, and bipolar disorder on families and society are profound. Though pathphysiologies and molecular mechanisms are not fully understood for any of these, they are areas of major research and interest.

●●● SINGLE-GENE DISORDERS

Neurofibromatosis

Until the 1970s, different forms of neurofibromatosis were not distinguished. Today several forms are recognized with the most common being neurofibromatosis type 1 (NF1) and type 2 (NF2).

NF1 is the most common form of the disease. It was originally called von Recklinghausen disease or peripheral neurofibromatosis. NF1 is a common disease with an incidence of 1 in 4500 and complete penetrance by age 5. It is inherited in an autosomal dominant manner, and most patients have café-au-lait spots, peripheral neurofibromas, and Lisch nodules (Table 8-1). Two thirds of individuals also have freckling in the axilla, base of the neck, groin, and submammary regions.

Café-au-lait spots, also found in other disorders, may be present at birth but invariably develop before 2 years of age. These pigmented regions demonstrate variable expressivity in size, number, and coloration, and while six or more are required for diagnosis the absolute number is not linked to the severity of the disease (Fig. 8-1).

TABLE 8-1. Comparison of Neurofibromatosis 1 and Neurofibromatosis 2

	Neurofibromatosis 1	Neurofibromatosis 2
Gene symbol	NF1	NF2
Gene location	17q11.2	22q12.2
Protein	Neurofibromin-1	Merlin (neurofibromin-2)
Incidence	1 in 4500	1 in 40,000 to 50,000
Mode of Inheritance	AD with variable expression, complete penetrance	
Age of onset	Before age 5 years	Between ages 15 to 25 years
Major Clinical Features		
Café-au-lait spots	>99%	Generally fewer than NF1
Freckling	67%	Generally absent
Peripheral neurofibromas	>99%	Yes
Lisch nodules	90% to 95%	Absent
Plexiform neurofibroma	25% to 30%	Yes
Vestibular schwannomas		
Bilateral		85%
Unilateral		6%
Hearing loss (bilateral)		35%
Cranial or spinal tumors		
Meningiomas		45%
Spinal meningiomas		26%
Peripheral schwannomas		68%
Ocular abnormalities		90%
Minor Clinical Features		
Macrocephaly	45%	
Short stature (below third percentile)	31.5%	

Peripheral neurofibromas begin to appear during the teen years and are found in nearly all adults with NF1. These neurofibromas are discrete nodules within the dermis and epidermis, found mainly on the trunk of the body, and may range in size from less than a centimeter to several centimeters in diameter. Although cosmetically unappealing, they are rarely painful (Fig. 8-2). One of the most common causes of morbidity in individuals with NF1 is the development of plexiform neurofibromas along large nerves. These may invade adjacent structures and impinge on organs.

Lisch nodules are asymptomatic hamartomas of the iris associated with NF1 in 90% to 95% of individuals with NF1 (Fig. 8-3). These nodules generally develop before peripheral neurofibromas.

The gene responsible for NF1 is neurofibromin. It is a large gene, and more than 500 mutations have been described that disrupt normal neurofibromin expression, but most germline mutations produce a truncated protein. This protein has a domain homologous to the GTPase-activating family. The protein also has a GAP-related domain (GRD) that interacts with the RAS proto-oncogene. Mutations that truncate neurofibromin in the GRD region inactivate the tumor suppressor function of neurofibromin. The large size of the protein and the large number of mutations identified indicate that many mutations are family specific and that carrier screening can yield many false negatives in a large population.

Neurofibromatosis type 2 (NF2) was previously referred to as *bilateral acoustic* or *central neurofibromatosis*. It shares several phenotypic similarities with NF1 such as café-au-lait spots and peripheral nerve tumors, but it is a distinct disorder. Morbidity and mortality are predominantly due to *vestibular schwannomas* (Fig. 8-4) and other cranial or spinal tumors (see Table 8-1). Because many schwannomas may be asymptomatic and symptoms leading to diagnosis such as tinnitus or vertigo may begin as vague complaints, diagnosis usually occurs much later than for NF1. Nearly all patients develop symptoms that lead to deafness, but this progression may take years.

Also inherited in an autosomal dominant manner, NF2 results from mutations in the merlin gene and has strong homology to protein 4.1, important in membrane cytoskeletons. There are differences in the presentation of mild and severe forms of the disease. Mild forms usually have an earlier onset (15 to 25 years vs 25 to 30 years) and slower

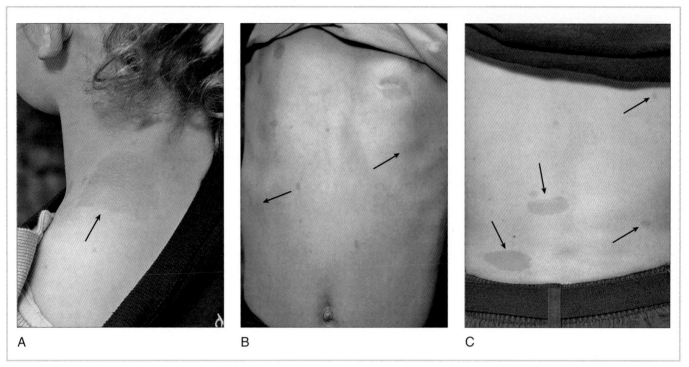

Figure 8-1. Isolated café-au-lait spots are found in many people without neurofibromatosis; however, individuals with more than five or six of these should be investigated further for NF, particularly if the spots appear within the first 5 years of life. These dizygotic twins are age 7.

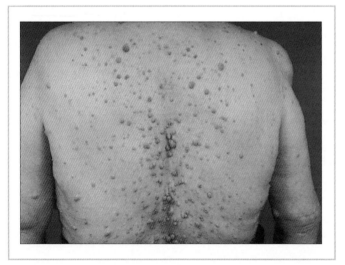

Figure 8-2. Cutaneous neurofibromas. There are four types of neurofibromas: cutaneous, subcutaneous, nodular plexiform, and diffuse flexiform. These cutaneous neurofibromas have no malignant potential. (From Feit J et al. *Hypertext Atlas of Dermatology*. Available at: http://www.muni.cz/atlases.)

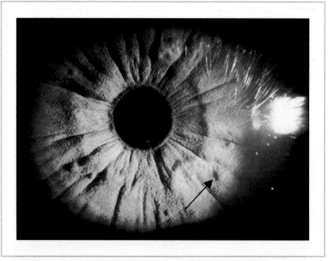

Figure 8-3. Lisch nodules (*arrow*) are associated with neurofibromatosis type 1. (From Digre K, Corbett JJ. *Practical Viewing of the Optic Disc*. Philadelphia, Butterworth Heinemann, 2003, p 223.)

progression of tumor development. Mild forms usually demonstrate vestibular schwannomas, whereas the more severe forms generally have meningiomas and other spinal tumors. Unlike NF1, which has an early age of onset with complete penetrance, onset of symptoms due to NF2 is generally in the late teens with almost complete penetrance by age 60.

Lesch-Nyhan Syndrome

Lesch-Nyhan syndrome is a metabolic disorder of purine and pyrimidine metabolism. It is a X-linked deficiency of the enzyme hypoxanthine-guanine phosphoribosyltransferase (HPRT) encoded by the *HPRT1* gene. More than 210 *HPRT1* mutations are associated with Lesch-Nyhan syndrome, and

GTPases, Components of the G-Protein Complexes

G proteins exist in an active or inactive state and participate in signal transduction. In the inactive state, GDP is bound to the G protein, which is composed of α-, β-, and γ-subunits. Ligand binding to a receptor allows interaction with a G protein, causing GDP to be replaced by GTP in the α-subunit of the G protein. This α-GTP complex dissociates from the β- and γ-subunits as well as from the receptor and interacts with an appropriate effector, such as adenylate cyclase, to produce cAMP.

To inactivate the active G protein, GTPase activity that is intrinsic to the complex converts GTP to GDP and the α-subunit recombines with the β- and γ-subunits. The rate-limiting step in this cycle is the GDP dissociation, since GTP cannot bind until GDP dissociates.

its severity correlates with the severity of the genetic lesion. Infants born with this disorder appear normal at birth, but symptoms begin to appear between 3 and 6 months of age. Enzyme deficiencies block the ability of hypoxanthine and guanine to form inosine 5′-monophosphate and guanosine 5′-monophosphate, respectively (Fig. 8-5), leading to increased de novo synthesis. This metabolic block results in the conversion of hypoxanthine and guanine to uric acid crystals that accumulate in joints, tissues, and the central nervous system (CNS). These crystals ultimately lead to kidney stones and impaired kidney function, blood in the urine, and swollen and painful joints.

The first symptom of this disease may be the observation of orange-colored crystals in the infant's diaper. Symptoms progress, however, and the child becomes hypotonic and hyperreflexic as spasticity of the limbs develops. Self-mutilation behavior develops and is demonstrated in children who bite and chew away fingertips, lips, and tongue. A mild form in which the enzyme has some activity is rare but when present lacks neurologic symptoms.

Lysosomal Storage Disorders

Lysosomes are cytoplasmic organelles that enzymatically degrade glycoproteins, glycolipids, and mucopolysaccharides. Deficiencies in the enzymes responsible for degradation of these substrates result in substrate accumulation. The substrate accumulates in the cytoplasm or is taken up by phagocytes, leading to clinical features. Lysosomal storage diseases represent a continuum of disease severity characterized by age of onset, clinical course, and whether the CNS is involved. Clinical symptoms in lysosomal storage disorders are variable with the disorder but all are progressive. The major sites affected by the accumulation of substrate are the brain, skeleton, and organs such as the heart, liver, and spleen. There are two major classes of lysosomal storage disorders: sphingolipidoses and mucopolysaccharidoses.

Sphingolipidoses

Sphingolipids are complex lipids and a major component of cell membranes. Sphingolipids include sphingomyelins and glycosphingolipids. This latter group includes cerebrosides (glucocerebrosides and galactocerebrosides) and gangliosides. Normally, phagocytic cells, particularly histocytes or

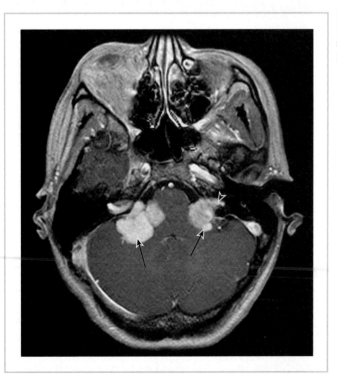

Figure 8-4. Bilateral vestibular schwannomas (*arrows*) shown by MRI with contrast. The arrowhead shows extension of the right schwannomas into the internal auditory canal. (Courtesy of Simin Dadparvar, MD.)

BIOCHEMISTRY

HPRT

Hypoxanthine-guanine phosphoribosyltransferase (HPRT) is a ubiquitous enzyme found in the cytoplasm. Its highest activity is in the brain and testes. HPRT catalyzes the transfer of the phosphoribosyl group of phosphoribosylpyrophosphate to hypoxanthine and guanine; this forms inosine monophosphate and guanosine monophosphate. In situations in which hypoxanthine and guanine cannot be recycled, there is a lack of feedback control of synthesis, resulting in rapid catabolism of these bases to uric acid.

PHARMACOLOGY

Allopurinol

Allopurinol is a xanthine oxidase inhibitor used to treat chronic gout. It is also administered with colchicine to prevent gouty arthritis. Xanthine oxidase oxidizes allopurinol to alloxanthine, which also inhibits xanthine oxidase and de novo purine synthesis.

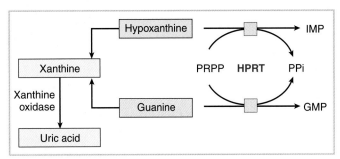

Figure 8-5. Hypoxanthine and guanine pathway. A deficiency in hypoxanthine-guanine phosphoribosyltransferase (HPRT) leads to the overproduction of uric acid and the symptoms associated with Lesch-Nyhan syndrome. IMP, inosine 5′-monophosphate; GMP, guanosine 5′-monophosphate; PP$_i$, inorganic pyrophosphate; PRPP, 5-phospho-α-D-ribosyl-1-pyrophosphate.

macrophages, degrade membranes. In the brain, there is normally rapid turnover of gangliosides, the most common sphingolipid, during development. Any accumulation of sphingolipid degradation products results in a sphingolipid disorder (Fig. 8-6). The entire degradation pathway occurs in the lysosome, where the pH of 3.5 to 5.5 is optimal for enzymatic activity.

Tay-Sachs Disease and Sandhoff Disease

Tay-Sachs disease occurs with a deficiency of the lysosomal enzyme hexosaminidase A and results in the accumulation of GM$_2$ gangliosides. These gangliosides accumulate in all tissues, but the clinical symptoms are seen in those cells with the greatest accumulation. As expected from the discussion above, these cells are neurons of the central and autonomic nervous systems as well as retinal cells.

Three gene products are required to form a complex resulting in the degradation of GM$_2$ gangliosides. Hexosaminidase A is composed of an α- and a β-subunit and an activator—each expressed from different genes. Proper binding of this complex to the ganglioside causes hydrolysis between N-acetylgalactosamine and galactose (Fig. 8-7). A mutation of the α-subunit leads to a deficiency of hexosaminidase A activity. The mutation has an autosomal recessive mode of inheritance.

Normal at birth, these children develop mental and physical deterioration, blindness, deafness, and muscle atrophy followed by paralysis. A *cherry red spot of the macula* is present in Tay-Sachs just as in other lipid storage diseases (Fig. 8-8). In this classical presentation that begins around the fifth or sixth month, death usually occurs by age 5. Tay-Sachs is common in the Ashkenazi Jewish population and French Canadians. Ninety-eight percent of Tay-Sachs results from

one of three mutations in the Ashkenazi Jewish population, thus providing a basis for carrier screening within this population.

Sandhoff disease results from a mutation in the β-subunit and thus causes a deficiency in hexosaminidase A and hexosaminidase B complexes, the latter being composed of two β-subunits and an activator. Tay-Sachs and Sandhoff diseases have similar presentations; however, individuals with Sandhoff disease have hepatosplenomegaly and the disease is not predominant in any particular population.

Fabry Disease

Among the enzymes in the sphingolipid degradation pathway, only α-galactosidase A is inherited in an X-linked manner, and mutations in the cognate *GLA* gene are specific for Fabry disease (see Fig. 8-6). Over 300 *GLA* mutations have been characterized in affected males. The substrate for this enzyme is globotriaosylceramide, a cerebroside containing glucose and galactose. Mutations in the enzyme cause substrate accumulation within endothelial cells, pericytes, smooth muscle cells, renal epithelial cells, myocardial cells,

PATHOLOGY & HISTOLOGY

Histiocytes

Histiocytes are fixed cells of the immune system found in many organs and connective tissue. They are phagocytic cells of the reticuloendothelial system and may also be known as macrophages or mononuclear phagocytes. Examples include:

- Gaucher cells: uniformly vacuolated mononuclear, kerasin-containing cells present in the bone marrow, spleen, liver, and lymph nodes in patients afflicted with Gaucher disease
- Kupffer cells: phagocytes located within the sinusoids of the normal liver
- Dust cells: macrophages located in the alveoli and interalveolar spaces of the lung
- Langerhans cells: dendrite-shaped cells found in the stratus spinosum of skin

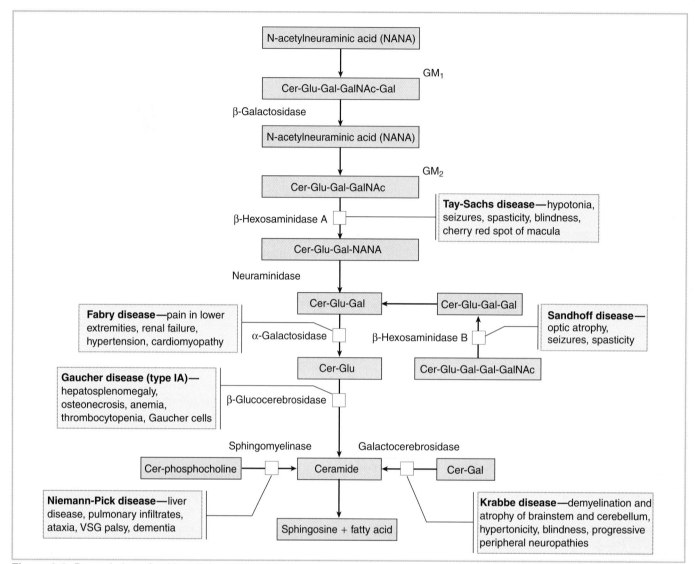

Figure 8-6. Degradation of sphingolipids by lysosomal enzymes. Fabry disease has X-linked inheritance. Other examples are autosomal recessive. VSG, vertical supranuclear gaze palsy.

peripheral nerves, and dorsal ganglia. The most conspicuous features of Fabry disease are angiokeratomas (Fig. 8-9) and acroparesthesia with recurrent episodes of severe neuropathic pain. Burning pain occurs in the distal extremities, particularly in the palms and soles of the feet. These episodes of pain may last from a few minutes to days and usually occur during exercise, emotional stress, fatigue, or rapid changes in temperature or humidity. Pain can be excruciating, and it is presumed that the acroparesthesia results from deposition of sphingolipid in small vessels supplying blood to the peripheral nerves.

There are three forms of Fabry disease: classical, a cardiac variant, and a renal variant. In the classical form of the disease, less than 1% of the enzyme is present. Cardiac and renal variants have greater than 1% activity. As expected, the most severe clinical presentation occurs with the classical form, and the life expectancy is 41 years. Onset of symptoms in the classical form is during childhood (4 to 8 years) rather than adulthood, as seen with the cardiac and renal variants, where onset is generally after ages 25 and 40 years, respectively. The variations in the later onset presentations often lead to delayed diagnosis and missed diagnosis. As a result, a correct diagnosis may not be made until more than a decade after the first symptoms appear. It has been estimated that 4% of individuals with hypertrophic cardiac disease may have the cardiac variant of Fabry disease. Similarly, 1.2% of

BIOCHEMISTRY

Gangliosides

Gangliosides are the most complex group of glycosphingolipids. These ceramide (a family of lipids composed of sphingosine and fatty acid) oligosaccharides are composed of a sugar and at least one sialic acid residue. They are the primary component of cell membranes and make up 6% of brain lipids.

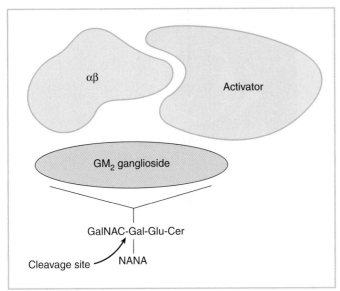

Figure 8-7. Hexosaminidase A complex is composed of three proteins: the α-subunit, the β-subunit, and an activator. A mutation in the α-subunit results in Tay-Sachs disease. GalNAC, *N*-acetylgalactosamine; Gal, galactose; Glu, glucose; Cer, ceremide; NANA, *N*-acetylneuraminic acid.

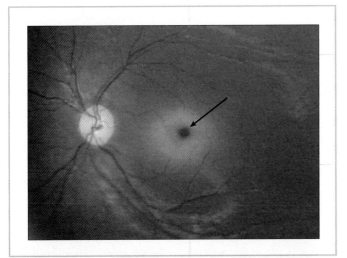

Figure 8-8. A cherry-red spot (*arrow*) in Tay-Sachs disease is due to glycolipid deposits in ganglion cells everywhere except in the macula, where there are no ganglion cells. (From Digre K, Corbett JJ. *Practical Viewing of the Optic Disc.* Philadelphia, Butterworth Heinemann, 2003, p 518.)

all dialysis patients with end-stage renal failure have been shown to have the renal variant of Fabry disease.

The development of recombinant α-galactosidase A has provided a treatment for Fabry disease worldwide. This enzyme effectively degrades the substrate and prevents accumulations leading to symptoms. Studies demonstrate treatment reduces or stabilizes general symptoms as well as stabilizing renal deterioration and improving cardiac function. Treatment should begin as early as possible in all males

with Fabry disease, even with end-stage renal disease, as well as female carriers with significant symptoms.

Gaucher Disease

Gaucher disease occurs from an inability to degrade a sulfatide to ceramide (see Fig. 8-6). A defect in *glucocerebrosidase* causes an accumulation of glucocerebroside in the spleen, liver, lung, bone marrow, and occasionally in the brain. Glucocerebrosides are a component of cell membranes, as are sphingolipids in general, and are released when cells are degraded; in the brain, glucocerebrosides arise from complex lipid turnover during brain development and the formation of myelin sheaths. When this substrate is not degraded, it accumulates in Gaucher cells (Fig. 8-10). The accumulation of Gaucher cells in bone marrow can cause pain and even fractures. Hepatosplenomegaly occurs from accumulation in the spleen and liver contributing to anemia, bruising, and impaired clotting. Neurologic damage occurs when Gaucher cells accumulate in the nervous system.

There are three clinical forms: adult, infantile, and juvenile, (Table 8-2) also characterized as types 1, 2, and 3. The most common form of Gaucher disease is type 1. This is a chronic nonneuropathic form and is responsible for 85% of cases. The onset of symptoms may be early or delayed until adulthood. These include easy bruising and fatigue, anemia, low platelets, hepatosplenomegaly, bone pain, and aseptic necrosis

PATHOLOGY

Angiokeratoma Corporis Diffusum

Angiokeratoma corporis diffusum is the hallmark of Fabry disease, causing red to blue-black cutaneous vascular lesions. Early lesions may be small and nonhyperkeratotic, but they tend to increase in number and size with age and are nonblanching with pressure. Lesions may occur anywhere but tend to concentrate between the umbilicus and the thighs; they rarely occur on the face, scalp, or ears.

NEUROSCIENCE

Pain

Pain receptors, called nociceptors, are free nerve endings in the periphery that initiate a pain sensation. Pain fibers enter the spinal cord in the lateral region of the dorsal root and divide into Lissauer's tract. Synapses occur in the substantia gelatinosa, located in the apical region of the posterior horn of the spinal cord gray matter and extending the entire length into the medulla oblongata. Pain is transmitted via a second-order neuron in the lateral spinothalamic tract and ascends in the contralateral quadrant of the spinal cord. From there it travels to the ventral posterolateral nucleus of the thalamus. A third-order neuron travels to the postcentral gyrus of cortex for conscious awareness of pain.

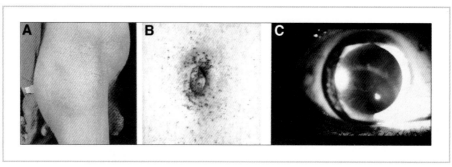

Figure 8-9. A, Angiokeratomas are characteristic dark red to blue-black angiectases. In Fabry disease, they are often found between the umbilicus and thigh. **B,** They become larger and more numerous with age. **C,** The whorled corneal opacity is seen with a slit-lamp and does not affect vision. It is found in almost all males and 70% to 90% of female carriers of Fabry disease. (From Desnick RJ, Brady R, Barranger J, et al. Fabry disease, an under-recognized multisystemic disorder: expert recommendations for diagnosis, management, and enzyme replacement therapy. *Ann Intern Med.* 2003;138:338–346.)

(Fig. 8-11). Unlike in other lipidoses, there is no brain involvement.

Type 2 Gaucher disease is an acute neuropathic disease. The clinical onset of hepatosplenomegaly is apparent by 3 months of age. There is extensive and progressive brain damage. Death occurs by age 2.

Type 3 Gaucher disease is a subacute neuropathic form with variable hepatosplenomegaly. Brain involvement, such as seizures, is gradual. Other than the neurologic symptoms, symptoms in type 3 may be similar to those in type 1. Life expectancy is generally three to four decades without treatment.

Gaucher disease is an autosomal recessive disorder caused by mutations in the gene for glucocerebrosidase (*GBA*). Although approximately 200 Gaucher-associated mutations have been characterized within the *GBA* gene, only four variants account for 90% of disease in the Ashkenazi Jewish population. These same mutations account for 50% to 60% of mutations in other populations. Type 1 affects 1 in 450 Ashkenazi Jewish individuals and is *the most common genetic disorder affecting this population.* Types 2 and 3 occur in 1 in 100,000 individuals and have no predilection for any particular ethnic group.

Treatment has dramatically reduced the symptoms of Gaucher disease since the introduction of enzyme replacement therapies for types 1 and 3 Gaucher's disease in 1991. The administration of a recombinant analog for human β-glucocerebrosidase eliminates the symptoms but does not cure the disease. This therapy reduces the size of the liver and spleen, reduces skeletal anomalies, and normalizes blood cell counts. Therapy must be maintained for the life of the individual or the symptoms will recur as substrate once again begins to accumulate. Bone marrow transplantation has been used in some patients to replace hemopoietic cells; however, the risks of graft-versus-host rejection may be high. Enzyme

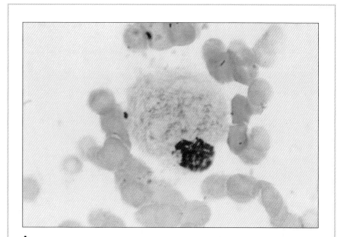

A

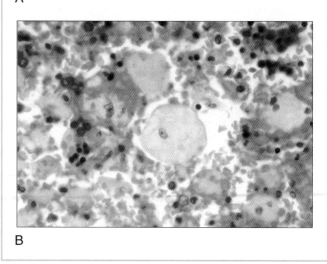

B

Figure 8-10. Gaucher cells in bone marrow **(A)** and spleen **(B)**. Note the fibrillar cytoplasm that looks like parchment or crumpled tissue paper. (Courtesy of Dr. Jerome Tift, Mercer University School of Medicine.)

PATHOLOGY & HISTOLOGY

Gaucher Disease

Gaucher disease is a group of autosomal recessive disorders with mutations in the gene encoding glucocerebrosidase. This defect causes glucocerebroside to accumulate in massive amounts within phagocytic cells throughout the body. These malfunctioning phagocytic cells (Gaucher cells) are distended and found in the spleen, liver, bone marrow, lymph nodes, tonsils, thymus, and Peyer's patches. In severe cases, Gaucher cells may displace bone marrow, causing bone to become demineralized and weakened, a situation that can lead to fractures. In the lung, these cells can lead to hypoxia, cyanosis, and clubbing.

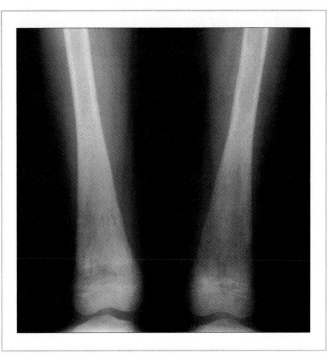

Figure 8-11. Children with type 1 Gaucher disease will develop hepatosplenomegaly early in childhood. Many will develop a characteristic "Erlenmeyer flask deformity" of the distal femur, reflecting thinned cortices and dilatation of the medullary cavity. (From GE Healthcare. Available at: http://www.medcyclopaedia.com.)

replacement therapy is a better choice of treatment. There is no treatment for the severe brain involvement seen with types 2 and 3. Treatment can increase the life expectancy of individuals significantly and it may even approach normal. However, while Gaucher disease is the most common lysosomal storage disorder in the general population, life-long enzyme replacement therapy and the annual cost of about $300,000 are not options for every family. Yet without this therapy, the options are limited.

Niemann-Pick Disease

Niemann-Pick disease is an autosomal recessive group of related neurologic disorders designated as A, B, and C. Both A and B have mutations in sphingomyelinase, causing sphingomyelin to accumulate rather than be degraded to ceramide (see Fig. 8-6). Type A is the most severe form and is seen in the majority of individuals with Niemann-Pick disease. There is less than 1% of the normal enzyme in type A, resulting in feeding difficulties, an enlarged abdomen within the first 3 to 6 months, a cherry red spot, and progressive loss of motor skills. These individuals usually die by 2 to 3 years of age.

Individuals with type B have more enzymatic activity, generally between 10% and 60%, and thus experience less severe symptoms. These symptoms may include hepatosplenomegaly and respiratory problems that can lead to cardiovascular stress, but there is little or no neurologic involvement. These individuals may survive into late childhood or adulthood. In addition to types A and B, some individuals may have an intermediate form of disease with more neurologic problems than type B but milder symptoms than type A.

TABLE 8-2. Comparison of the Three Forms of Gaucher Disease*

Type	Signs and Symptoms	Incidence	Life Expectancy
I, Adult form (most common)	Anemia, bruising, fatigue, low platelets, hepatosplenomegaly, bone pain and aseptic necrosis, growth retardation	1 in 450 in Ashkenazi Jewish population	Variable; in general, the later in life symptoms appear, the less severe the disease
II, Acute or infantile form	Rapid, progressive development of neurologic symptoms	1 in 100,000—no ethnic focus	2 years
III, Subacute or juvenile form	Slowly developing neurologic symptoms beginning in childhood; other symptoms similar to type I	1 in 100,000—no ethnic focus	3 to 4 decades

*There is also a perinatal form that is lethal and associated with skin abnormalities or with nonimmune hydrops fetalis. A cardiovascular form is characterized by calcifications of the aortic and mitral valves, supranuclear ophthalmoplegia, corneal opacities, and splenomegaly.

Complications of Bone Marrow Transplantation

Graft-versus-host (GVH) reaction is the major complication of bone marrow transplantation. The reaction occurs when the immunocompetent cells contained in the bone marrow graft recognize the host tissue as foreign and initiate rejection.

During the afferent phase of the disease, alloreactive donor T cells recognize major and minor histocompatibility antigens of the host. The efferent phase follows, and inflammatory effector cells are activated. Cytopathic molecules, including cytokines, are also secreted and induce pathology in the skin, gastrointestinal tract, liver, lung, and immune system. GVH reaction symptoms include rash, jaundice, hepatosplenomegaly, diarrhea, and infection. Cyclosporine may be used to decrease the GVH reaction.

Type C Niemann-Pick disease has a different genetic defect that may lead to a secondary deficiency of sphingomyelinase due to the large accumulation of lipids. The total sphingomyelinase may be normal but inadequate. Two genes are responsible for type C—*NPC1* and *NPC2. NPC1* is a member of a gene family of membrane-bound proteins with a sterol-sensing domain. Mutations in *NPC1*, which occur in 95% of type C disease, disrupt transport of cholesterol and other lysosomal products, leading to neuronal degeneration.

The second gene, *NPC2*, produces a cholesterol-binding protein. Mutations in this protein decrease cholesterol binding, causing it to accumulate in the cell. NPC1 and NPC2 therefore work together to transport lipids. Mutations in NPC1 prevent proper transport of lipids out of the cell, whereas mutations in NPC2 affect lipid movement within the lysosome and perhaps between lysosomes and other organelles such as the endoplasmic reticulum.

Cholesterol enters the cell normally, but in Niemann-Pick disease cholesterol and other unmetabolized lipids accumulate in cells of the liver, spleen, and brain. Infants often have jaundice at or shortly after birth, followed by the progressive development of hepatosplenomegaly, ataxia, dystonia, dysarthria, and dementia. Vertical supranuclear gaze palsy is highly suggestive of type C. Individuals with type C disease generally die before age 20.

Some populations are more affected than others with a specific type of Niemann-Pick disease. For example, types A and B occur more frequently in the Ashkenazi Jewish population. Type B is also prevalent among North African populations. Type C is more likely to occur among Hispanic Americans in southern New Mexico and Colorado.

Krabbe Disease

Krabbe disease results from a mutation in *galactocerebrosidase* (see Fig. 8-6). This enzyme is responsible for the degradation of galactocerebroside to ceramide and galactosylsphingosine, also known as psychosine, to sphingosine. Galactocerebroside is a major component of myelin. Myelin is not abnormal in these individuals, but the enzyme deficiency causes an accumulation of substrates. This is particularly critical during the first 18 months of life when myelin formation and turnover are high. It is the increased galactosylsphingosine levels that are toxic and lead to the *destruction of oligodendroglia* and *impaired Schwann cell function* in the CNS and to demyelination. The undegraded substrates accumulate in multinucleated macrophages in demyelinated regions of the brain. These "globoid" cells characterize this disease, which is also known as *globoid cell leukodystrophy*.

Symptoms begin at 3 to 6 months age in the classical infantile form (85% to 90% cases) with irritability, unexplained crying, fever, limb stiffness, seizures, feeding difficulties, vomiting, and decreased mental and motor development. Unlike in the other sphingolipidoses, lipid storage clinically differs in that the galactosylceramide and total brain lipids are actually reduced because myelinogenesis fails following the loss of myelin-producing cells. As noted above, individual globoid cells, however, accumulate galactosylceramide. As may be anticipated from this description, Krabbe disease is a disease of white matter because of the presence of myelin; gray matter is relatively unaffected. Many mutations have been defined in the galactocerebrosidase gene. Some are associated with a later onset and milder adult form.

In the infantile form of Krabbe disease, a 30-kb deletion is responsible for 45% and 35% of cases occurring in individuals of European and Mexican ancestry, respectively. This differs from late-onset disease, which often has a G809A mutation. Compound heterozygotes with both mutations demonstrate late-onset disease.

Mucopolysaccharidoses

Mucopolysaccharidoses (MPS) are caused by excessive intralysosomal accumulation of glycosaminoglycans, specifically heparan sulfate and dermatan sulfate (Table 8-3). Mucopolysaccharides, more appropriately called glycosaminoglycans (GAGs), are unbranched polysaccharides made up of repeating disaccharide units that may be sulfated. Glycosaminoglycans linked to protein are called proteoglycans, the major component of ground substance in connective tissues (see

Vertical Supranuclear Gaze Palsy

Supranuclear and internuclear pathways are involved with voluntary conjugate eye movement. Nuclear refers to cranial nerve nuclei. The pathways originate in the middle frontal gyrus and require bilateral activation of nuclei for movement. The principal pathway controlling coordinated eye movement is the internuclear pathway, which is linked to the third, fourth, and sixth cranial nerve nuclei via the medial longitudinal fasciculus. The supranuclear pathway feeds into the medial longitudinal fasciculus.

BIOCHEMISTRY

Psychosine

Galactosphingosine, also called psychosine, is a constituent of cerebrosides. It is synthesized by direct galactosylation of sphingosine. The accumulation of psychosine leads to the formation of "globoid cells" that may lead to cytotoxity of oligodendrocytes. These multinuclear, globular giant cells are derived from macrophages and microglia. Although the complete mechanism is still unclear, it has been shown that psychosine acts through a G protein–coupled receptor—perhaps composed of unknown heterotrimeric proteins—to block cytokinesis but not mitosis. The observation of cytoplasmic filamentous structures suggests that psychosine affects vesicle transport, actin reorganization, or both, resulting the abnormal cytokinesis.

TABLE 8-3. Comparison of Heparan, Heparan Sulfate, and Dermatan Sulfate

Glycosaminoglycan*	Distribution
Heparan	Component of intracellular granules of mast cells; lining of arteries of the lungs, liver, and skin
Heparan sulfate	Basement membranes, components of cell surfaces
Dermatan sulfate	Skin, blood vessels, heart valves

*Heparin sulfate contains more acetylated glucosamine than heparan, and heparan is more sulfated than heparan sulfate.

Chapter 7). Similarly to the sphingolipidoses, defects in lysosomal enzyme activity results in the accumulation of partially degraded molecules; however, rather than sphingolipids, GAGs accumulate and are secreted in urine.

There are at least 14 known types of lysosomal storage diseases affecting glycosaminoglycan degradation. It is the accumulation of GAGs, or mucopolysaccharides, that leads to the commonly associated clinical features of coarse facies, thick skin, corneal clouding, and organomegaly. The accumulation also results in defective cell function represented by mental retardation, growth deficiencies, and skeletal dysplasias. Because GAGs are such important constituents in the extracellular matrix, hernias and joint contractures may also be seen. As noted, the most commonly known disorders of GAG degradation involve heparan sulfate and dermatan sulfate (Fig. 8-12). Among these Hurler syndrome, Hunter syndrome, Scheie syndrome, and Sanfilippo syndrome will be described (Table 8-4). Each of these, with the exception of Hunter syndrome, is inherited in an autosomal recessive manner; Hunter syndrome is an X-linked recessive disorder.

MPS I: Hurler, Scheie, Hurler-Scheie Syndromes

The most severe of the mucopolysaccharidoses is Hurler syndrome, also known as MPS-IH. A mutation in iduronidase, encoded by the *IDUA* gene, leads to the accumulation of heparan and dermatan sulfate (see Fig. 8-12). The Hurler phenotype—coarse facies, enlarged skull, corneal clouding, hepatosplenomegaly, thickened skin, hernias, and contractures—become evident by the age of 1. Mental deterioration is progressive. Heparan sulfate and dermatan sulfate accumulate in the coronary artery, leading to ischemia and cardiac insufficiency. Other problems are the potential for large hernias, respiratory infections, and thickening of the meninges, leading to decreased cerebrospinal fluid circulation and increased cranial pressure.

Scheie syndrome is a milder form of MPS, designated as MPS-IS. Intermediate to Hurler and Scheie is MPS-IH/S. MPS-IH and MPS-IS forms are allelic. The intermediate form, MPS-IH/S, is a compound heterozygote. The milder form has no CNS involvement (Table 8-5).

Both enzyme replacement and bone marrow transplantation have been used to treat MPS-I. Recombinant α-L-iduronidase has been approved for treatment. Individuals with severe disease may be treated with bone marrow transplantation (BMT) or umbilical cord blood transplantation to

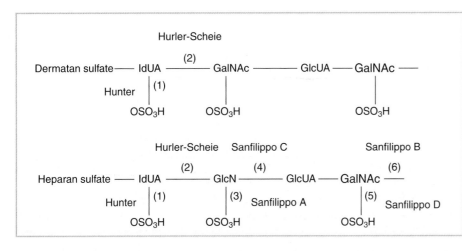

Figure 8-12. Structures of dermatan sulfate and heparan sulfate. Disease occurs when these glycoaminoglycans are not degraded and permitted to accumulate. Hurler and Scheie syndromes are allelic. Shown here are the resulting mucopolysaccharidoses that occur when specific enzymes are absent or have reduced activity. The numbers in parentheses refer to enzymes that hydrolyze the bonds: (1) iduronate sulfatase; (2) α-L-iduronidase; (3) heparan sulfamidase; (4) acetyl-CoA: α-glucosaminide acetyltransferase; (5) *N*-acetylglucosamine-6-sulfatase; (6) *N*-acetylglucosaminidase.

TABLE 8-4. Summary of Mucopolysaccharidoses

MPS Type	Disease	Life Expectancy	Enzyme Deficiency	Accumulated Product
I	Hurler Hurler-Scheie	<10 Years (teens to 20s) Normal expectancy	α-L-Iduronidase	Heparan sulfate and dermatan sulfate
II	Hunter	15 Years (severe) Normal expectancy (mild)	Iduronate sulfatase	Heparan sulfate and dermatan sulfate
III-A	Sanfilippo A		Heparan-N-sulfatase	Heparan sulfate
III-B	Sanfilippo B	20 Years	α-N-acetylglucosaminidase	Heparan sulfate
III-C	Sanfilippo C		Acetyl-CoA: α-glucosaminide acetyltransferase	Heparan sulfate
III-D	Sanfilippo D		N-acetylglucosamine-6-sulfatase	Heparan sulfate

BIOCHEMISTRY

Proteoglycans

Proteoglycans are found in the extracellular matrix and on cell surfaces. These large and complex molecules consist of a protein core with covalently bound glycosaminoglycans (GAGs) or mucopolysaccharides. Several types of GAG are dermatan sulfate, heparan sulfate, heparan sulfate, and chondroitin sulfate. These GAGs are removed from the protein core in lysosomes by 10 specific enzymes. Defects in any of these enzymes leads to an accumulation of GAG metabolites, with clinical consequences.

TABLE 8-5. Comparison of MPS-I Types

Severe Form	Intermediate Form	Mild Form
Hurler	Hurler-Scheie	Scheie
MPS-IH	MPS-IH/S	MPS-IS
• Severe developmental and mental delay • Severe respiratory disease • Obstructive airway disease • Progressive	• Normal or near normal intelligence • Respiratory disease • Obstructive airway disease • Joint stiffness, contractures • Skeletal abnormalities • Decreased vision	• Normal intelligence • Less progressive physical problems • Corneal clouding • Valvular disease of the heart

modify disease progression and improve survival. This treatment may improve some of the physical features and decrease the CNS deterioration. Because of the morbidity and mortality risks associated with transplants, BMT is generally not used in milder forms of the disease.

MPS-II: Hunter Syndrome

MPS-II, also known as Hunter syndrome, is an X-linked disorder. The wide spectrum of clinical severity correlates with the amount of iduronate sulfatase activity present. Like MPS-I, this is a progressive disorder. Typically, symptoms begin between ages 2 and 4 years. Clinical features are similar to those in MPS-I. Atypical retinitis pigmentosa or retinal degeneration may occur without the corneal clouding seen in MPS-I. Progressive loss of hearing also occurs.

MPS-III: Sanfilippo Syndromes

There are four types of MPS-III; each results from a defect in a different enzyme (see Fig. 8-12). The four enzymes affected are heparan-N-sulfatase, α-N-acetylglucosaminidase, acetyl-CoA:α-glucosaminide acetyl transferase, and N-acetylglucosamine-6-sulfatase. These enzymes participate in the degradation of heparan sulfate but not of dermatan sulfate. As expected, heparan sulfate accumulates in tissues and is found in the urine of these individuals (see Table 8-4). Sanfilippo type A, MPS-IIIA, has the most severe presenta-

tion; types IIIB to IIID have decreasing severity with MPS-IIID the least severe.

The physical changes of Sanfilippo syndromes tend to be mild when compared with MPS-I and MPS-II. Infants are normal at birth. The first changes may appear in a child between the ages of 2 and 6 years presenting as developmental delay, particularly of speech, and behavioral changes such as sleep disturbances, short attention span, and impulsiveness. The facies are coarse with thickened eyebrows that meet, also called synophrys. Individuals may also have coarse, thick hair that is often blond or light brown. Diarrhea is common.

Skeletal changes are similar to those seen in MPS-I. Typically, the calvarium is thickened, vertebral bodies are oval shaped (Fig. 8-13), and hypoplasia of the pelvis may occur. It is not uncommon for individuals with MPS-III to be shorter than the mean. Joint stiffness is not uncommon, and in some individuals contractures may occur.

Intellectual changes become evident, followed by mental retardation, progressive neurologic disease, and severe CNS degeneration. Eventually the individual is unable to speak and

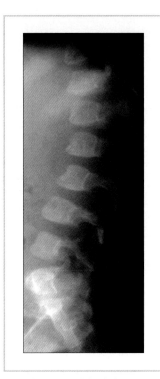

Figure 8-13. Mucopolysaccharidosis is accompanied by many skeletal abnormalities. Oval-shaped vertebrae and hook-shaped spinous processes result from defective development, leading to a gibbus deformity and lumbar kyphosis. (From GE Healthcare. Available at: http://www.medcyclopaedia.com. Used with permission.)

progressively loses all motor skills. Life expectancy is about two decades although BMT treatment may extend this.

Triplet Repeats

The mechanism of triplet repeat expansion and inheritance was discussed in Chapter 3. As noted, the expansions are parent-of-origin specific and occur within or near particular genes. Two examples will be discussed to better illustrate these features in neurologic disease: fragile X syndrome and Huntington disease.

Fragile X Syndrome

Fragile X syndrome is the most common type of inherited mental retardation and has been called the second most common *chromosomal* cause of mental retardation after Down syndrome; however, it is questionable whether this disorder should be classified as having a chromosomal etiology in the usual sense. Fragile X is not caused by nondisjunction, chromosomal translocations, or deletions. Rather, the DNA is greatly expanded at one particular region of the DNA on the X chromosome. It is inherited just as other genes are by independent assortment. However, the expansion, or amplification, resulting in fragile X occurs during maternal meiosis. No change occurs to the expanded region in males. Expression of the gene affected by amplification is dependent upon the extent of amplification.

DNA analysis revealed an unstable region of DNA characterized by a long, repeating sequence of three nucleotides: CGG. The CGG repeat localizes with the brain-expressed *fragile-X mental retardation gene,* or *FMR1* gene. Four categories of CGG repeats are recognized: normal, intermediate, premutation, and full mutation. *Normal* alleles range from approximately 5 to 44 and are stably transmitted without a change in number. There is a threshold of CGG repeat copies (about 44 to 58 copies, or about 50 on average) at which the DNA segment becomes prone to DNA expansion. Repeats within the *intermediate* range (approximately 45 to 58 repeats) are usually transmitted stably by females with occasional minor increases or decreases in the repeat number. *Premutation* alleles range from approximately 59 to 200 repeats and are not associated with mental retardation. Premutations may become full mutations during oogenesis, but remain stable during spermatogenesis. Women with alleles in this range are at risk for having affected children owing to the instability of the alleles. The upper limit of the premutation range is sometimes noted as approximately 230 repeats. Both 200 and 230 are approximations from laboratory data. *Full mutations* have more than 250 repeats and often expand to several hundred to several thousand repeats. Once expansion extends beyond 200, hypermethylation of deoxycytidylate residues usually occurs. Any person with a full mutation—100% of males and as high as 50% of female carriers—will be mentally impaired, whereas the risk is very low (about 3%) in carriers of a premutation.

The CGG repeat is located within the 5′ untranslated region of the *FMR1* gene. Loss of expression of the *FMR1* gene is associated with methylation. One region of particular note is characterized by a high density of cytosine phosphate guanine (CpG) dinucleotides, belonging to a class of regulatory sequences called CpG islands. These CpG islands frequently identify the promoter regions of eukaryotic genes. DNA methylation in such regions generally down-regulates expression of adjacent genes. It is likely that expression of the

FMR1 gene is repressed by methylation of the CpG islands, since amplification of the CGG sequences can down-regulate the production of *FMR1* mRNA transcripts. The inability to produce a protein from the gene results in the expression of fragile X syndrome. This protein has been called FMRP for "fragile-X mental retardation protein."

Males affected with fragile X syndrome have moderate to severe mental retardation and show definitive facial features (Table 8-6) The classical physical phenotype of a fragile X male includes a long narrow face, large and protruding ears, and a prominent jaw (Fig. 8-14). Additional features include velvet-like skin, hyperextensible finger joints, and double-jointed thumbs. There are other problems, which may be briefly mentioned, such as eye disturbances, otitis, orthopedic conditions, skin problems, and cardiac involvement (mitral valve prolapse). As one might suspect, these phenotypic features are generally not observed until maturity.

A striking feature of most adult fragile X males is the enlarged testicular volume *(macroorchidism)*. Normal adult males have a mean testicular volume of 17 mL, whereas the testicular volume in fragile X patients ranges from 40 to 140 mL. Fragile X men are fertile and offspring have been documented, but those with significant mental retardation rarely reproduce. The hormonal basis for the oversized testis is unclear; the levels of testosterone are normal, but there may be excessive gonadotropin stimulation. Table 8-6 lists the predominant clinical findings in fragile X males.

BIOCHEMISTRY

Methylation

Methylation of DNA occurs primarily at cytosines of CpG dinucleotides, called CpG islands, and is important in imprinting. About 70% of CpG sequences are methylated, and this occurs on both strands. Methylation of cytosine residues forms 5-methylcytosine. Methylation of CpG islands in promoter regions correlates with a lack of transcription. Methylation also correlates with deacetylation of histones and decreased transcription.

BIOCHEMISTRY

FMRP Protein

FMRP protein transports mRNAs to the cytoplasm for translation. It is very abundant in the brain, and contains two receptor-binding sites known as the nuclear localization signal (NLS) and the nuclear export signal (NES).

Once FMRP mRNA is translated in the cytoplasm, an NLS receptor binds to the protein and allows it to return to the nucleus. This FMRP-NLS complex then binds an NES protein. This complex interacts with specific mRNAs, which bind to the NES, and becomes a messenger ribonuclear protein (mRNP). The mRNP is transported to cytoplasm, where it binds to the 80S ribosome for translation.

TABLE 8-6. Predominant Clinical Features of Fragile X Syndrome in Males

Prepubertal	Postpubertal
Delayed developmental milestones	Mental retardation
Sit alone, 10 months	Pronounced
Walk, 20.6 months	craniofacies
First clear words, 20 months	Macroorchidism
Developmental delay	
Abnormal behavior	**Additional Features**
Tantrums	Strabismus
Hyperactivity	Joint hyperextensibility
Autism	Mitral valve prolapse
Mental retardation: IQ 30 to 50	Soft, smooth skin
Abnormal craniofacies	
Long face	
Prominent forehead	
Large ears	
Prominent jaw	

Despite being X-linked, fragile X syndrome can manifest in females. About 50% of heterozygous females show some degree of mental impairment, and as many as 30% are mentally retarded (IQ range is 55 to 75). The prevalence of mentally impaired females is one in every 2000 to 2500. The high rate of heterozygous expression is unprecedented for X-linked inheritance. The fact that carrier females may be affected is consistent with random inactivation of one of the two X chromosomes. If the active chromosome is the fragile one in the majority of the affected female's brain cells, then brain function is affected, with results comparable to that of fragile X males. It has been surmised that the degree of mental retardation is correlated with the percentage of cells in which the fragile X allele is active. Hence, the fragile X mutation predisposes affected females to a characteristic cognitive profile deficit. In addition to the neurologic features, recall that heterozygous females also have a different clinical profile that includes premature ovarian failure and features of fragile X-associated tremor/ataxia syndrome (FXTAS; see Chapter 3).

Huntington Disease

Huntington disease (HD) is a progressive disorder of motor, psychiatric, and cognitive functions resulting from selective neuronal death. It is a particularly devastating disease for the patient and family because there is no cure and because symptoms of HD usually begin in midlife between the ages of 35 and 45. This later age of onset is significant, since the mutated allele may have already been passed on to offspring before symptoms begin to appear. It is inherited as an autosomal dominant disease with complete penetrance. Mean survival time after onset of symptoms is 15 to 18 years.

Like fragile X syndrome, HD results from the expansion of a triplet repeat. Fragile X and Huntington disease differ by the triplet that amplifies—CGG for fragile X and CAG for

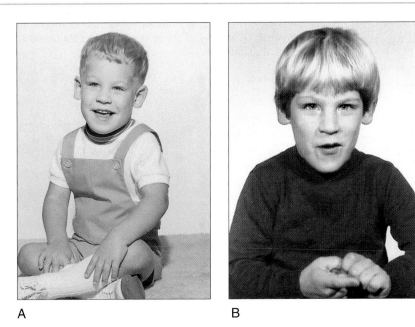
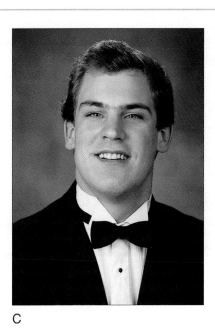

Figure 8-14. Fragile X syndrome. **A,** Two-year-old male with a full mutation exhibiting a relatively normal appearance with an elongated face and prominent ears; also note tapering fingers, a minor anomaly. **B,** At age 5 years, his head is large with large ears and a prominent jaw. **C,** At age 22 years. (From Scriver CR, Beaudet AL, Sly WS, et al. *Metabolic and Molecular Bases of Inherited Disease,* 8th ed, vol. 1. New York, McGraw-Hill, 2000, p 1269, Fig. 64-7.)

Huntington—and the number of repeats necessary for pathogenesis. The number of CAG triplets normally present in the *HD* gene is 10 to 26. Unlike the fragile X repeat that expands during maternal gametogenesis and lies outside the gene, the HD repeat is found in the first exon of the gene and is inherited from the father. The disease displays *anticipation,* in which a larger expansion is associated with an earlier onset of the disease and more severe symptoms. De novo mutation of this gene has never been reported.

The initial effects of the disorder are subtle, with minor difficulties of coordination, slight adventitious movements of the fingers, and abnormal darting eye movements. The motor disturbances are generally accompanied by behavioral changes, including chronic depression, impulsiveness, and irritability. Until the diagnosis is made, individuals with this disease can be mistakenly thought to abuse alcohol or drugs. The movement disorders gradually worsen, with more frequent and exaggerated chorea and abnormal posturing. Speech becomes disturbed, and memory is disrupted. Depression and apathy are heightened. Extreme weight loss occurs. Eventually, the victim of HD is totally incapacitated and the choreic movements give way to dystonia and rigidity.

Aggregates of the *HD* gene protein, huntingtin, are seen in brains of HD patients. Recent results suggest that the polyglutamine tract resulting from the CAG repeats inhibits the normal movement of huntingtin between the cytoplasm and nucleus, causing it to accumulate within the nucleus. This decreases the transport of brain-derived neurotrophic factor (BDNF) along microtubules, resulting in increased neuronal

toxicity and progressive death of medium spiny GABAergic neurons of the striatum and in the deep layers of the cortex. In later stages, degeneration extends to a variety of brain regions, including the hypothalamus and hippocampus (Fig. 8-15).

●●● COMPLEX DISEASES OF THE BRAIN

Single-gene disorders follow the rules of Mendelian segregation and inheritance. The special characteristics of triplet repeat amplification provide better explanations for inheritance and the pathogenesis of gene action. For many common disorders, however, inheritance patterns are more complex, and the genes affecting susceptibility and disease conditions are more slowly identified. It is expected that for diseases such as Parkinson disease and Alzheimer disease multiple and quite possibly a combination of genetic and environmental factors may be involved.

Alzheimer Disease

Alzheimer disease is typically a late-onset disorder with symptoms appearing after the age of 65. The predominant clinical feature of Alzheimer disease is progressive dementia, but the disorder is most readily identified by its neuropathologic effects evident in postmortem brain tissue—the formation of neuritic plaques containing insoluble spherical amyloid deposits and of intracellular neurofibrillary tangles composed

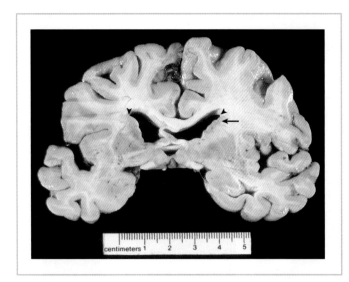

Figure 8-15. Huntington disease brain showing reduced caudate nucleus (*arrow*) and abnormal lateral ventricular angle (*arrowheads*). (Courtesy of Dr. Jerome Tift, Mercer University School of Medicine.)

of the cytoskeletal protein termed tau (τ). The degeneration and death of neurons in the hippocampus and portions of the cerebral cortex shackle the minds of victims in confusion. Studies of the epidemiology of Alzheimer disease indicate that the disease is present in 2% of the over-65 population and at least 8% of the over-85 population worldwide. The prevalence of Alzheimer disease is lower than expected because of the competing causes of death. That is to say, many individuals destined to express geriatric genetic disease will not express symptoms because they fail to survive to the age of onset.

Attention was initially focused on a small subset of clinical cases in which the patients showed an early onset of symptoms in the fourth and fifth decades. Although appearing relatively early in life, the symptoms are clinically and neurologically indistinguishable from the later onset Alzheimer disease. Since the early-onset patients are clustered in large pedigrees, the early-onset form is generally referred to as familial Alzheimer disease (FAD). In FAD families, the disorder segregates as an autosomal dominant trait over multiple generations.

There is genetic heterogeneity in the etiology of FAD, which means early-onset disease can be caused by mutations in different genes. Four known genes—*PS1, APP, PS2,* and *APOE*—contribute to Alzheimer disease, which is the most commonly occurring dementia, affecting almost half of all individuals with dementia.

PS1 Gene

The presenilin 1 (*PS1*) gene at chromosome 14q24.3 has been associated with FAD by linkage studies. More than 70% of FAD pedigrees show linkage to this locus and not to the *APP* locus. This gene codes for a protein localizing mainly in the endoplasmic reticulum. *PS1* mutations apparently disrupt Ca^{++} regulation in the endoplasmic reticulum and result in impaired mitochondrial function, the formation of reactive O_2 species, and an increased vulnerability to apoptosis. This suggests that aberrant APP processing in cells with mutant presenilins may be secondary to disturbed Ca^{++} homeostasis and increased oxidative stress.

APP Gene

The major proteinaceous constituent of neuritic plaques is amyloid β-peptide. This is a proteolytic fragment of the larger transmembrane protein precursor β-amyloid precursor protein (APP). This cell-surface protein is expressed in many cell types, with the highest expression in the brain. The cerebral cortex and limbic structures, which are particularly vulnerable to senile plaque formation in Alzheimer disease and Down syndrome, exhibit disproportionately large amounts of mRNA encoding APP. *APP* gene mutations are a rare cause of early-onset FAD, accounting for no more than 10% to 15% of cases.

The clinical hallmarks of FAD—amyloid plaques and neurofibrillary tangles—also occur in Down syndrome (trisomy 21). Plaques and tangles appear as early as the third decade of life in Down syndrome patients and affect virtually all patients by the fourth decade of life. However, in spite of these similarities, there is no evidence of association of chromosome 21 markers with late-onset AD.

PS2 Gene

A second presenilin gene (*PS2*) is located at chromosome 1q31-242. It has a greater than 80% homology to *PS1* and is localized to the same regions of the brain as *PS1*. Mutations in this gene account for less than 5% of FAD cases.

APOE Gene

There is compelling evidence that the apolipoprotein E (*APOE*) gene predisposes individuals to late-onset Alzheimer disease. This "susceptibility" locus is on chromosome 19. A susceptibility gene is one that affects the risk of developing a disease; it is not causal. The APOE protein product plays a critical role in triglyceride-rich lipoprotein metabolism and

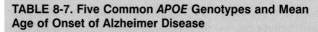

cholesterol homeostasis. APOE is a known risk factor for cardiovascular disease and was not initially considered as a risk factor for AD.

There are three variant alleles at the APOE locus—APOE ε2, APOE ε3, and APOE ε4—which occur in 6%, 78%, and 16% of Caucasian populations. These alleles result in different protein isoforms and therefore can occur in different allelic combinations, such as ε2/ε3 or ε3/ε3, reflecting the inheritance of one allele from each parent. Different allelic combinations demonstrate differences in age-specific predisposition to AD (Table 8-7). Generally speaking, the ε4 allele increases the risk and decreases the age of onset of AD. In a study of 42 families with late-onset AD, 91% of the AD individuals had ε4/ε4 alleles; this combination normally occurs in only 2% of the population. Table 8-7 also reveals that individuals with this genotype demonstrate symptoms earlier than those with a single ε4 allele. The two alleles provide a protective effect by apparently slowing the rate of the process leading to AD.

The ε4 allele is not a reliable predictor that a person will develop AD. In the United States, 64% of individuals with AD have at least one ε4 allele. This is twice the frequency observed in the general population, and the remaining 36% have no ε4 allele.

Oxidative insults associated with an age-related increased frequency of mutations in mitochondrial DNA apparently represent a risk factor in the pathogenesis of AD. Excess O_2 radicals result in a cascade of neuronal dysfunction, including membrane alterations, perturbed calcium homeostasis, vascular damage, and apoptosis. By reducing the level of oxidative stress, the development and progression of AD may slow.

Parkinson Disease

One of the most common progressive degenerative diseases affecting individuals over the age of 60 is Parkinson disease. Most of the causes of this disease are unknown; however, oxidative damage, environmental toxins, and accelerated

TABLE 8-7. Five Common *APOE* Genotypes and Mean Age of Onset of Alzheimer Disease

Genotype	Age of Onset (years)		Percentage of U.S. Population
	Mean	Range	
ε2/ε2	Unknown	Unknown	<1
ε2/ε3	>90	50 to 140	11
ε2/ε4	80 to 90	50 to >100	5
ε3/ε3	80 to 90	50 to >100	60
ε3/ε4	70 to 80	50 to >100	21
ε4/ε4	<70	50 to <100	2

aging processes have been discussed as possible contributors. As expected, the complex nature of Parkinson disease etiology makes diagnosis difficult and often imprecise until the disease has advanced. Diagnosis is based on the clinical presentation of bradykinesia, tremor, and rigidity.

Although most commonly associated with aging, Parkinson has several forms: *juvenile-onset* disease occurring before age 20 years, *early-onset* disease occurring before age 50 years, and *late-onset* disease occurring after age 50 years. Each of these is expected to have a different etiology, but they all share the cardinal feature of the disease: dopaminergic neurons are lost in the substantia nigra and Lewy bodies are present in the remaining, intact nigral neurons (Fig. 8-16). As many as 80% of the dopaminergic neurons may be lost before clinical symptoms are apparent in affected individuals.

Underlying the complexity of Parkinson disease are seven genes implicated in its etiology. Four have an autosomal

BIOCHEMISTRY & PHYSIOLOGY

Adverse Effects of Oxygen

Oxygen is a biradical that can form toxic reactive oxygen species (ROS), such as superoxide (O_2^-), hydroxyl radical (OH), and hydrogen peroxide (H_2O_2). Oxidative stress occurs when ROS are produced faster than they are removed, particularly for the respiratory, cardiovascular, nervous, and gastrointestinal systems. Damage arises from the mitochondria, where O_2^- is the final acceptor of electrons in oxidative metabolism. These ROS leak out of the mitochondria into the cytoplasm and initiate oxidative damage, or oxidative stress tissue and cells in DNA, proteins, and polyunsaturated fats.

Oxidative stress caused by O_2 toxicity may have adverse effects on virtually every organ of the body. This has been most extensively demonstrated in neonates, in whom O_2 toxicity has long been linked to *retrolental fibroplasia* and *bronchopulmonary dysplasia.* In adults, prolonged exposure to hyperbaric O_2 can cause CNS toxicity, atelectasis, pulmonary edema, and seizures.

PHYSIOLOGY & BIOCHEMISTRY

APOE and Cardiovascular Disease

In general, lipoproteins are complex molecules that transport nonpolar lipids in an aqueous environment, and each lipoprotein contains one or more apolipoproteins on its surface that have a variety of functional or structural roles. Apolipoprotein E is the main apoprotein of intermediate-density lipoprotein (IDL) and remnants to LDL receptors and LDL receptor–related proteins. It is synthesized in the brain, spleen, lung, adrenals, ovary, kidney, and liver. The presence of APOE mediates the uptake of IDL by the liver and conversion of IDL to LDL. Individuals who either lack APOE or are homozygous for variants that bind less efficiently to receptors will have elevated IDL and chylomicron remnants. These situations result in hypercholesterolemia and hypertriglyceridemia.

dominant mode of expression, and three have an autosomal recessive mode (Table 8-8). Originally, these genes had other abbreviations but as they became more closely associated with Parkinson disease the gene term was changed to *PARK*. In addition to these loci, there are at least three susceptibility genes. Most twin studies across a broad spectrum of ages and focusing on late-onset disease have been ambivalent in distinguishing a genetic influence. However, the best association indicates that disease onset before age 50 may be better related to genetic factors, suggesting that environmental influences in association with other genes have a stronger association with later onset disease.

It is important to note that clinical signs of bradykinesia, tremor, and rigidity may be associated with other neurologic diseases that mimic true Parkinson disease. Included among these are Alzheimer disease, Lewy body dementia, progressive supranuclear palsy, and others. Parkinson disease may also accompany diseases such as Huntington disease, spinocerebellar ataxia, and Wilson disease. These co-occurrences underscore the need for critical assessment of family history, laboratory findings, and individual presentation of symptoms for correct diagnosis. The correctness of the diagnosis can have familial consequences for diagnoses and management of other members of the family and future generations.

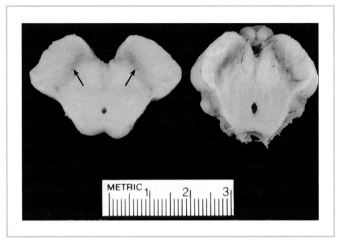

Figure 8-16. Parkinson disease midbrain showing decreased substantia nigra neurons (*arrows*) compared with normal (*right image*). (Courtesy of Dr. Jerome Tift, Mercer University School of Medicine.)

PATHOLOGY

Lewy Bodies

Lewy bodies are characteristically found within the pigmented neurons of the substantia nigra. They are abnormal aggregates of protein in nerve cells. The major component of Lewy bodies is α-synuclein, which has an altered shape: it is changed from a β-structure into filamentous sheets. The cells stain for α-synuclein and for ubiquitin, which conjugates with proteins prior to degradation. Lewy bodies are also found in dementia with Lewy bodies, Alzheimer disease (Lewy body variant), and Hallervorden-Spatz syndrome.

Studies of Behavioral Genetics

For many years the study of behavior has been very much a quantitative science and the classical methods employed by scientists are twin and family studies to associate the degree of relatedness with behavioral expression. These studies consistently demonstrate that complex disorders, such as Alzheimer disease, Parkinson disease, schizophrenia, and bipolar affective disorder run in families. They remain excellent tools for studying complex diseases caused by a constellation of predisposing variant alleles acting in concert with environmental influences to convert a vulnerability to a personality disorder.

Twin Studies

Twin studies are based on the genetic identity that occurs in monozygotic (MZ), or identical, twins and the dissimilarity that occurs between dizygotic (DZ) twins, also called nonidentical twins. In the latter, the genetic similarity is

TABLE 8-8. Comparison of Several Genes Implicated in Parkinson's Disease

Gene	Protein	Location	Mode of Inheritance	Pathogenesis
PARK1	α-Synuclein	4q21	AD	Neurotoxic aggregates of α-synuclein
PARK2 (juvenile form)	Parkin	6q25	AR	Impaired protein degradation
PARK3	Unknown	2p13	AD	Unknown
PARK5	Ubiquitin carboxyterminal esterase L1	4p14	AD	Impaired C-terminal hydrolysis of ubiquitin
PARK6	PTEN-induced putative kinase 1	1p36	AR	Mitochondrial dysfunction
PARK7	DJ-1	1p36	AR	Impaired oxidative stress response
PARK8	Leucine-rich repeat	12q12	AD	Unknown

similar to that of siblings. The basic assumption in these studies is that differences in gene expression result in phenotypic behavioral differences between the twins, since the prenatal and postnatal environments are either identical or very similar. Comparisons provide estimates of genetic variability for a particular trait.

The earliest twin studies focused on intelligence, mental illness, and personality. Perhaps the most startling finding is that MZ twins are more than twice as similar as DZ twins. This finding led to three laws of behavioral genetics, presented by Irving Gottosman and Eric Turkheimer:

First Law: Behavioral traits are heritable.

Second Law: The effect of being raised in the same family is smaller than the effect of genes.

Third Law: A substantial portion of variation in complex behavioral traits is not accounted for by the effects of genes or families.

Although seemingly straightforward, each of these laws actually interacts with each other in ways that are not fully understood. What is becoming clearer is that even minor variations in allele expression, both temporally and physically, may affect function and alter the cascade of following events in profound ways.

Association Studies

Association studies are a common tool for genetic epidemiology studies and employ both case-control studies and case-parent trio studies. More recently, they have also been used to determine the frequency of a particular trait in a population occurring with a particular polymorphism; in other words, they have been used as a mapping tool. It is possible to use a population-based association study, and many of these have been reported; however, there are far fewer problems with family studies where variables, which may alter results, can be minimized. The greatest difficulty with these studies is *ascertainment bias* in which there is a difference in the likelihood that affected relatives of the case individual will be reported compared with affected relatives of the controls. Family members of an affected individual are more likely to know of other relatives who are affected than relatives or controls. The relatives of affected individuals are also more likely to respond to questionnaires than relatives of controls.

However, the advent of molecular tools affected the study of behavior just as it did other areas of science. Now the focus has turned more to the effect of gene expression on behavior. The greatest area of interest is the area of psychiatric genetics. Tremendous efforts are being made in the areas of schizophrenia and bipolar disorder, the two most intensely studied psychiatric illnesses. However, the task of identifying susceptibility genes and gene interactions is extremely challenging and perhaps even daunting.

Schizophrenia

Schizophrenia is a neurologic disorder afflicting about 2.2 million people in the United States and more than 51 million people worldwide (Table 8-9). It is characterized by delusions, hallucinations, reduced interest and drive, altered emotional reactivity, and disorganized behavior. Structural brain abnormalities observed in individuals with schizophrenia include decreased volume, loss of gray matter (Fig. 8-17), and ventricular enlargement. The clinical features are often not recognized until late in the second decade or early in the third. Retrospectively, cognitive and behavioral signs are present from early childhood in individuals with schizophrenia.

Twin studies, family studies, and adoption studies all demonstrate a strong genetic component to schizophrenia. These studies show conclusively that the risk of schizophrenia increases among close relatives. Figure 8-18 reveals the morbid risk for relatives of schizophrenics. The morbid risk is the probability that a person who survives through the period of greatest manifestation, in this case 18 to 45 years of age, will develop schizophrenia. The morbid risk in the general population is approximately 1%. This serves as a benchmark for comparing the risk of schizophrenia in relatives of schizophrenics. As shown, the risk for relatives is considerably higher than for the general population, and the risk varies as a function of the degree of genetic relatedness to the affected individual. The risk declines sharply as one moves from near to distant relatives.

In samples of parents of a schizophrenic child, the risk of a given parent developing schizophrenia is 6%. This value is of dual importance: *the majority of schizophrenics do not have affected parents, and the lack of schizophrenia in parents cannot be used to exclude the diagnosis in the child.* The risk to a child of a schizophrenic parent is, on the average, 13%. When both parents are schizophrenic, the risk to their offspring rises sharply to 46%.

The risk of siblings of a proband (affected child) is influenced by the status of the parents' mental health. When the parents are free of schizophrenia, the risk to a sibling of an affected individual is 9%. When one parent is also affected, the risk increases to 17%.

Both classical and modern studies concur that the concordance rate in MZ twins—the proportion of co-twins who are affected—is 48% (see Table 8-8). This concordance rate holds even when MZ twins are reared apart. This rate differs appreciably from that of DZ twins, which is 17%. The con-

TABLE 8-9. Prevalence Rates for Schizophrenia

Country	Affected Individuals*
Australia	285,000
Britain	250,000
Canada	280,000
China	6 to 12 million (estimate)
India	4.3 to 8.7 million (estimate)
United States	2.2 million
Worldwide	51 million (estimate)

*Approximately 1.1% of the population over 18 years of age.

Rate of Gray Matter Loss

Normal Adolescents   Schizophrenic Subjects

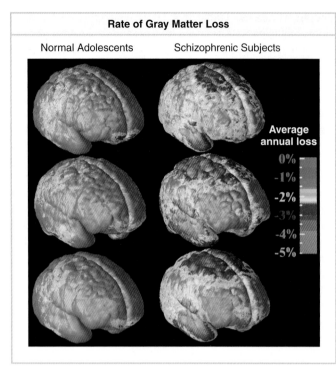

Average annual loss

0%
-1%
-2%
-3%
-4%
-5%

A

Figure 8-17. Three-dimensional maps of brain changes in childhood-onset schizophrenia derived from high-resolution magnetic resonance images. **A,** Average rates of gray matter loss in normal adolescents and in schizophrenia reveal profound, progressive gray matter loss in schizophrenia. Average rates of gray matter loss from 13 to 18 years in the same subjects show severe loss (red and pink; up to 5% annually) in parietal, motor, and temporal cortices, whereas inferior frontal cortices remain stable (blue; 0 to 1% loss). Dynamic loss is also observed in the parietal cortices of normal adolescents, but at a much slower rate. **B,** Deficits occurring during the development of schizophrenia are detected by comparing average profiles of gray matter between patients and controls at their first scan (age 13; *upper*) and their last scan 5 years later (age 18; *lower*). Although severe parietal, motor, and diffuse frontal loss has already occurred (*upper*) and subsequently continues, the temporal and dorsolateral prefrontal loss characteristic of adult schizophrenia is not found until later in adolescence (*lower*), where a process of fast attrition occurs over the next 5 years. The color code shows the significance of these effects. (Reprinted with permission from Thompson PM, Vidal C, Giedd JN, et al. Mapping adolescent brain change reveals dynamic wave of accelerated gray matter loss in very early-onset schizophrenia. *Proc Natl Acad Sci U S A.* 2001;98: 11650–11655.)

Early and Late Gray Matter Deficits in Schizophrenia

Earliest deficit

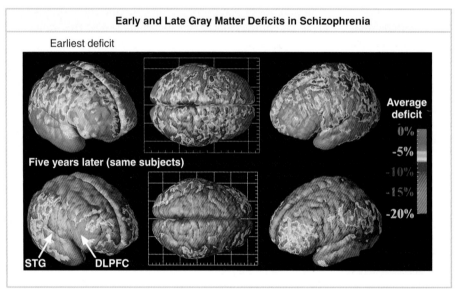

Five years later (same subjects)

STG   DLPFC

Average deficit

0%
-5%
-10%
-15%
-20%

B

cordance rate in DZ twins is in good agreement with family studies showing a 9% to 17% rate of schizophrenia among nontwin siblings. Therefore, as stated earlier, the twin data favor a significant genetic component in the etiology of schizophrenia, but since 52% of MZ twins are discordant, environmental factors are also strongly implicated.

Numerous studies have associated environmental factors with schizophrenia. The most common study design for these studies is the case-control study in which individuals with the disorder are compared with individuals not experiencing the disorder. These groups are matched for as many variables as possible such as age, sex, race, weight, background for different diseases, and geographic area. Statistical analysis demonstrates the strength of proposed associations. For schizophrenia, previous associations include illegal drug use, winter and spring birth, pregnancy and delivery complications, delayed development, low IQ, immigration status, and urban birth and domicile. The biggest disadvantage of case-control studies is that they provide little information about the absolute risk of the disorder.

The overarching implication of twin and family studies along with case control studies is that genes and environmental factors

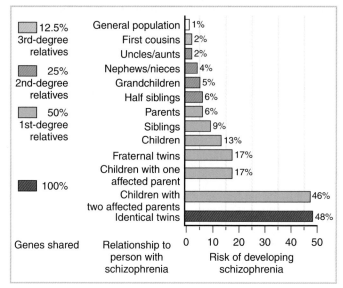

Figure 8-18. Risks of schizophrenia for relatives of individuals with schizophrenia.

involved in the etiology of schizophrenia most likely affect neurologic development (Fig. 8-19). Many studies have substantiated the role of genetics and heritability in brain morphology. In general, brains of individuals with schizophrenia are smaller than brains of controls and cerebral ventricles are larger. Several areas of the brain are specifically implicated in the schizophrenic phenotype including the basal ganglia, areas of the frontal lobe, Wernicke's area, the occipital lobe, the hippocampus, and the limbic system (Fig. 8-20). As might be expected. these are the areas of intense investigation for candidate genes involved in the pathophysiology of the disease.

The mechanism of inheritance for schizophrenia is complex. The number of specific susceptibility loci, the risks associated with these, and their interaction with each other and other genes is clearly unknown. It is even possible that schizophrenia is not a single disorder but a group of disorders with overlapping presentations that remain to be clearly delineated. Several susceptibility genes have strong associations with schizophrenia.

DTNBP1 Gene

The dystrobrevin-binding protein 1 gene (*DTNBP1*) is localized on chromosome 6p22.3. This protein, also known as dysbindin, has a strong association with schizophrenia by SNP and haplotype association studies. It localizes primarily in axon bundles, particularly at termini, of mossy fiber synaptic terminals in the cerebellum and hippocampus. This protein is ubiquitously expressed and binds to dystrobrevins seen in the dystrophin-associated protein complex (see Fig. 7-13). Dysbindin is also expressed in the hippocampus in the presynaptic termini of glutaminergic pathways. In individuals with schizophrenia, protein expression in the hippocampus is reduced and the expression of vesicular glutamate transporter proteins is increased. Thus, glutamate release may be decreased and may be related to decreased cognitive function.

NRG1 Gene

A strong association between the neuregulin gene and schizophrenia exists according to several population studies. However, different studies have demonstrated different haplotype associations. This gene is located at chromosome 8p21-22. This region is also deleted in individuals with velo-cardiofacial syndrome (VCFS), a disorder highly associated with an increased risk for schizophrenia. Twenty to thirty percent of individuals with this disorder develop schizophrenia. The *NRG1* gene spans more than 1.1 Mb and contains 21 alternatively spliced exons that produce at least 14 isoforms. Neuregulins and their receptors, the ERBB protein kinases, are essential for neuronal development and are important in expression and activation of neurotransmitter receptors such as the glutamate receptors. Neuregulin signaling from the axon is essential for Schwann cell survival, and these cells are essential for axon maintenance.

DAO and DAOA Genes

The D-amino acid oxidase gene (*DAO*) and D-amino acid oxidase activator gene (*DAOA*) are located at different loci, chromosome 12q24 and chromosome 13q34, respectively, but interact together. The exact functions of these two genes are unknown, but they are involved in glutamate receptor

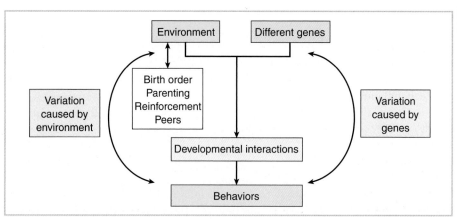

Figure 8-19. Behavior is dependent on both genes and environmental factors.

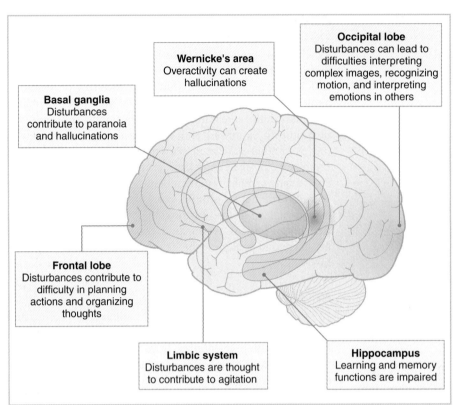

Figure 8-20. Regions of the brain affected by schizophrenia.

In the figure:

Wernicke's area
Overactivity can create hallucinations

Occipital lobe
Disturbances can lead to difficulties interpreting complex images, recognizing motion, and interpreting emotions in others

Basal ganglia
Disturbances contribute to paranoia and hallucinations

Frontal lobe
Disturbances contribute to difficulty in planning actions and organizing thoughts

Limbic system
Disturbances are thought to contribute to agitation

Hippocampus
Learning and memory functions are impaired

activation and four specific single nucleotide polymorphisms are associated with schizophrenia in case-control studies.

Other Candidate Genes

Several chromosomal regions have strong linkage and associations with schizophrenia. At least nine regions associated with schizophrenia have been identified; these include chromosomes 6p22-p24, 6q21-q25, 1q42, 1q21-q22, 13q32-q34, 8p21-p22, 22q11-q12, 5q21-q33, and 10p11-p15. Two of these are supported in multiple studies: chromosomes 8p and 22q. Chromosome 8p21-22 has been discussed above with neuregulin. Deletions of chromosome 22q11 account for associations in a smaller set of individuals with schizophrenia. Candidate genes in this region include catecholamine-O-methyl transferase (COMT), proline dehydrogenase (PRODH), and a zinc finger–DHHC domain (ZDHHC8). COMT participates in catecholamine degradation. A V158M mutation affects the activity and stability of the enzyme and is seen in decreased frontal lobe function tests for some individuals. Data are mixed for schizophrenic individuals, but data continue to support this finding in certain populations. SNP haplotype analysis (see Chapter 13) demonstrates strong association within specific populations for this gene.

The focus of many hypotheses about the etiology of schizophrenia and bipolar disorder is that there is a defect in GABAergic signaling. Studies demonstrate that down-regulation of two genes, reelin (RELN) and glutamic acid decarboxylase (GAD1) in telencephalic GABAergic neurons of schizophrenic patients correlates with increased expression of a DNA-methyltransferase (DNMT1) responsible for methylating cytosines in promoter CpG islands. Decreased expression of RELN and GAD1 leads to decreased conversion of glutamic acid to GABA. However, it is unclear whether these results are contributory to schizophrenia or a consequence of the disease.

Another area of focus is the metabolism of dopamine by catechol-O-methyltransferase in schizophrenia and bipolar disorder, since an imbalance of dopamine is considered key in the pathogenesis of psychosis. As noted above, COMT is located in a region deleted in VCFS, a syndrome with increased risk for schizophrenia. This enzyme catalyzes the transfer of a methyl group from S-adenosylmethionine to catecholamines, including the neurotransmitters dopamine, epinephrine, and norepinephrine (Fig. 8-21). Genetic variation producing reduced levels of this enzyme is also

BIOCHEMISTRY

D-Amino Acid Oxidase (DAO) Is a Peroxisomal Enzyme

The reaction

D-Amino acid + H_2O + O_2 = a 2-oxo acid + NH_3 + H_2O_2

requires an FAD coenzyme and catalyzes oxidative deamination of histamine, putrescine, or both. It is ubiquitous and highly expressed, especially in the brain, where it oxidizes D-serine—an activator of N-methyl-D-aspartate-type glutamate receptor.

associated with decreased prefrontal cortical function, a finding in both schizophrenia, bipolar disorder, ADHD, panic disorder, phobias, obsessive-compulsive disorder, and anorexia nervosa. Other similarities or related dissimilarities are seen in studies of families with independently occurring schizophrenia and bipolar disorder. Chromosomal studies implicate similar abnormalities in both disorders. Dopamine expression is similarly affected in both disorders, and several genes in the dopamine pathway are being investigated intensely. Likewise, interest in the dopaminergic pathway is of considerable interest to investigators for other disorders. Along with Parkinson disease, which has already been discussed, dopamine is hypothesized to play a role in ADHD and Tourette syndrome as well. Both schizophrenia and bipolar disorder demonstrate elevated levels of vesicular monoamine transporter (VMAT2 protein; *SLC18A2* gene) in the brainstem. This protein regulates neurotransmitter transport but is distributed differently in brains affected by the two disorders. Its proper function is essential for correct activity of the monoaminergic systems, and it is the site of action of several drugs including reserpine and tetrabenazine. Finally, the left side of the hippocampus is larger in brains affected with bipolar disorder, but the hippocampus is smaller in schizophrenia-affected brains.

Bipolar Disorder

Bipolar disorder, or manic-depressive illness, is a major illness characterized by mood swings between periods of mania, or hypomania, and depression. The two major forms of this disorder are bipolar disorder I and bipolar disorder II (Table 8-10). The similarities have suggested to some that these disorders may be variations of the same underlying etiology; however, sufficient differences exist to warrant separation (Table 8-11).

Bipolar disorder affects 1 to 2 million people in the United States per year and more than 121 million worldwide. It is the most common psychotic disorder, affecting approximately 1% to 1.5% of individuals in all age groups. Several biological factors are observed in bipolar disorder, but the role they play is unclear. They include oversecretion of cortisol, an efflux of calcium into brain cells, abnormal hyperactivity of prefrontal cortical glulamatergic system of the brain, and a change in circadian rhythm.

The effort to identify susceptibility genes for major psychiatric disorders, including schizophrenia and bipolar affective disorder, has been difficult and certainly lags behind other complex diseases such as diabetes mellitus and Alzheimer disease for both of which vulnerability genes have been identified. As noted above, advances in gene

NEUROLOGY

γ-Aminobutyric Acid (GABA)

GABA is a neurotransmitter. It acts at inhibitory synapses in the CNS. Inhibition results from hyperpolarization of the transmembrane potential when GABA binds to receptors. It is highly concentrated in the substantia nigra and globus pallidus nuclei of the basal ganglia, the hypothalamus, the periaqueductal gray matter, and the hippocampus. GABAergic neurons use GABA as a neurotransmitter.

PHARMACOLOGY

Monoamine Oxidase (MAO) Inhibitors

MAO inhibitors were the first drugs used as antidepressants. They inhibit MAO and prevent catabolism of catecholamines. They work more rapidly than tricyclic antidepressants, which prevent uptake of norepinephrine and serotonin. MAO inhibitors also block tyramine catabolism, which results in increased blood pressure.

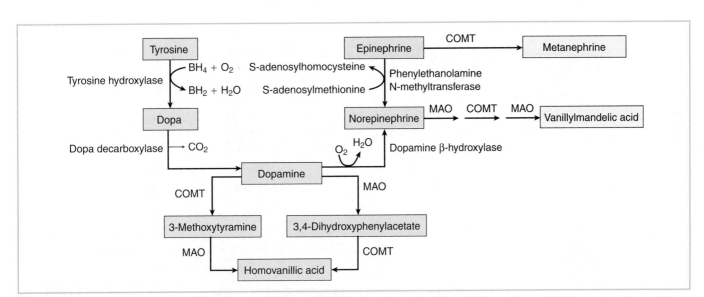

Figure 8-21. Biosynthesis and metabolism of dopamine. COMT, catecholamine-*O*-methyl transferase; MAO, monoamine oxidase.

identification are occurring with schizophrenia, but they have not provided a clear picture of how the disease develops and progresses. The greatest obstacles to progress with identification of genes involved in psychiatric disorders include the following:

- Incomplete penetrance and nonmendelian inheritance
- Inadequate definition of phenotypes
- Etiologic heterogeneity and diagnostic comorbidity
- Insufficient standards in valid diagnostic definitions

As a result of these types of challenges, many studies have been unable to corroborate loci associated with the disease that are easily supported in other studies.

Notwithstanding these difficulties, MZ studies strongly support a genetic component for about 60% of cases of bipolar disorder. The interpretation of data is complicated, however, by the co-occurrence of other psychiatric diseases at a higher rate in families with bipolar disorder. These include anxiety disorders, schizophrenia, attention-deficit/hyperactivity disorder (ADHD), and major depression. In fact, proper diagnosis may be masked because symptoms of these may be similar. For example, bipolar disorder symptoms may be confused with ADHD in children. To complicate the diagnosis further, some of these disorders may coexist, such as ADHD and bipolar disorder or schizophrenia and bipolar disorder.

The first-degree relatives of individuals with bipolar I disorder are seven times more likely to have the disease than the general population (1% to 1.5%). The offspring of an affected parent have a 50% risk of having a major psychiatric disorder. Studies have not implicated a specific gene association in this disease although a few have been suggested in a general mechanism shared between several disorders such as schizophrenia and bipolar disorder.

Association studies have demonstrated that an increased incidence of bipolar disorder occurs in individuals born during the winter and with complications at birth. Bipolar disorder also occurs more frequently among individuals with higher socioeconomic status. Additionally, there is an increased incidence among individuals who lost a parent in early childhood. Diabetes is diagnosed three times more often in individuals with bipolar disease. Table 8-12 shows that not only is diabetes more prevalent in individuals with bipolar disorder but migraines, suicides, hypothyroidism, and substance abuse are also commonly seen in these affected individuals.

Disturbances in neurotransmitter function have been studied using several of the methods already described. A gene of particular interest has been the dopamine D4 receptor (DRD4) located on chromosome 11p15.5. This gene contains an unusual 48-bp repeat that is present 2 to 11 times, yielding different functional polymorphisms; the most common allele contains four repeats (DRD4.4). The gene is expressed in many areas of the body but is highly expressed in the frontal area of the brain and nucleus accumbens, areas that are associated with a lack of motivation and affective and emotional behaviors. Early association studies were often contradictory and highlighted the issues apparent with small sample sizes. More recent *meta-analysis* studies, or the combination of data from other studies to yield a larger sample

TABLE 8-10. Classification of Bipolar Disorders

Type	Description
Bipolar I	Mania and major depression
Bipolar II	Hypomania and major depression
Bipolar III	Cyclothymia
Bipolar IV	Antidepressant-induced hypomania
Bipolar V	Major depression with a family history of bipolar disorder
Bipolar VI	Unipolar mania

TABLE 8-11. Distinguishing Features Between Bipolar I and Bipolar II

	Bipolar I	Bipolar II
Manic episodes	At least one with or without depression	At least one episode of hypomania and at least one episode of major depression
	In 60% to 70% of cases, manic episodes precede or follow depressive episodes	Most function normally between episodes
	Average of four episodes per year	More chronic course than bipolar I—more depressive episodes, shorter periods of wellness than bipolar I
	Significant negative effects on social and work life	
	Duration of 1 week to months, if untreated	Highly associated with risk for suicide
Depressive episodes	Duration of 6 to 12 months, if untreated	Difficult to distinguish between unipolar (major) depression and bipolar II depression
		Typically lasts 2 to 3 months
		Depressive episodes tend to develop gradually

TABLE 8-12. Commonly Seen Associations with Bipolar Disorders Compared with Prevalence in the General Population

Associations with Bipolar Disorder	Prevalence in Patients with Bipolar Disorder	Prevalence in General Population
Diabetes	10% to 11%	3.4%
Suicide	15% to 20% overall with no treatment Bipolar I: >50% Children: 25%	0.01% (USA)
Migraines	Bipolar I: 14% Bipolar II: 77%	11% overall (USA, western Europe) 6% males 15% to 18% females
Substance abuse	>60% Most commonly alcohol followed by marijuana or cocaine	10% (U.S. adults) 20% (estimated; physicians' patients)
Hypothyroidism	10.4% (lithium-associated) 4.5% males 14% females	4.6% (USA) 2% to 5% (iodine deficiency worldwide)

TABLE 8-13. Major Types of Mania

Type	Characteristics
Hypomania	Euphoria
Severe mania	Euphoria, grandiosity, high levels of sexual drive, irritability, volatility, psychosis, paranoia, aggression
Extreme mania	Most of the displeasures; few pleasures

BIOCHEMISTRY

B-Cell CLL/Lymphoma 2 (*BCL2*)

There are 25 members of the *BCL2* family of genes classified into three subgroups:

- Anti-apoptotic: *BCL2*, *BCLxL*, and others
- Proapoptotic: *BAX*, *BAK*, *BOK*
- Proapoptotic: *BID*, *BAD*, and others

BCL2 regulates cytochrome c release and mitochondrial membrane permeability.

PHARMACOLOGY

Lithium

Lithium is effective in 60% to 80% of all hypomanic and manic episodes. It acts on signal transduction mechanisms such as G protein, glycogen synthase kinase–3β, protein kinase C, adenylyl cyclase, and phosphoinositide hydrolysis, to change neuronal signaling patterns.

Lithium affects the function of NMDA receptors by regulating glutamate-induced calcium entry by an unknown mechanism. Suppression of receptor function may occur by inhibition of glycogen synthase kinase. Lithium is concentrated in the thyroid by active transport against a concentration gradient and inhibits secretion of T_3 and T_4 and can lead to hypothyroidism and goiter.

PHARMACOLOGY

Valproate

Valproate is an anti-seizure agent that is also effective for many individuals with bipolar II disorder and mania. Some studies show better compliance with valproate than with lithium. It increases GABA available to the CNS and prolongs recovery of inactivated Na^+ channels. In neurons, it inhibits repetitive firing through interaction with voltage-sensitive Na^+ channels. Valproate will also alter fatty acid metabolism, impair β-oxidation in mitochondria, and disrupt the urea cycle, leading to hyperammonemia.

with stronger statistical power, demonstrate that the *DRD4.2* polymorphism (the *DRD4* gene with two 48-bp repeats) is significantly associated with unipolar depression and combined unipolar and bipolar depression. Stated differently, individuals with the *DRD4.2* allele have a higher risk of depression. The *DRD4.7* allele is associated with ADHD and schizophrenia. How the dopamine receptor is regulated is not fully understood. However, one function of the receptor is the inhibition of adenylyl cyclase, causing a reduction in ATP to cAMP conversion. Some reports suggest the DRD4.2 receptor, as well as other allelic forms, functions less effectively than the normal receptor, resulting in a blunted intracellular response to dopamine, and thus accounts for the clinical features of depression.

Early-onset disease occurs in individuals with first symptoms occurring during childhood or adolescence. Disease in children differs slightly from adult disease. The initial events of early-onset disease are general depression that develops later into bipolar I or bipolar II disorder. Manic events usually begin at an average age of 18 years (Table 8-13). Early-onset disease is associated with a family history of bipolar disorder, a higher incidence of comorbidity, and a more severe disease in children than in adults. Adult-onset disease may appear at age 40 or later. It is also possible for adult-onset disease to occur after years of repeated unipolar major depression or to accompany other medical or neurologic problems. An example is the development of bipolar disorder following a stroke. Adult-onset disease is less likely to be associated with a positive family history of bipolar disorder than is early-onset disease.

Two effective treatments for bipolar disorder are the use of lithium and valproate. These drugs up-regulate *BCL2* expression, which has an anti-apoptotic function, in the frontal cortex and hippocampus. Since neuroimaging studies suggest cell loss in these regions of the brain, one hypothesis is that bipolar disorder occurs from abnormal apoptosis in these regions of the brain. Thus, lithium and valproate may stabilize mood by stimulating alternative cell survival pathways and increasing neurotrophic factors.

Cardiopulmonary Disorders 9

This chapter presents an overview of the major heritable cardiopulmonary disorders in humans. Inherited disease among the cardiopulmonary disorders with well-characterized genetics is uncommon relative to that in other organ systems, perhaps reflecting a high degree of mortality associated with severe heart or lung disease. Here, both classical, common monogenic diseases, such as familial hypercholesterolemia and cystic fibrosis (CF), and rare disorders with complex and heterogeneous genetic etiologies, represented by long QT

syndrome and α_1-antitrypsin deficiency, are featured. When possible, a discussion on therapeutic intervention is included although no cures currently exist for these diseases.

●●● CARDIAC AND VASCULAR-RELATED DISORDERS

Familial Hypercholesterolemia

Familial hypercholesterolemia (FH) is caused by a mutation altering the structure and function of a cell surface receptor that is specific for low-density lipoprotein (LDL). When this receptor is reduced, absent, or malfunctioning, it results in persistently elevated levels of cholesterol in the blood, ultimately leading to early coronary heart disease.

LDL Receptor

The LDL receptor gene (*LDLR*) is found on chromosome 19 p13.1-13.3 and spans 45 kb. The gene contains 18 exons constituting a 5.3-kb mRNA and encodes a single-chain glycoprotein that consists of 839 amino acids (Fig. 9-1). Exons 2 through 6 make up the ligand-binding site, which is composed of seven

PATHOLOGY

Classifying Lipoproteins

There are several ways to classify lipoproteins. The most widely used systems recognize the differences in densities during ultracentrifugation and electrophoresis. $\downarrow\downarrow$ = greatly decreased; $\uparrow$ = increased; $\uparrow\uparrow$ = greatly increased.

Type	Elevated Lipoprotein	Laboratory Findings	Serum TC	Serum TG	Example
I	Chylomicrons	Very high triglycerides	Normal	$\downarrow\downarrow$	Lipoprotein lipase deficiency
IIa	LDL	High cholesterol	$\uparrow\uparrow$	Normal	Familial hypercholesterolemia, familial apolipoprotein B
IIb	LDL and VLDL	High cholesterol and triglycerides	$\uparrow\uparrow$	$\uparrow$	Familial hypercholesterolemia, familial combined hyperlipidemia
III	IDL	High cholesterol and triglycerides	$\uparrow$ or normal	$\uparrow$	Dysbetalipoproteinemia
IV	VLDL	High triglycerides	$\uparrow$	$\uparrow\uparrow$	Familial hypertriglyceridemia
V	Chylomicrons and VLDL	Very high triglycerides and high cholesterol	$\uparrow$	$\uparrow\uparrow$	Severe hypertriglyceridemia

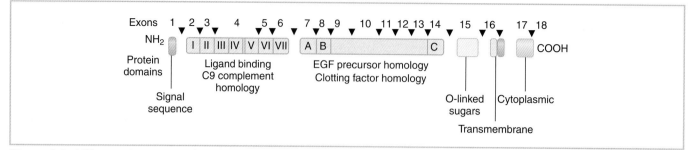

Figure 9-1. LDL receptor gene and protein structure. The domains of the protein are shown and are labeled in the lower portion. The seven cysteine-rich, 40-amino-acid repeats in the LDL binding domain are assigned numerals I to VII. Repeats IV and V are separated by eight amino acids. The three cysteine-rich repeats in the domain that is homologous with the EGF precursor are lettered A to C. Arrowheads indicate the positions where introns interrupt the coding region. Exon numbers are shown between the arrowheads.

tandem repeats of roughly 40 amino acids. Each repeat harbors six cysteine residues. Also, the C-terminal ends of each repeat are characterized by a group of negatively charged amino acids that play a direct role in binding basic amino acid–rich segments of apolipoprotein B-100.

An interesting feature of the *LDLR* gene is that it shares exons with other genes. Exons 7 to 14 of the *LDLR* gene encode a region homologous with the epithelial growth factor (EGF) precursor. In fact, the EGF precursor contains the same eight exons. Other *LDLR* exons have been found in members of at least three different gene families. The sharing of exons between the LDL receptor gene and the other genes is referred to as *exon shuffling*. Exon shuffling hypothesizes that introns permit functional domains encoded by discrete exons to shuffle between different proteins, thereby allowing proteins to evolve as mosaic combinations of preexisting functional units. The LDL receptor is a vivid example of such a mosaic protein.

LDL Metabolism

LDL receptors are localized in clathrin-coated pits found primarily in liver cells and bind the apolipoprotein B-100 ligand—the only protein found in LDL. As cholesterol-rich LDL molecules are endocytosed into the cell, they dissociate from the receptor, and the detached receptor protein is recycled to the cell surface (Fig. 9-2). The LDL molecule is incorporated into a lysosome and degraded. The resulting free cholesterol can then be incorporated into cell membranes or metabolized into bile salts or steroids.

An important aspect of the normal processing of LDL is the mechanism by which the surface receptors mediate feedback control of cholesterol synthesis. Excessive levels of free cholesterol inhibit cholesterol synthesis and LDL receptor synthesis, thus reducing LDL uptake and promoting cholesterol storage. Free cholesterol represses 3-hydroxy-3-methylglutaryl coenzyme A (HMG-CoA) reductase, the rate-limiting step in cholesterol synthesis. One consequence of restricting the cell's uptake of LDL molecules is that serum cholesterol levels remain high with a risk of accumulating in arterial walls. Serum LDL appears to be the major source of cholesterol in atherosclerotic plaques, and the two most

devastating sequelae of atherosclerotic plaques in arterial walls are myocardial infarction and stroke.

Genetics of Familial Hypercholesterolemia

FH is a single-gene disorder due to mutations in the *LDLR* gene that result in either absent or defective receptors. It is a common autosomal dominant disease that spares no racial or ethnic group. More than 420 mutations have been identified that disrupt LDLR function. Phenotypic expression is variable owing in part to the many different mutations that

PHYSIOLOGY

Acute Myocardial Infarction

Most acute myocardial infarction (AMI) occurs from thrombotic occlusion and coronary atherosclerosis. Atherosclerosis may preexist for years, but precipitation of acute thrombotic occlusion occurs because of the instability of plaques. AMI can be seen with hemorrhage, fissuring, and plaque rupture. In more than 90% of patients, Q-wave infarcts, characterized by an elevated S-T segment, result when occlusive thrombi persist and a large area of the myocardium is blocked. Non-Q-wave infarcts, characterized by S-T segment depression, result from incomplete thrombi where less of the myocardium is affected and necrosis is not elicited.

PHYSIOLOGY

Stroke

A cerebral infarction, or stroke, occurs when there is an interruption of blood flow to the brain.

Ischemic stroke occurs when a blood vessel is blocked, reducing the flow of O_2 and nutrients to areas beyond the blockage, and waste material beyond the blockage cannot be removed. This is the most common cause of stroke.

Hemorrhagic stroke occurs when a blood vessel ruptures causing hemorrhaging that reduces blood flow and leading to decreased mean arterial pressure and thus reduced blood flow to tissues.

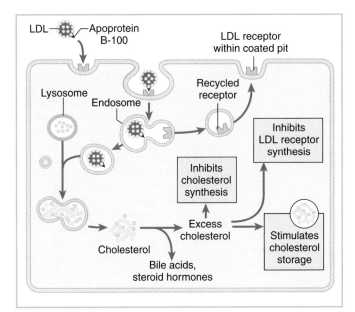

Figure 9-2. Circulating LDL binds to specific receptors synthesized in the cell. The receptors localize in depressions ("coated pits") in the cell surface. LDL particles are engulfed by endocytosis, and the coated pit pinches off to form a vesicle (endosome). LDL dissociates from the receptor, and the latter is recycled to the cell surface. The LDL is delivered to a lysosome, where enzymatic action results in free cholesterol that is used to meet cellular needs (such as steroid hormone production). The cellular level of cholesterol is controlled by at least three feedback loops. Excessive levels of cholesterol serve to (1) inhibit cholesterol synthesis, (2) inhibit receptor synthesis (hence, inhibit LDL uptake), and (3) stimulate the storage of cholesterol in the form of cholesteryl esters.

occur at the *LDLR* locus. Point mutations or deletions in the gene may render a nonfunctional *or* an absent protein depending on the location of the point mutation or extent of the deletion. LDLR protein may be normal in certain respects (e.g., its binding capacity for LDL is normal in vitro) but unable to escape from the endoplasmic reticulum and therefore unable to reach the plasma membrane (Fig. 9-3). Alternatively, the protein may insert into the plasma membrane, but its capacity to bind LDL will be severely impaired or nonexistent.

Phenotypic effects are manifested in *both* heterozygotes and homozygotes with FH. Heterozygotes have half the number of normal LDL receptors while FH homozygous individuals have no or exceedingly few receptors. Notably in this disease, there is a direct correlation between the number and activity of functioning LDL receptors, levels of plasma LDL-cholesterol, and the age of onset and severity of the resulting atherosclerosis. The clinical manifestations of each scenario are described below.

Heterozygous Familial Hypercholesterolemia

Heterozygous FH is the second most common single gene–determined disorder in humans, affecting 1 in 500 persons in the United States (Table 9-1). As a rule,

PATHOLOGY

Atherosclerotic Lesions

Atherosclerosis is responsible for the majority of cases of myocardial and cerebral infarction, and it exists in two forms. Fatty streak, or early, lesions are the more common form. They usually are confined to the intima, creating flat, yellow areas on the artery surface. Initially, they are composed of foam cells, macrophages, and T cells but later also can include smooth muscle cells.

Fibrous plaque, or advanced lesions, also exist in the intima, creating raised, pearly gray areas on the surface and leading to narrowing and thickening of artery. The plaque is covered by dense connective tissue at the luminal surface (fibrous cap) and composed of lipid-laden smooth muscle cells, macrophages, and T cells. The plaque covers an area of foam cells, necrotic debris, and cholesterol. Fibrous plaques become a *complicated lesion* once there is extensive degeneration and calcification.

TABLE 9-1. Incidence of Common Single-Gene Disorders

Single Gene Disorder	Incidence
Hemochromatosis	1 in 200 to 1 in 500
Hypercholesterolemia	1 in 500
Sickle cell anemia	1 in 600 (African ancestry)
Cystic fibrosis	1 in 1600 (European ancestry)
Tay-Sachs disease	1 in 3500 (Ashkenazi Jewish ancestry)
Huntington disease	1 in 5000
Phenylketonuria	1 in 10,000

heterozygotes remain asymptomatic until the third to fourth decade, although hypercholesterolemia is present from birth. With no reduced reproductive fitness the persistence of the high disease allele frequency is explained. Manifestations of the condition include xanthomas of the tendons, particularly the Achilles and tendons around the knees and elbows (Fig. 9-4) and in the hand. The tendon xanthomas are deposits of cholesterol and are virtually pathognomonic. Their incidence increases with age and they eventually manifest in about 80% of heterozygotes. Less specific signs, found also in persons with normal lipid levels, are xanthelasma (palpebral xanthomas) and arcus cornealis (Fig. 9-5).

Far more serious are symptoms of coronary disease, which develop in most patients during the third to fourth decades of life. Frank infarctions begin to occur in the fourth decade and peak in the fifth and sixth decades. By age 60, as many as 85% of affected individuals have sustained an infarction.

FH heterozygotes are expected to produce defective or absent LDLR protein from one allele but normal LDLR

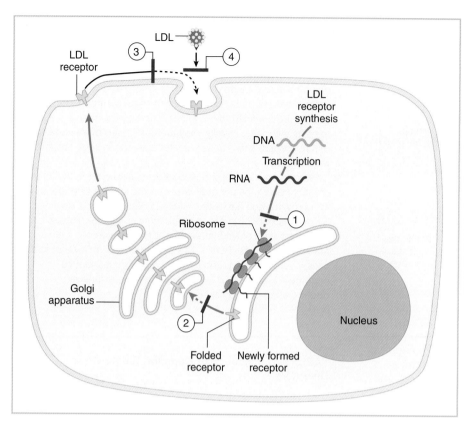

Figure 9-3. Familial hypercholesterolemia is caused by several genetic defects, all involving the gene for the LDL receptor molecule. Sometimes the gene is either missing or so damaged that the receptor is not transcribed and processed into a functional mRNA (1). Alternatively, the receptor may be translated and folded but is still sufficiently abnormal that it is not transported to the cell surface (2) or, if it reaches the surface, cannot migrate along the cell membrane to the coated pits, which are the only sites where LDL can be internalized (3). In still other defects, the receptor reaches the coated pits, but its capacity to bind LDL is reduced (4). In all cases, the ultimate result is the same: reduced cellular intake of LDL, leading to higher serum LDL levels and atherogenesis.

proteins from the other allele. It is possible, however, especially with the high incidence of heterozygosity, for two individuals carrying different mutant alleles to produce a child carrying both mutations. The mutant alleles may be unable to complement each other in the *compound heterozygote*, leading to a severe form of FH.

Homozygous Familial Hypercholesterolemia

Homozygous FH is a rare disease, occurring in approximately 1 in 1 million persons born with the complete absence of functional receptors. These patients have severe hypercholesterolemia (600–1000 mg/dL; normal, 150–230 mg/dL) at birth and develop raised, yellowish, cutaneous xanthomas by age 4. Tendon xanthomas and arcus cornealis are typically present in childhood. Severe, persistent atherosclerosis leads to early-onset coronary heart disease; death from myocardial infarction before age 30 is common.

Although homozygosity is rare, homozygous FH has been an important paradigm of human lipoprotein metabolism from several different perspectives. First, this condition established the role that LDL plays in human atherosclerosis. Second, FH established the first genetic basis for atherosclerosis. Third, this disease has emerged as a model for understanding the variable phenotypic expression of a complex disorder. Finally, FH has played a key role in developing new therapies for forestalling, if not preventing, human atherosclerosis.

Experimental Therapies for Familial Hypercholesterolemia

FH heterozygotes are treated with more conventional therapies than FH homozygotes: diet plus a combination of niacin, an inhibitor of HMG-CoA reductase, and a bile acid sequestrant can reduce the total cholesterol and LDL cholesterol concentrations in FH heterozygotes by as much as 50%. Because 50% to 70% of LDL receptors are located

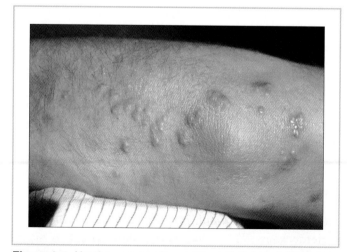

Figure 9-4. Xanthomas on elbow. (From Feit J et al: *Hypertext Atlas of Dermatology*. Available at: ttp://www.muni.cz/atlases.)

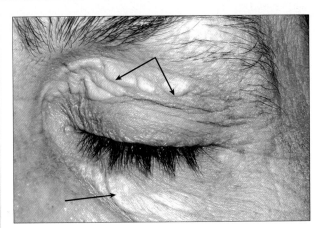

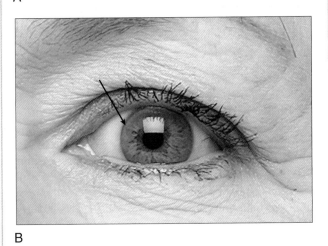

A

B

Figure 9-5. Xanthelasma (**A**) and corneal arcus (**B**). (From Feit J et al: *Hypertext Atlas of Dermatology*. Available at: http://www.muni.cz/atlases.)

in the liver, the most efficacious modern therapeutic option for FH homozygotes has been liver transplantation, which provides cells with normal, active LDL receptors. The profound effect of liver transplantation has been to normalize the plasma lipoprotein concentrations as well as to induce regression of the tissue deposition of cholesterol. Cholesterol levels decrease postoperatively to normal or near-normal levels, and many patients require no additional pharmacologic intervention, such as therapies with statins, to further reduce and maintain cholesterol levels. Within 5 years after successful liver transplantation, xanthomas in many patients have regressed and coronary artery lesions have stabilized. Some lesions may even have regressed. Transplantation is most successful when done prior to the onset of cardiovascular complications resulting from the course of the disease.

Development of novel gene therapy protocols will benefit from efficient routine means of delivering genomic DNA to cells. Several gene therapy strategies have been investigated in animal models with varying levels of success. A limitation of some earlier strategies was that vector systems carrying

BIOCHEMISTRY

Niacin

Niacin is a vitamin. It is pyridine-3-carboxylic acid, which is a component of the coenzymes NAD and NADP. More than 200 enzymes require these coenzymes for electron transfer in redox reactions. NAD frequently functions in catabolic reactions to produce energy; NADP functions more often in anabolic reactions such as cholesterol and fatty acid synthesis. Most niacin comes from the diet, since synthesis from tryptophan is inefficient. A mild deficiency causes glossitis; a marked deficiency causes pellagra.

PHYSIOLOGY

Bile Acids Are End Products of Cholesterol Metabolism

Cholesterol is excreted in bile as free cholesterol and bile acids. Bile acids and phospholipids solubilize cholesterol in bile. When bile acids cannot be recycled, they can be synthesized in the liver and stored in the gallbladder. Those bile acids that are transferred to the small intestine but not reabsorbed at the portal vein are then converted to secondary acids. Some secondary acids are reabsorbed in the colon.

Some drugs, such as colestipol, which cause decreased bile acid reabsorption in the intestine, will cause an increase in plasma cholesterol conversion to bile acids. This, in turn, increases cholesterol synthesis.

PHARMACOLOGY

Statins

The statin family of drugs inhibits HMG-CoA reductase in the liver. They are the most commonly used cholesterol-lowering drugs. Lovastatin and simvastatin are prodrugs, whereas others are in the active form. Statins may be used in combination with other drugs for greater effect.

Statins are metabolized by the cytochrome P-450 3A4 system. Drugs inhibiting P-450 3A4 increase plasma statin concentration and can increase the toxicity risk. Grapefruit juice contains a substance that acts as a natural statin inhibitor for some statins. Drugs that induce P-450, such as barbiturates, will increase statin metabolism.

Statins are teratogenic.

DNA into cells could incorporate only small fragments of DNA while entire genes often exceed this limitation. This was coupled with low efficiencies of delivering large (>100 kb) DNA inserts to cells. Original vector systems relied on viruses, such as adenovirus, lentivirus, or retrovirus, with limited capacity for additional DNA incorporation or unacceptable immunogenicity. Newer systems employ bacterial artificial chromosomes (BACs) that will accept large DNA inserts needed to replace entire genes. The efficiency of the BAC DNA delivery is still low, but progress is being made to improve efficiency and demonstrate stable incorporation and expression of genes in human cells.

One approach to improve efficiency has been to modify a BAC to become infectious. A BAC was identified containing the complete 45-kb *LDLR* genomic DNA locus within a 135-kb insert. The insert contains all 18 *LDLR* exons, the introns, and the promoter. Immediately adjacent to the promoter are three steroid response elements (SREs) critical for promoter regulation by steroids. This BAC was converted by molecular manipulation to an infectious vector incorporating elements from herpes simplex virus (HSV-1) and Epstein-Barr virus (EBV). The modified BAC was then used to infect human fibroblasts in culture from receptor-negative FH patients. Transfection of the infectious BAC containing the *LDLR* gene, promoter, and controlling elements was highly efficient compared with the noninfectious BAC construct. In addition, and most importantly, the *LDLR* gene insert restored LDLR expression to appropriate levels.

Familial hypercholesterolemia is a classical monogenic loss-of-function disease, and homozygous FH has long been considered a candidate for a gene replacement strategy. The application of molecular genetics to BACs and the *LDLR* gene provides several advantages for gene therapy strategies. First, the gene is controlled by its own promoter, which will drive expression at a physiologically relevant level. Second, the gene is expressed from a genomic DNA sequence, including all intron sequences. This allows alternative splicing to occur that can produce alternative forms of the protein in a tissue-specific or developmentally regulated fashion. Third, the critical noncoding elements that control gene expression at a transcriptional level are present and correctly oriented toward the promoter to control expression. These three features can be easily combined in a gene delivery vector with the capacity to deliver other complete genomic DNA loci.

BIOCHEMISTRY

Steroid Response Elements

Two different response elements have been identified for steroids. The SRE with a consensus sequence of 5'-GGTACAnnnTGTTGT-3' is bound by the androgen receptor (AR), glucocorticoid receptor (GR), progesterone receptor (PR), and mineralocorticoid receptor (MR).

The estrogen response element (ERE) with a consensus sequence of 5'-AGGTCAnnnTGACCT-3' is recognized only by the estrogen receptor.

The mechanism of transmission of cues from receptors to response elements is unknown.

Long QT Syndrome

The long QT (LQT) syndromes are a collection of related cardiac ion channel defects that alter myocardial repolarization, culminating in prolonged electrocardiographic QT intervals and a form of ventricular tachycardia (Fig. 9-6) termed *torsades de pointes* (TdP). Prolonged QT may occur from either a decrease in repolarization of cardiac currents or an increase in depolarizing cardiac currents, although the former occurs more commonly owing to reductions in potassium currents (IKr or IKs). The ion channel abnormalities predispose a person to arrhythmia that may result in sudden syncope, or to a sudden drop in blood pressure resulting in temporary loss of consciousness. This is perhaps the most common clinical sign seen in the LQT syndromes. The syncopal events can be solitary and rare or recur frequently. If not corrected, the TdP may degenerate to ventricular fibrillation and sudden death. In the United States, the LQT syndromes have a prevalence of 1 in 7000

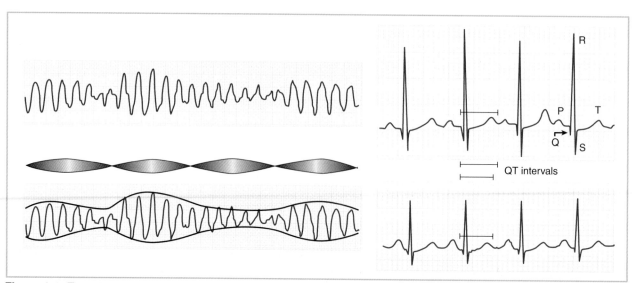

Figure 9-6. Torsades de pointes (French, "twisting of points") is a cardiac arrhythmia seen with prolonged QT intervals in long QT syndrome (LQTS).

PHYSIOLOGY

Cardiac Action Potentials

Differences in cardiac action potential occur in different areas of the heart. These differences are caused by the different types and distribution of channels, and they reflect differences seen in initiation time, shape, and duration of the potential. Four major time-dependent and voltage-gated membrane currents are seen in cardiac action potentials:

- The Na$^+$ current (I_{na}) is responsible for rapid depolarization of the action potential in the atria, ventricles, and Purkinje fibers.
- The Ca^{++} current (I_{ca}) is responsible for rapid depolarization of the action potential in the sinoatrial (SA) and atrioventricular (AV) nodes. This current also initiates contractions in cardiomyocytes.
- The K$^+$ current (I_K) is responsible for repolarization of the action potential in cardiomyocytes.
- The "pacemaker current" (I_f) is partially responsible for the pacemaker activity of the SA and AV nodal cells and Purkinje fibers.

PHYSIOLOGY

QT Interval

The time in seconds between the start of the Q wave and the end of the T wave on an ECG is the QT interval. It represents the time it takes ventricles to contract and recover. Heart rate is dependent on the QT interval. Bazett's formula is the most popular clinical method to describe QT interval/heart rate relationship:

$$QTc = QT/\sqrt{RR}$$

where QTc is the QT interval corrected for heart rate and RR (heart rate) is the interval (measured in seconds) from the onset of one QRS complex to the onset of the next complex. The formula overcorrects at high heart rates and undercorrects at slow heart rates. Normal values range from 0.30 to 0.44 seconds (0.45 seconds in women).

individuals. Indeed, it is estimated that congenital LQT syndrome may be responsible for nearly 4000 cases of sudden childhood death annually. Accordingly, LQT syndromes may also account for a percentage of sudden infant death syndrome (SIDS) cases.

Seven genes are associated with LQT syndrome (Table 9-2). Five of the genes are associated with two syndromes: Romano-Ward (RW) syndrome and Jervell and Lange-Nielsen (JLN) syndrome. Prior to molecular characterization of the gene mutations within individuals and families with LQT syndrome, the two syndromes were recognized as unique, thus underscoring the phenotypic heterogeneity that has become clearer with molecular studies. Both syndromes present with LQT syndrome but differ in the presence or

PHARMACOLOGY

Acquired Long QT Syndrome

Acquired LQTS generally results from drug use or metabolic abnormalities. Common causes include the following:

- Drugs: all block the IKr current mediated by the *KCNH2*-encoded potassium channel (HERG protein). This is not apparent before exposure to the drug. Major classes of drugs that can cause LQTS are antiarrhythmic drugs, certain nonsedating antihistamines (terfenadine and astemizole have been removed from the market), macrolide antibiotics, antipsychotics, and antidepressants.
- Electrolyte abnormalities: hypokalemia and hypomagnesemia.
- Eating disorders.
- Stroke.

absence of hearing and in the mechanism of inheritance. Normal hearing and autosomal dominant transmission characterize RW syndrome, whereas JLN syndrome features sensorineural hearing loss and autosomal recessive inheritance. The two additional LQT syndromes have been proposed as candidates for RM but currently have not been designated as such. In RW and JLN syndromes, four genes produce potassium channel proteins. A Na$^+$ channel protein gene is involved with LQT3, also a member of the RW syndrome family.

Romano-Ward Syndrome

The most common forms of LQT syndrome are LQT1, LQT2, and LQT3. Among these, LQT1 is the most common and represents more than 60% of cases. LQT2 represents about 35% of cases, and LQT3 less than 5% of cases. The other forms are quite rare.

The autosomal dominant forms of LQT syndrome are responsible for the majority of cases. Three distinct ST-T wave phenotypes associated with five different genes are recognized as RW syndrome (see Table 9-2). As with most forms of LQT syndrome, *characteristic "triggering" events are associated with precipitating cardiac events.* LQT1, for example, seems to be triggered by exercise, particularly swimming, and emotional stress. Incredibly, 99% of cardiac events occurring while swimming involve individuals with LQT1.

LQT2, representing approximately 35% of cases, is due to mutations in the *KCNH2* gene on chromosome 7. Auditory stimuli such as telephone ringing or an alarm clock may provoke LQT2 onset. Over 80% of cardiac events associated with auditory stimuli occur in individuals with LQT2.

LQT3, associated with 10% of cases, is due to a mutation in the *SCN5A* gene on chromosome 3. This gene codes for the cardiac Na$^+$ channel. Sleep or undisturbed rest apparently triggers LQT3, suggesting that slowed heart rate is a risk factor.

As mentioned above, RW syndrome accounts for most LQT syndrome cases. Although greater than 200 different

TABLE 9-2. Comparison Between Long QT Syndromes

Type	Syndrome AD	Syndrome AR	Gene Name	Protein	Chromosome	Initiating Factors
LQT1	RW	JLN1	KCNQ1	KVLQT1	11p15.6	Exercise, such as swimming, and emotional stress; responds to β-blockers
LQT2	RW		KCNH2	HERG	7q35-36	Startled by noise, such as alarm clocks and ringing telephone
LQT3	RW		SCN5A	Nav 1.5	3p21-24	Occurs during sleep; more likely to be fatal than LQT1 or LQT2; responds best to mexiletine than other forms; also called Brugada syndrome
LQT4	Sick sinus syndrome with bradycardia		ANKB	Ankyrin-B	4q25-27	Exercise and emotional stress
LQT5	RW	JLN2	KCNE1	Mink	21q22.1-22.2	Sympathetic stimulation
LQT6	RW		KCNE2	MiRP1	21q22.1-22.2	Certain medications and exercise
LQT7	Andersen		KCNJ2	Kir2.1	17q23	Hypokalemia; also known as Andersen syndrome; patients can develop periodic paralysis (usually associated with hypokalemia) and skeletal developmental abnormalities

mutations have been associated with RW syndrome, nearly 30% of clinically diagnosed RW individuals do not have mutations in one of the five genes described above. Hence, additional genetic loci, representing genetic heterogeneity of the syndrome, appear to be involved in the etiology. Penetrance is also incomplete in RW syndrome, and 30% to 50% of individuals harboring a disease-causing mutation in one of the five RW genes show no symptoms. Overall, LQT syndrome is a genetically heterogeneous and mechanistically complex disorder.

Jervell and Lange-Nielsen Syndrome

JLN syndrome is a rare, autosomal recessive form of LQT syndrome that features congenital bilateral sensorineural hearing loss. The estimated prevalence for JLN syndrome is 3 in 1 million individuals. Whereas heterozygous mutations in the *KCNQ1* gene result in the LQT1 phenotype of RW syndrome, the *homozygous* (or compound heterozygous) mutations precipitate JLN syndrome. In keeping with the relative frequencies of the gene defects found for RW syndrome, roughly 90% of all JLN syndrome cases are due to mutations in the *KCNQ1* gene. Because of the incomplete penetrance found in the heterozygous state, it is possible that the parents of a child with JLN syndrome are asymptomatic.

Another gene, *KCNE2*, is involved in 10% of JLN syndrome. Both forms of JLN feature autosomal recessive inheritance. *KCNE1* encodes a "minimal potassium ion channel" protein, MinK. These proteins are β-subunits that coassemble with α-subunits, KvLQT1, produced by *KCNQ1*. The β-subunits are ancillary proteins that modulate the gating

kinetics and enhance stability of multimeric channel complexes. Different mutations within the *KCNE1* gene result in LQT5 that presents either as RW or JLN. In JLN syndrome, the mutations affect both inner ear and cardiac channels.

LQT4 and LQT7

The last two genes associated with LQT syndrome but not RW or JLN include a potassium channel protein and the ankyrin-B protein. LQT7, also known as Andersen syndrome, is characterized by periodic paralysis, prolongation of the QT interval, cardiac arrhythmias, and mildly dysmorphic features such as low-set ears, micrognathia, hypertelorism, syndactyly, short stature, and clinodactyly. It is unique among the channelopathies in that it may affect both cardiac and skeletal muscle, thus explaining the co-occurrence of periodic paralysis and LQT in the same individual. For LQT7, the *KCNJ2* gene produces the K+ channel 2 protein, Kir2.1, found in both skeletal and cardiac muscle. Mutations reducing Kir2.1 prolong the terminal phase of the cardiac action potential; by reducing the extracellular setting of K+, there are delayed-after-depolarizations (DADs) and spontaneous arrhythmias. Ventricular arrhythmias are common but only rarely degenerate into a hemodynamically compromising rhythm, such as torsades de pointes or ventricular fibrillation. Unlike with other forms of LQT syndrome, sudden death is not associated with LQT7.

It is suggested that mutated ankyrin B in cardiomyocytes causes an abnormal cytoskeleton arrangement resulting in fewer functional Na+ channels with altered kinetics and prolonged cardiac repolarization. In both LQT3 and LQT4, Na$^+$ channels reopen late, but the plateau potentials differ at –20 mV and –40 to –50 mV, respectively.

Management for Long QT Syndrome

For many individuals, those with no syncope or complex arrhythmias, no treatment is required. However, for individuals with syncope, complex arrhythmias, or a family history of sudden cardiac death, β-adrenergic blockers, such as propranolol and atenolol, are recommended. These drugs slow the heart rate and can prevent syncope in about 90% of individuals with LQT syndrome. LQT3, the Na$^+$ channel defect, responds best to the Na$^+$ channel blocker mexiletine.

Individuals who have not been responsive to medications and are at risk of suffering serious or sustained abnormal arrhythmias may receive an implantable cardioverter defibrillator (ICD). The ICD is usually implanted in the left pectoral region and monitors the cardiac rate. When the heart rate exceeds a programmable rate, a biphasic shock wave is delivered to restore normal rhythm.

●●● PULMONARY-RELATED DISORDERS

Cystic Fibrosis

Cystic fibrosis (CF) is a disease that affects the epithelia of several organ systems including the respiratory tract, exocrine pancreas, male gonads, intestinal tract, hepatobiliary tract, and sweat glands. It is caused by defects in the CF transmembrane regulator protein (CFTR). Congenital bilateral absence of the vas deferens (CBAVD) without other clinical signs is a related, milder manifestation of the same pathophysiologic mechanism.

Clinical Features of Cystic Fibrosis

Clinically, CF is identified by a triad of abnormal conditions primarily manifested as pulmonary problems, gastrointestinal problems, and elevated Cl$^-$ in sweat (>60 mEq/L) (Table 9-3). In addition, reproductive problems are significant in males—more than 95% of whom may be sterile.

The most commonly affected organs in CF are the lungs and pancreas. However, lung disease is the primary cause of morbidity and mortality (Fig. 9-7). In general, classical CF patients manifest early symptoms of dry, hacking, nonproductive cough with wheezing. Later symptoms include a productive cough, rales, wheezing, repeated infections, decreased appetite, failure to grow, and clubbing. These symptoms increase progressively without proper management of infections and nutritional status.

Male infertility, seen as azoospermia, is nearly universal in male patients with CF and most often takes the form of CBAVD. Sperm ducts degenerate or atrophy as a consequence of prolonged blockage by thick mucus secretions. In females, fertility is reduced because of thick desiccated cervical mucus. Meconium ileus is found at birth in nearly 20% of all patients. Other problems commonly encountered with

TABLE 9-3. Problems Associated with Cystic Fibrosis

Site	Associated Problem

Pulmonary system	Mucus-obstructed airways
	Bacterial infections
	Early symptoms
	  Dry, hacking, nonproductive cough
	  Increased respiratory rate (wheezing)
	Intermediate symptoms
	  Productive cough with rales, wheezing
	  Repeated infections
	  Decreased appetite, weight loss
	  Failure to grow
	  Clubbing
	Advanced symptoms
	  Chronic, productive cough
	  Exertional dyspnea
	  Cyanosis
	  Lung abscess
	  Bone pain
	Osteoarthropathy

Gastrointestinal system	Mucus-obstructed pancreatic ducts Decreased pancreatic enzymes Intestinal blockage Poor weight gain Easy bruising secondary to vitamin K deficiency Chronic diarrhea in infancy Rectal prolapse Hypoproteinemia Pancreatitis Diabetes
Sweat gland	Hyponatremia Hypochloremia Heat exhaustion and dehydration during exercise, ↑ hot weather, and fever
Reproductive system	Blocked or absent vas deferens and aspermia Cervical polyps

CF include nasal polyps, rectal prolapse, cirrhosis, and diabetes mellitus (Box 9-1). Whereas CF used to be a fatal childhood disease, aggressive symptom monitoring and treatment has raised the overall median age of survival to 32 years (Fig. 9-8).

Molecular Pathophysiology of Cystic Fibrosis

The basic defect expressed in CF is a failure of Cl$^-$ transport across cell membranes. Figure 9-9 depicts transport of ions across cell membranes forming the epithelial lining of the airways. In normal airway cells, the ion traffic utilizes two

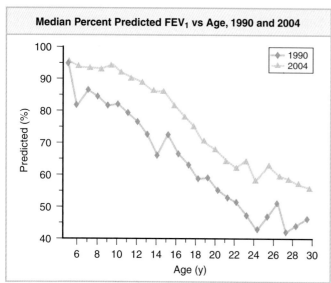

Figure 9-7. Lung function in individuals with CF, measured as forced expiratory volume per 1 second (FEV₁), decreases by about 2% per year. The lower a person's FEV₁, the more severe the lung disease. (From the Cystic Fibrosis Foundation. Patient Registry 2004 Annual Report, Bethesda, MD, 2004.)

Box 9-1. DIFFERENTIAL DIAGNOSES FOR CYSTIC FIBROSIS

Cystic fibrosis should be considered in:
- Infants with
  Meconium ileus
  Hypoproteinemia and anemia
  Hyponatremia of unknown etiology
- Older children with
  Rectal prolapse
  Failure to thrive, poor growth and weight gain, nutritional problems, chronic diarrhea, malabsorption
  Recurrent and refractory respiratory disorders, including nasal polyps
- Adolescents and adults with
  Recurrent pancreatitis
  Recurrent sinusitis/bronchitis
  Recurrent bronchiectasis
  Nasal polyps
  Male infertility

MICROBIOLOGY

Cystic Fibrosis and Respiratory Infections

Respiratory infections are a major concern for individuals with CF. Infection and swelling damage the lungs and cause lung function (FEV₁) to decrease. Infections occur more often in damaged lungs.

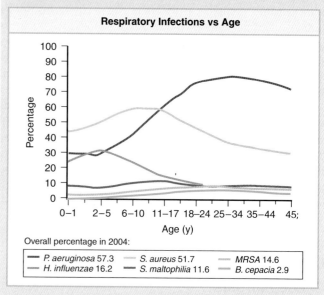

Overall percentage in 2004:

P. aeruginosa 57.3	S. aureus 51.7	MRSA 14.6
H. influenzae 16.2	S. maltophilia 11.6	B. cepacia 2.9

Figure from the Cystic Fibrosis Foundation. Patients Registry 2004 Annual Report, Bethesda, MD, 2004.

---

channels of Cl⁻ conductance at the luminal surface. One channel is dependent on cyclic AMP (cAMP), and the other is activated by Ca⁺⁺. CFTR governs the cAMP channel.

CFTR is a large chloride ion channel composed of 1480 amino acids. It comprises five functional domains including two membrane-anchoring segments each characterized by six membrane-spanning portions that form the core of the ion channel, two nucleotide-binding domains capable of binding ATP to modulate channel function, and a regulatory (R) domain, whose multiple capacities for phosphorylation

suggest that it serves as a switch that governs CFTR function. As might be expected from the clinical manifestations, CFTR is expressed on the apical surface of epithelia in the lungs, pancreatic ducts, intestines, and sweat gland ducts.

Defective CFTR proteins result in an impaired ability to secrete chloride ions (see Fig. 9-9). The disturbance of Cl⁻ transport across the luminal surface is associated with a compensatory influx of Na⁺ ions to retain electrical neutrality. The accompanying water influx causes dehydration at the cellular surface, leading to the sticky mucus characteristic of the disease. The sticky mucus in the lung causes mechanical obstruction and chronic inflammation of the airways.

Inheritance of Cystic Fibrosis

CF is one of the most common autosomal recessive disorders in Caucasians. It is the most common lethal monogenic disease. One infant in 3200 is born with the recessive disorder, and there are approximately 30,000 affected individuals in the United States. This means that approximately 1600 affected newborns may be expected each year in the United States. Almost all patients with CF are Caucasians; blacks (1 in 15,000) and Asian Americans (1 in 31,000) are rarely afflicted.

As seen with other autosomal recessive disorders, the frequency of heterozygous carriers is greater than the frequency of affected homozygous individuals. One in 22 to 28 Caucasians is a carrier of CF. The majority of affected

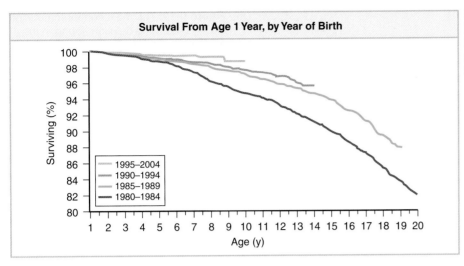

Figure 9-8. Mean survival age of individuals with CF. (From the Cystic Fibrosis Foundation. Patient Registry 2004 Annual Report, Bethesda, MD, 2004.)

children—more than 99%—come from marriages of two normal parents, both of whom are heterozygous carriers. A reproductive advantage for the heterozygote (*Aa*) over the normal homozygote (AA) would account for the high frequency of the lethal recessive gene for CF in white populations. The hypothesis currently favored is that heterozygous carriers are more resistant to infantile gastroenteritis than noncarriers, and thus a single mutant allele might protect the carrier from profuse diarrhea and fluid loss. This describes a *heterozygote advantage* that is seen in several disorders in which the heterozygous genotype has a higher relative fitness than either the homozygous dominant or homozygous recessive genotype. One of the best known examples of heterozygote advantage is sickle cell trait (see Chapter 6).

CF Gene and CFTR

The *CFTR* gene, responsible for CF, is located on the long arm of chromosome 7. The gene is large, containing more than 230,000 base pairs, and it has 27 exons, producing a 6.5-kb mRNA. More than 1000 different mutations have been described at the CF locus. The most common is an in-frame 3-bp deletion (termed ΔF508) that causes omission of a single phenylalanine at amino acid 508 within one of the ATP binding domains. CFTR protein harboring the ΔF508 mutation does not fold properly and hence fails to move through the endoplasmic reticulum to the Golgi, where it would normally undergo posttranslational maturation (Fig. 9-10). Accordingly, the defective protein is absent from its final destination on the surface of luminal epithelial cells in CF patients. The inability of the altered CFTR to move beyond its intracellular location to the cell membrane surface explains why heterozygous carriers with this mutation have only normal cell surface channels and no interference in Cl⁻ transport.

Most of the CF mutations are single-base changes or small deletions in the *CFTR* gene. Remarkably, the ΔF508 deletion accounts for 70% of classical CF cases in Caucasians. Overall, it can be found in approximately 30% to 80% of the patients, depending on the ethnic group. The

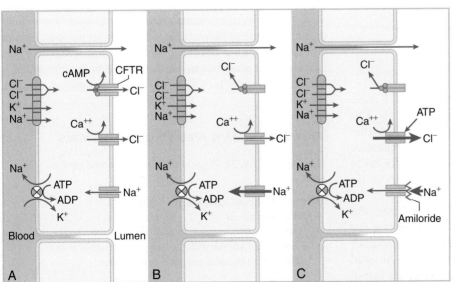

Figure 9-9. Ion transport across epithelium. **A,** In normal airway cells, there are two Cl⁻ channels for conductance. One channel is dependent on cyclic AMP, and the other is activated by Ca^{++}. CFTR governs the cAMP channel. **B,** In individuals with CF, the defective CFTR protein results in an ability to secrete Cl⁻ ions and a compensatory influx of Na ions to retain electroneutrality. The accompanying water influx causes dehydration at the cellular surface and leads to the sticky mucus characteristic of the disease. **C,** Two strategies are shown to normalize the electrolyte imbalances in CF: amiloride to lessen the Na⁺ influx and ATP (or UTP) to stimulate the Ca^{++}-dependent Cl⁻ input.

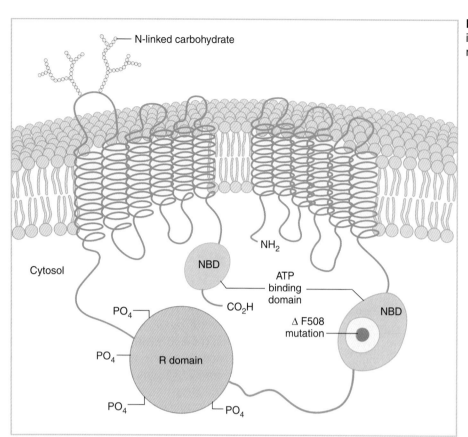

Figure 9-10. The most common mutation in CF is the Δ508 deletion, found in the nucleotide-binding domain (NBD).

TABLE 9-4. Classification of CFTR Mutations

Mutation Class	Effect of Mutation of CFTR Protein	Mechanism
I	Reduced or absent synthesis	Nonsense, frameshift, or splice-junction mutations
II	Block in protein processing	Missense mutations, amino acid deletions
III	Block in regulation of CFTR chloride channel	Missense mutations
IV	Altered CFTR chloride channel conductance	Missense mutations

mutations in 97% of Ashkenazi Jewish, 88% of other white, 69% of black, and 57% of Hispanic patients. Hence, for the great majority of CF patients, genetic testing is highly informative.

The F508 deletion is a severe mutation, whereas other mutational changes appear to be less severe, since the clinical course can range from mild to severe. This is best seen with regard to pancreatic dysfunction, where certain severe mutations consistently predict pancreatic insufficiency and other base changes prescribe some pancreatic function. Such a genotype-phenotype relationship is less readily apparent with the pulmonary symptoms. In fact, even individuals sharing the same deleterious CFTR genotype may exhibit differences in lung disease progression and symptomology, indicating that other factors—either genetic or environmental—may have a role in CF lung disease expression. Finally,

remaining mutations occur at other sites in the CF gene and are classified by the type of mutation (Table 9-4). This profusion of "private mutations" occurring at low frequencies has increased the difficulty of devising a comprehensive strategy to screen for CF. Such *allelic heterogeneity* helps explain the variations seen in the qualitative and quantitative phenotypic expression of CF.

In an effort to both standardize and maximize the efficiency of DNA-based diagnoses and carrier testing for CF, the American Academy of Medical Genetics recommends that a panel of the 25 most common CF mutations be used for genetic testing (Table 9-5). This panel detects the causal

Box 9-2. CBAVD AND *CFTR* MUTATIONS

Mutations of the *CFTR* gene may be suggested by the following:

- Absence of vas deferens on palpation
- Azoospermia
- Low ejaculated semen volume
- Evidence of abnormalities of seminal vesicles or vas deferens on rectal ultrasound examination

TABLE 9-5. CF Screening Panel and Mutation Detection Rates

Alleles Recommended for Carrier Screening (25)

1078delT	3120+1G>A	A455E	G85E	XR334W
1717-1G>A	3659delC	ΔF508	I148T	R347P
1898+1G>A	3849+10kbC>T	ΔI507	N1303K	R553X
2184delA	621+1G>T	G542X	R1162X	R560T
2789+5G>A	711+1G>T	G551D	R117H	W1282X

Mutation Detection Rate Population

Ashkenazi Jewish	85%
North American white	80% to 85%
Hispanic	75%
Black	64%
Mexican	58%
Colombian	46%
Venezuelan	33%
Other	Variable

CBAVD is nearly universal in males with CF but may also occur in males without other CF symptoms (Box 9-2). These individuals harbor one mild and one severe CFTR mutation. In the absence of two severe mutations, CF is not clinically observed. This suggests that derivatives of wolffian duct structures are very sensitive to CFTR dysfunction.

Mutations in the *CFTR* gene may overlap phenotypes presented by other disorders, not only CBAVD. Chronic rhinosinusitis (CRS) is a consistent feature of individuals with CF. In some patients, the severe ΔF508 mutation on one allele combined with a less deleterious mutation presents a clinical picture of chronic rhinosinusitis without other CF features. Similarly, CRS is also seen in individuals who have a single *CFTR* allele mutation but who do not meet other criteria required for diagnosis of CF. For these reasons, practitioners should consider *CFTR* mutations when evaluating other CF-like and CF-associated presentations such as recurrent sinusitis, bronchitis, bronchiectasis, nasal polyps, recurrent pancreatitis, refractory asthma in children, recurrent pneumonia, hypoproteinemia and anemia in infants, and children with rectal prolapse.

Molecular Testing for Cystic Fibrosis

In genetic counseling programs, an important consideration is the development of simple, inexpensive means of unambiguously detecting heterozygous carriers of inherited recessive disorders. CF testing has largely been achieved by DNA-based molecular genetic testing for common disease alleles. Such testing is invaluable in population screening programs and to at-risk relatives and their reproductive partners. Ideally, carrier screening should be offered to couples before they become pregnant to allow time to consider options if they are carriers. Studies show, however,

that individuals are more likely to seek testing if there is a family history of CF *or* after a pregnancy occurs.

As suggested, many but not all CF mutations can be detected in screening panels, and particular panels can be designed to recognize the most common mutations in a particular population. A negative report for one or both members of a couple does not exclude the possibility of an affected offspring. The risk, known as the residual risk, is dependent on other factors such as racial or ethnic background of each parent, the specific mutations being tested, and whether both parents are tested.

Gene Therapy for Cystic Fibrosis

Since the pulmonary complications of CF are life threatening, the lung is the principal target of gene therapy. Although lung transplantation has become more common, it is not a viable option for all CF patients and it carries significant risks that restrict the number of individuals considered for this surgery. Currently, the 1-year survival rate for lung transplantation is 80% to 90% and 5-year survival is 60%

MICROBIOLOGY

Viral Gene Therapy Vectors

Viruses are efficient at transferring DNA into a host cell. Viral vectors must be modified to avoid eliciting an immune response—the greatest disadvantage of viral vectors—by the host. Commonly used vectors are retrovirus, adenovirus, adeno-associated virus, herpes simplex virus, and lentivirus. The size of the insert is a limiting factor for choice of vector.

to 70%. Successful outcomes of transplantation depend on timing of surgery, medical status of other organs, and psychosocial support systems. Infections present a special problem for CF transplant patients. It would be desirable to target pulmonary epithelial cells—and not other cells—for corrective gene therapy because the long-term consequences of overexpression of a cAMP-regulated Cl^- channel in other cell types are not yet known. Targeting is facilitated by the fact that the airway epithelium is contiguous with the external environment. For this reason, gene delivery by viruses with tropism for the airways, such as adenoviruses, currently has the most appeal.

Adenovirus-based vectors have been used to introduce normal human cDNAs of CFTR into the lung epithelium of animal models and normal expression of membrane-lined CFTR has been demonstrated. Since the adenovirus does not integrate into the genome of the lung epithelial stem cells, it is lost with cellular turnover. Reinfection therefore is necessary but can cause immunologic reactions. There also may be the risk of a replication-competent infectious virus being generated as a result of recombination with ubiquitous wild-type virus. In general, the possible risk factors have excluded application of the strategy of gene therapy in humans by adenovirus vectors.

A nonviral gene transfer vector has been used to transfer a normal *CFTR* gene to epithelial cells. Compacted DNA nanoparticles containing only the *CFTR* gene sequences are used to more efficiently cross the cell membrane and enter the nuclei, where recombination can occur. These nanoparticles have shown few immunogenic or toxic effects in animals and humans and extend the strategies being used to develop new gene therapies designed to correct defective genes in situ.

α₁-Antitrypsin Deficiency

One of the etiologies for chronic obstructive pulmonary disease (COPD) and emphysema is unrestrained proteolytic activity in the connective tissue of the lungs, especially the elastin component. The gradual destruction of pulmonary elastic tissue results from a diminished presence of α₁-antitrypsin (AAT).

BIOCHEMISTRY

Nonviral Gene Vectors
Nonviral vectors avoid some problems seen with viral vectors.
- DNA vaccination: recombinant gene is injected into tissues (i.e., muscle).
- Liposomes: gene fused with liposomes; can cross blood-brain barrier.
- Poly-cation conjugates: DNA condensed into nanostructure; can pass through membranes; cells can be targeted by use of conjugated receptor ligands.
- Bacteria: *Salmonella* with altered genes targets cells (i.e., macrophages) to deliver DNA.

AAT is a major serum serine protease inhibitor produced in the liver. The 394-amino-acid protein is the most abundant antiprotease in the lung, constituting roughly 95% of all alveoli antiprotease activity. In blood, AAT is associated with the α₁-globulin fraction and accounts for 90% of the antiprotease activity based on its reactivity with trypsin. Human antitrypsin actually inhibits the activity of a broad spectrum of proteins, including trypsin, chymotrypsin, elastase, skin collagenase, plasmin, thrombin, and bacterial proteases. Because of this, the protein is more accurately labeled α₁-antiprotease, but by convention, most biomedical scientists, physicians, and patients refer to the protein as AAT. Unequivocally, however, the key physiologic role played by AAT in the lungs is the inhibition of *neutrophil elastase*, an enzyme that normally destroys bacteria. In the absence of AAT, neutrophil elastase will destroy elastic fibers in lung connective tissue.

COPD and emphysema were originally believed to occur from an imbalance between protease and antiprotease activity. When a marked genetic deficiency of AAT became associated with severe pulmonary disease, it became clear that AAT deficiency was a risk factor for lung disease. However, because the onset, rate of progression, and severity of pulmonary disease varies among individuals with severe AAT deficiency, it is also clear that additional genetic or environmental factors are etiologically relevant.

AAT Gene

The *AAT* gene is found at chromosome 14q32.1, is 12.2 kb in length, and contains seven exons. The gene has at least three different names in the literature including *AAT*, *PI*, and *SERPINA1*; all can be used interchangeably.

The *AAT* gene is highly polymorphic. More than 125 different mutations have been identified in the gene, and a subset of these impacts serum AAT levels. Three codominantly expressed AAT alleles—M, S, and Z—are primarily important to lung, as well as liver, disease. By convention, these variants have been assigned the symbol *Pi*, designating protease inhibitor, followed by a superscript capital letter (Pi^M, Pi^S, and Pi^Z) to define the allele. Historically, the capital letter indicates the relative electrophoretic mobility of the mutant protein, where M represented moderate, S slow, and Z the slowest gel mobility.

The Pi^M, or M, allele is the normal allele. There are actually a number of M alleles that do not reduce the serum AAT concentration, which normally is 20–53 μmol/L. Hence, they are simply neutral polymorphisms of the *AAT* gene. The M allele is the most common form in Caucasians with an allele frequency of 95% and a homozygote (MM) frequency of approximately 90% (Table 9-6). The S and Z alleles are more rare and are associated with reduced levels of AAT activity and hence account for AAT-deficient disease. The S variant results from a valine for glutamate substitution at amino acid 264, V264E, of the *AAT* gene. The Z form is defined by a glutamate to lysine substitution at position 342, E342K, and represents the most severely impaired AAT variant. Homozygosity of the Pi^Z (ZZ) has the greatest deficiency

TABLE 9-6. AAT Genotype Frequencies in Whites of Northern European Ancestry and Associated AAT Serum Activities

AAT/Pi Genotype	Frequency	Enzyme Activity (% Control)
MM	0.90	100
MZ	0.038	60
SS	0.001	50–60
SZ	0.0012 (1/800)	30–35
ZZ	0.0004 (1/2500)	10–15

of protease inhibitor (serum levels of 3.4–7 μmol/L, indicating 10% to 15% of the activity found in the normal, or MM, state). This form is associated with nearly all AAT-deficiency disease. However, emphysema also occurs with moderate frequency in individuals heterozygous for the Pi^S and Pi^Z alleles, designated SZ. Because the *AAT* genes are *codominant*, any combination of a deficiency allele and an M allele (*MS* or *MZ*) results in at least 50% AAT activity and, accordingly, is not associated with pulmonary disease.

Several families have been reported in which a "silent," or *null*, allele appears to be present. The rare silent allele (designated Pi^{Null}) results in the complete absence of synthesis of AAT; individuals homozygous for the null allele develop emphysema by their mid-twenties. Affected individuals are generally homozygous for a deletion that results in a frame shift and premature termination of translation.

ZZ Genotype

The frequencies of molecular variants show considerable variation among ethnic groups and geographic areas. The ZZ genotype has the highest incidence in Scandinavia, where approximately 1 in 1700 persons (0.06%) is homozygous for this defective allele. DNA haplotype analysis suggests that the original Z mutation arose in Scandinavia. This detrimental Z allele is essentially absent in African blacks, Asians, and Native Americans, indicating that the deleterious homozygous state, and thus AAT deficiency, is largely a disorder of whites.

In the United States, 0.01% to 0.05% of the Caucasian population is ZZ homozygotes. Although one person in 2500 has α_1-antitrypsin deficiency, about one person in 25 is a heterozygous carrier. Thus, there are 100 times as many heterozygous carriers as there are affected individuals, a scenario similar to that seen in CF.

The Z variant of AAT differs from the normal M protein in interesting ways. This single-amino-acid substitution (E342K) affects the folding and ultimately the conformation of the molecule. Most misfolded Z antitrypsin aggregates near the end of the endoplasmic reticulum, where newly synthesized proteins ordinarily bud off and pass into the

Golgi apparatus to be packaged for transport. The basic defect, accordingly, is a blockage in Z antiprotease processing in the endoplasmic reticulum, resulting in the intracellular accumulation and polymerization of mutant AAT with subsequently lowered levels of circulating antiprotease. Presumably because of the accumulation of AAT polymers, liver disease, characterized by abnormal liver enzymes, fibrosis or cirrhosis, occurs in a minority of patients.

Additionally, the Z protein isolated from hepatocytes contains carbohydrate side chains that differ markedly from normal. The Z protein has an increase in mannose and a decrease in both sialic acid and galactose residues. Apparently, the excess of mannose residues on the carbohydrate side chains prevents the final formation of carbohydrate side chains with terminal sialic acid residues. Finally, there is evidence that, in addition to the abnormalities in protein processing and secretion, Z protein has a reduced ability to inhibit elastase. Overall, the ZZ genotype typically results in an AAT activity of only 10% to 15% of normal values (see Table 9-6). Such individuals with familial emphysema are highly susceptible to the development of lung disease as early as age 35 years.

Pathogenesis of Lung Disease in ZZ Individuals

Not all ZZ individuals with severe AAT deficiency develop emphysema. Interestingly, serum levels of AAT in ZZ asymptomatic and emphysema-symptomatic individuals may

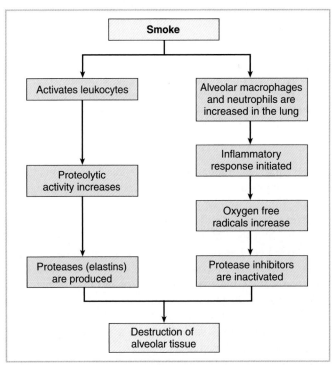

Figure 9-11. Tobacco smoke activates leukocytes to increase proteolytic activity. It also causes alveolar macrophages and neutrophils to release chemotactic substances that initiate an inflammatory response. This response creates oxygen free radicals that inactivate protease inhibitors. Thus alveolar tissue damage proceeds unchecked.

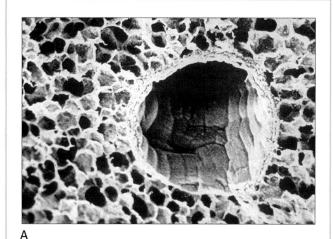

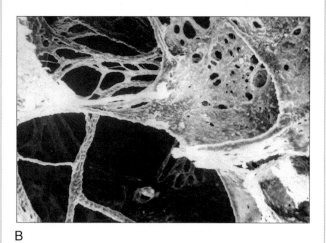

Figure 9-12. AAT deficiency leads to an increased risk of emphysema. Alveolar walls break down, resulting in overinflation and permanent enlargement. **A**, normal lung; **B**, emphysema lung. (Reproduced by permission of Talecris Biotherapeutics, Inc., http://www.prolastin.com.)

MICROBIOLOGY

Macrophages and Inflammation

Macrophages have an important role in inflammatory responses initiated by foreign substances. They are recruited from surrounding tissues or derived from monocytes that migrate to the site. At the site, macrophages are exposed to stimuli, such as gamma interferon, cytokines, and lipopolysaccharides from bacteria, and morphologic and functional changes occur. Macrophages secrete proteases (collagenase, elastase) and plasminogen activator. They are known as activated macrophages when phagocytosis and microbicidal activity increase. Activated cells produce IL-8, a neutrophil chemotaxin. Leukotrienes and superoxide may also be released.

The heavy cigarette smoker with an AAT deficiency is in double jeopardy because macrophages are found in greater numbers in the lungs of smokers than of nonsmokers. Macrophages release a chemotactic factor that attracts neutrophils to the lungs, resulting in an increased concentration of proteases. Further, macrophages release a variety of substances that provoke an inflammatory response with a concomitant increase in oxidative metabolism. Consequently, the release of freely diffusible O_2 free radicals from macrophages and neutrophils react with the active site of AAT—a methionine-serine peptide bond at AAT methionine residue 358. The inhibition of elastase by AAT depends on the integrity of the methionine-serine bond in the active site. Cigarette smoke leads to the oxidation of the methionine residue in the active site, which effectively destroys the bond between methionine and serine. The cleaved, ineffective AP molecule is eventually catabolized in the liver and spleen.

Overall, cigarette smoke can be implicated in many ways in the pathogenesis of COPD and emphysema, including activation of macrophages, recruitment of neutrophils, enhanced release of proteolytic enzymes by macrophages and neutrophils, and oxidative inactivation of the protease inhibitors.

Therapy for α₁-Antitrypsin Deficiency

The presence of methionine at the reactive site of AAT renders the molecule more susceptible to inactivation by oxidants present in cigarette smoke or released by phagocytes. Using recombinant DNA technology, the methionine residue at position 358 could be replaced by valine in the *AAT* gene (Table 9-7). It has been demonstrated that the genetically modified *AAT* is more resistant to oxidant damage than the native molecule. In principle, *ZZ*-susceptible individuals can be given transfusions of the modified AAT with its enhanced capacity to inhibit neutrophil elastase. Several constructs have shown promising results in preclinical and early clinical trials.

The most successful treatment strategies begin with life-style alterations, such as discontinuing smoking, bronchodilation,

be the same. The manifestations of clinical illness evidently require exposure to certain precipitating environmental factors. Tobacco smoke is a major and unambiguous trigger for overt pulmonary disease in *ZZ* individuals (Fig. 9-11). Characteristically, *ZZ* emphysema-symptomatic individuals have been heavy smokers for many years. The smoking habit seems to subtract an average of at least 10 years from their life span. In *ZZ* patients, the onset of dyspnea occurs at a median age of 40 in *ZZ* smokers compared with 53 years in *ZZ* nonsmokers. The insidious onset of shortness of breath in smokers progresses relentlessly to a typical presentation of pulmonary emphysema.

In health, the neutrophil elastase is continually inhibited by AAT and, to a lesser extent, by α₂-macroglobulin. AAT enters lung tissue by simple diffusion from the serum. In the absence of AAT, the unrestrained action of proteolytic enzymes damages the lung parenchyma and vascular bed (Fig. 9-12).

TABLE 9-7. Modification of ATT Reactive Site by Change of Methionine to Valine to Decrease Inactivation by Oxidants

Protease Inhibitor		Target
α_1-Antitrypsin	Pro-Met*-Ser-Ile-Pro-Pro	Elastase
Engineered oxidation resistant mutant	Pro-Val*-Ser-Lie-Pro-Pro	Elastase

*Reactive site.

MICROBIOLOGY

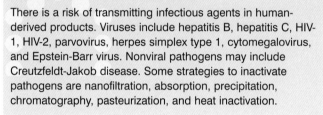

Risks of Human-derived Products

There is a risk of transmitting infectious agents in human-derived products. Viruses include hepatitis B, hepatitis C, HIV-1, HIV-2, parvovirus, herpes simplex type 1, cytomegalovirus, and Epstein-Barr virus. Nonviral pathogens may include Creutzfeldt-Jakob disease. Some strategies to inactivate pathogens are nanofiltration, absorption, precipitation, chromatography, pasteurization, and heat inactivation.

ANATOMY & PHYSIOLOGY

Estimating Static Lung Volume Following Lung Volume Reduction Surgery

Lung volume reduction surgery (LVRS) removes diseased lung tissue—usually 20% to 30%—because disease alters the mechanics of breathing. This allows the remaining lung to function with more normal mechanics. In emphysema, it is important to remove the diseased lung because the disease destroys elastin in the extracellular matrix.

$$C = \frac{\Delta V_L}{\Delta P_{TP}}$$

Therefore, for the above equation, static compliance (C) is greatly increased with the same transpulmonary pressure (P_{TP}); the diseased lung enlarges (V_L) greater than a normal lung but has less elastic recoil. A graph of emphysema and normal static pressure volume will show a greater slope for emphysema.

oxygen therapy, and pulmonary rehabilitation. As the disease progresses, AAT replacement therapy is available for those with signs of emphysema to minimize lung damage and to slow the progression of the disease. Human AAT is obtained from serum and administered intravenously. As the disease approaches the severe state, surgery options such as lung volume reduction surgery and lung replacement become the best options.

There is compelling evidence that the ZZ individual is more susceptible to cirrhosis of the liver and liver cancer than are normal individuals in the general population. Liver disease apparently relates to the sustained aggregation of the Z-type AAT in the liver, where AAT is primarily synthesized. Even with a modicum of success of the current genetically engineered AAT, it will be necessary to prevent accumulation of the Z protein in the liver. Current research efforts are directed at deactivating, or "turning off," the Z form of the *AAT* gene, as well as fostering secretion of the abnormal protein. Replacement of the diseased liver with a liver transplant remains a feasible option.

Hepatic, Renal, and Gastrointestinal Systems

10

●●● OVERVIEW

The hepatic, renal, and gastrointestinal systems are linked by function, and considering them together provides an opportunity to view several disorders that affect more than one organ either primarily or secondarily. This chapter begins by addressing renal development and a few disorders that may cause kidney development to fail or occur inappropriately. A metabolic disorder affecting reabsorption within the kidney and intestine draws attention to the fact that transport across membranes may occur by similar mechanisms in different organs, causing similar or different problems.

A well-known disorder of intestinal development, Hirschsprung disease, emphasizes the role of progenitor cell function; in this case, the progenitor cells are neural crest cells. Although the hallmark of Hirschsprung disease is megacolon, this disease may occur in association with syndromic disorders and as such is a concern of physicians evaluating children with chromosomal abnormalities. Equally interesting is that the gene that causes Hirschsprung disease is the same gene involved in normal development of the kidney and other organs; however, when mutated, it may also result in several forms of multiple endocrine neoplasia.

Finally, several disorders of the liver are discussed. The intestine must absorb metal ions correctly or an overload or deficiency may occur as discussed for iron and copper. Both are toxic if not transported correctly and excreted properly. Some of the same genes are involved in the transport of both metals.

●●● RENAL DISORDERS

Urinary tract abnormalities are present in approximately 40% of all congenital abnormalities and are frequently associated with syndromes. Likewise, there is an increased risk for urinary tract abnormalities with structural anomalies of most organ systems. Chronic renal failure in infants and children results from inborn errors of development in a majority of cases (Box 10-1). With complex adult phenotypes associated with renal failure, such as hypertension, more subtle defects of development are suggested. Among the many disorders described in the intestine are more than 250 syndromes and single gene disorders that confer an increased risk for urinary tract abnormalities.

Renal Agenesis

Organogenesis of the kidney is initiated when the ureteric bud forms as an outgrowth of the wolffian duct. The failure of the kidney to develop—agenesis—differs from atrophy of renal tissue although the latter may mimic agenesis. True agenesis results from failure of the ureteric bud to develop or maldevelopment of the metanephric blastema between the 25th and 29th days of development. Along with failure of the kidney to develop, both ureters and renal arteries are absent.

Box 10-1. CLINICAL FEATURES ASSOCIATED WITH A RENAL ANOMAY

Edema	Oligohydramnios
Exstrophy of the bladder	Imperforate anus
Anuria-oliguria	Ambiguous genitalia
Aniridia	Hemihypertrophy
Supernumerary nipples	Preauricular pits and ear tags
Hypertension	Polydypsia
Recurrent urinary infections	Prune belly abdomen
Abdominal mass	Polyuria

ANATOMY & EMBRYOLOGY

Kidney Abnormalities

Kidney anomalies in shape and size occur in 3% to 4% of newborns and include:

- Renal agenesis
- Malrotated kidneys: the kidney maintains its embryonic position; often associated with an ectopic kidney
- Ectopic kidneys: most are located in the pelvis and result from a failure to "ascend"
- Horseshoe kidney: the poles of the kidney fuse; usually asymptomatic
- Duplications of the urinary tract: duplications of the abdominal part of the ureter and renal pelvis are common; a supernumerary kidney is rare
- Ectopic ureter: the ureter opens anywhere except into the bladder
- Ureteric ectopia: the ureter is not incorporated into the posterior part of the bladder
- Cystic disease

Renal agenesis may be associated with chromosomal abnormalities such as trisomy 21, trisomy 22, trisomy 7, trisomy 10, and Turner and Klinefelter syndromes. It also has been associated with microdeletions of chromosome 22q11 (Box 10-2) and chromosome 11p13; the latter deletion contains the Wilms tumor gene (*WT1*) that produces an essential transcription factor for proper urogenital development.

The molecular mechanisms determining kidney formation are complex, and although they are not well understood, it is becoming increasingly clear that inductive signaling pathways direct the process. Several pathways important in kidney development are important in other organs. Some will be recognized as proto-oncogenes that were discussed in Chapter 5 (Table 10-1). Of the known genes involved in development, mutations in the human *SPRY2* gene result in complete agenesis, reduced size, or lobularization or cystogenesis of the ureteric bud. In one case, inappropriate SPRY2-

Box 10-2. CLINICAL CONDITIONS ASSOCIATED WITH DIFFERENTLY NAMED CHROMOSOME 22p11 DELETIONS

Velocardiofacial syndrome
DiGeorge sequence
CATCH-22 (cardiac defect, typical facial dysmorphism, mental deficiency, and chromosome 22q11.2 deletion)
Conotruncal anomaly face syndrome
Opitz G/BBB syndrome
CHARGE association with Cayler cardiofacial syndrome

mediated signaling was identified in an ectopic organ with a complete ureteric bud.

The incidence of renal agenesis varies, ranging from 0.4 in 10,000 to 3.9 in 10,000 births for *bilateral* renal agenesis and from 0.4 in 10,000 to 4.9 in 10,000 births for *unilateral* renal agenesis. Obviously, bilateral agenesis is fatal, and the infant is either stillborn or dies within a few hours of birth. Unilateral agenesis may be asymptomatic and an incidental finding (Fig. 10-1). In these cases, the adrenal gland is absent in less than 10% of cases. However, the ipsilateral fallopian tube in females and the seminal vesicle in males may be absent. Most cases of renal agenesis are spontaneous although a few reports offer evidence of autosomal dominant or recessive inheritance.

In addition to failure of the kidney and ureters to develop, oligohydramnios occurs and leads to other deformations such as a constricted chest cavity, underdeveloped lungs, and pulmonary hypoplasia. This occurs because amniotic fluid is mainly derived from fetal urine. This *deformation* sequence presents as *Potter's facies*, characterized by hypertelorism, low-set ears, receding chin, tapering fingers, and infraorbital folds (Fig. 10-2). Potter's facies is not pathognomonic for renal agenesis, since any abnormality causing oligohydramnios may cause this presentation.

TABLE 10-1. Examples of Genes Important in Kidney Development

Genes	Protein	Function
GDNF	Glial cell—derived neurophic factor	Binds to RET-GFRα_1 and regulates ureteric development
WNT Family		*WNT4*—expressed in mesenchymal pretubular aggregates; required for nephrogenesis *WNT6, WNT7, WNT11*—expressed in ureteric bud *WNT11*—involved in ureteric bud branching
BMP Family	Bone morphogenic protein	*BMP4*—expressed in mesenchyme; may antagonize ureteric bud development; controls *GDNF* expression
Foxd1		Expressed in renal stroma and required for ureteric branching and nephrogenesis
WT1	Wilms tumor protein	Crucial for nephrogenesis; regulates *SPRY1*
SPRY family	Sprouty	Expressed in ureteric bud

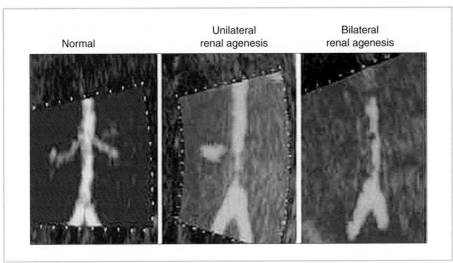

Figure 10-1. Unilateral and bilateral renal agenesis. (Courtesy of Dr. Philippe Jeanty, Women's Health Alliance, Nashville, TN.)

Normal | Unilateral renal agenesis | Bilateral renal agenesis

Multicystic Renal Dysplasia

The most common cause of an abdominal mass in a newborn results from unilateral or bilateral multicystic kidneys. Normally, the metanephric blastema differentiates into renal parenchyma under the influence of the ureteric bud. In the absence of normal induction of the metanephric blastema, multicystic dysplasia occurs (Fig. 10-3). For unknown reasons, the left kidney is involved more often than the right.

Most cases of unilateral multicystic renal dysplasia (MRD) undergo spontaneous involution for unknown reasons although it is suspected that cystic fluid is reabsorbed. In other cases, unilateral MRD may be asymptomatic until adulthood. Bilateral MRD is usually associated with oligohydramnios and Potter's facies and usually results in stillbirth or death within the first few days. Numerous nonrenal malformations may be associated with MRD involving the

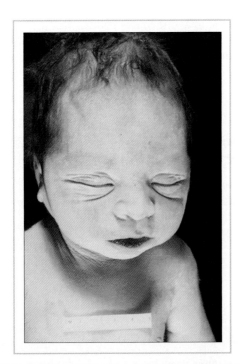

Figure 10-2. Potter's facies. (Courtesy of Edward Klatt, MD, Florida State University, College of Medicine. Used by permission of the Spencer S. Eccles Health Sciences Library, University of Utah Health Sciences Center; http://www-medlib.med.utah.edu.)

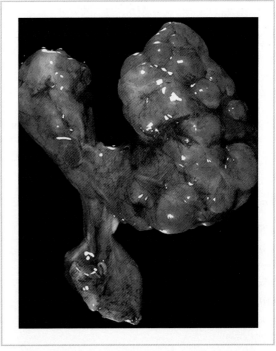

Figure 10-3. Multicystic renal dysplasia. The kidneys are asymmetric with variably sized cysts. Small ureters lead to a hypoplastic bladder. (Courtesy of Edward Klatt, MD, Florida State University, College of Medicine. Used by permission of the Spencer S. Eccles Health Sciences Library, University of Utah Health Sciences Center; http://www-medlib.med.utah.edu.)

TABLE 10-2. Malformations and Anomalies Reported with Multicystic Renal Dysplasia

System	Features
Urogenital	Bladder wall diverticulum
	Contralateral renal agenesis
	Hypoplasia
	Fused renal ectopia
	Cystic dysplasia of the testis
	Ectopic kidney
	Fibromuscular dysplasia
	Horseshoe kidney
	Patent urachus
	Seminal vesicle abnormalities
	Ureterocele
Gastrointestinal	Duodenal atresia
	Esophageal atresia
	Hirschsprung disease
	Imperforate anus
	Inguinal hernia
	Omphalocele
	Tracheoesophageal fistula
Neurologic	Anencephaly
	Caudal agenesis
	Caudal regression syndrome
	Congenital deafness
	Hydrocephalus
	Mental retardation
	Microcephaly
	Microphthalmia
	Myelomeningocele
	Spina bifida
Cardiovascular	Aortic stenosis
	Coarctation of the aorta
	Patent ductus arteriosus
	Pulmonary stenosis
	Truncus arteriosus
	Ventricular septal defect
Musculoskeletal	Clinodactyly of the fifth finger
	Congenital dislocation of the hip
	Flexion deformities of the fingers
	Syndactyly
	Talipes equinovarus

Dysmorphic Features

Bipartite uterus

Cleft palate

Epicanthal folds

Hymenal atresia

Hypertelorism

Low-set ears

Macroglossia

Macrosomia

Micrognathia

Preauricular pits

Pigment defects of iris and hair

Short neck

gastrointestinal, neurologic, cardiovascular, and musculoskeletal systems. Dysmorphologies may also be identified (Table 10-2).

The incidence of unilateral MRD is 1 in 4300 live births. Together, unilateral and bilateral MRD have an incidence of 1 in 3600 live births. Familial multicystic renal dysplasia has been described several times. An example of such a family is the occurrence of two children affected with unilateral MRD and a father who was also discovered to have unilateral MRD. The mother had terminated one pregnancy because of bilateral MRD with a Potter anomaly. Neither the two children nor the father nor the aborted fetus had any additional malformation. This and other cases support an autosomal dominant inheritance, but most cases are associated with chromosomal abnormalities (Box 10-3).

Cystinuria

Historically, cystinuria was one of the original inborn errors of metabolism identified by Sir Archibald Garrod in 1908. Cystine is produced endogenously from the metabolism of dietary methionine, as seen in Chapter 4 (see Fig. 4-5). It is transported across the epithelial cells of the gastrointestinal tract and reabsorbed at the brush border of the proximal renal tubules. Amino acids are readily filtered by the glomerulus and undergo nearly complete reabsorption by proximal tubular cells. Only 0.4% of the filtered cystine normally appears in the urine. A common pathway exists for cystine, lysine, arginine, and ornithine, and therefore a defect results in failure of reabsorption for all four amino acids. However, cystine is the least soluble of these amino acids, and as a result it is the only one that is pathogenic.

Dietary cystine is absorbed from the small intestine in a manner similar to that of the kidneys. Therefore, a defect is

Box 10-3. SYNDROMES ASSOCIATED WITH MULTICYSTIC RENAL DYSPLASIA

Beckwith-Wiedemann syndrome
Trisomy 18
Waardenburg syndrome
Joubert syndrome
VACTERL (vertebral, anal, cardiac, tracheal, esophageal, renal and limb) association

PATHOLOGY & ANATOMY

VACTERL Association

The VACTERL association is a combination of vertebral defects, anal atresia, cardiovascular anomalies, tracheoesophageal fistula, renal anomalies, and limb defects.

expected to affect intestinal absorption as well as reabsorption from the kidneys. However, in the absence of cystine absorption, cysteine may still be synthesized from methionine and homocysteine metabolism. The consequence of increased and insoluble cystine in the urinary tract is the formation of renal stones—nephrolithiasis. Onset can occur at any time beginning after about age 1 year, but most stones present with the painful symptoms of urinary obstruction in the second to third decade. Twenty-five percent of affected individuals first have stones in the first decade of life; 30% to 40% of affected individuals experience stones during the second decade. Although renal calculi, or kidney stones, are often the only presentation, several uncommon manifestations may also occur such as frequent urinary tract infections, chronic backache, and hematuria.

As noted for other metabolic disorders, cystinuria is an autosomal recessive disorder. Originally, three types of cystinuria were distinguished. In cystinuria type I, all four amino acids—cystine, lysine, arginine, and ornithine—are excreted in the urine in high concentration. Types II and III demonstrate an incomplete recessiveness in which heterozygotes have elevated amino acid excretion and variable intestinal absorption. All three forms were thought to be allelic and expressed from the *SLC3A* gene (solute carrier family member 3A) on chromosome 2 until a second gene was identified in a different cohort of individuals. The second gene encodes a subunit that associates with the active transporter produced by *SLC3A*; this gene, *SLC7A9*, is now recognized as being responsible for all non–type I cystinuria. A new terminology has been proposed to classify cystinuria as type A, formerly type I, and type B, formerly types II and III (Table 10-3).

Cystinuria is one of the most common errors in amino acid transport, occurring at a frequency of 1 in 7000 individuals. Most of these individuals have type A cystinuria. Type B disease is relatively rare although an increased incidence of cystinuria exists among individuals of Libyan Jewish ancestry resulting from a founder effect. *Founder effects* occur in small populations originating from very few founders that recruit few newcomers to the community, preferring instead to marry within the community. Approximately 1 in 2500 persons of Libyan Jewish descent has type B disease (Fig. 10-4). The carrier frequency in this population is around 1 in 25, the same as the frequency for cystic fibrosis, which is the most common autosomal recessive disorder among whites.

GASTROINTESTINAL DISORDERS

As demonstrated for cystinuria, mutations in a single gene may have effects in organs within different systems, such as intestine and kidney, because the proteins function in different places. Similarly, disorders such as multicystic renal dysplasia can be associated with different disorders including several that involve the gastrointestinal system. In this section, a disorder of intestinal function is discussed.

Hirschsprung Disease

Hirschsprung disease, or aganglionic megacolon, is a congenital disorder characterized by the absence of neural crest–derived neurons along part of the distal large intestine. This is also referred to as a neurocristopathy—a term used to describe lesions related to aberrations in neural growth, migration, or differentiation that occur during embryologic development. The abnormalities or dysfunctions of neural crest cells include carcinoid tumors, neuroblastoma, neurofibromatosis, pheochromocytoma, and Hirschsprung disease. Normally, neural crest cells originating primarily at the vagal level of the hindbrain and sacral regions of the spinal cord migrate to regions of the intestine and rectum. Failure of these cells to migrate or differentiate properly results in the disease.

Typically, newborns and infants with Hirschsprung disease have intestinal obstruction and subsequent colon distention resulting from a lack of peristalsis. The disease is variable, and the region of the colon affected varies. Aganglionosis is

TABLE 10-3. Classification of Cystinuria

Type	Gene	Location	Clinical Feature of Heterozygote	
			Urinary Excretion	Intestinal Absorption
I or A	*SLC3A1*	Chr 2p16.3	Normal	Normal
II, III or B	*SLC7A9*	Chr 19q13.1	Moderate increase in amino aciduria	Nearly normal to severely impaired

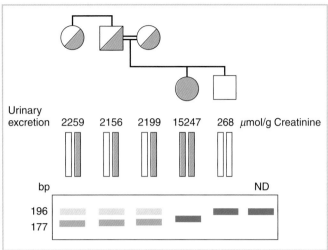

Urinary
excretion   2259   2156   2199   15247   268   µmol/g Creatinine

bp   ND
196
177

Figure 10-4. Mendelian inheritance of mutation G259R of SLC7A9 in a non–type I cystinuria consanguineous family. Haplotypes (vertical open and filled bars) were obtained with markers from cystinuria non–type I locus on chromosome 19. Open chromosomes are normal but not necessarily identical, and filled chromosomes are identical cystinuria-transmitting chromosomes. The sum of the urinary excretion of cystine, lysine, arginine and ornithine is reported for each individual as µmol/g of creatinine. Shown is detection of mutation G259R by the *Dde*I site generated using BR1 and the forward mutagenesis primer BF2 (5′-CTGCCTTTGGCCATTATC<u>C</u>TC-3′; the underscored character indicates the mutated nucleotide). The undigested (ND) band is 196 bp, which results in two bands of 177 bp and 19 bp (not shown) after the mutated allele is digested by *Dde*I.

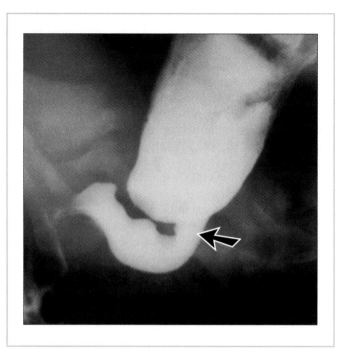

Figure 10-5. Long-segment Hirschsprung disease. The arrow indicates the area of the transition zone between the enlarged area that has ganglion cells (normal) and the small area that does not (Hirschsprung disease). Following barium enema and radiography, a biopsy confirms the presence or absence of ganglion cells. (From Moore KL, Persaud TVN. *The Developing Human*, 7th ed. Philadelphia, WB Saunders, 2003, p 282.)

PATHOLOGY & PHYSIOLOGY

Hirschsprung Disease

Owing to improper neural crest cell development in the intestine, Meissner submucosal and Auerbach myenteric plexuses are missing. Functional obstruction and dilatation proximal to the affected segment occurs with dilatation occurring proximal to the aganglionic segment. Mucosal inflammation or stercoral ulcers may also occur. Constipation, leading to an enlarged colon, is secondary to failure of the aganglionic segment to relax in response to proximal distention of the internal anal sphincters following rectal distention.

The rectum is always affected, and the intestinal submucosa fails to stain with acetylcholinesterase

restricted to the rectosigmoid colon, also referred to as *short-segment disease*, in 80% of individuals and extends proximally to the sigmoid colon in 15% to 20%. Total intestinal aganglionosis with the absence of ganglion cells from the duodenum to the rectum is rare, representing only 5% of cases; this is referred to as *long-segment disease* (Fig. 10-5).

Hirschsprung disease is the most common form of functional intestinal obstruction in infants, with an incidence of 1 in 5000 in live births. The disease is more common in males,

with a ratio of 4 to 1, and most of this is short-segment disease. In contrast, for long-segment disease, the male-to-female ratio is only 1.5 to 2. In 70% of cases, Hirschsprung disease occurs as an isolated disease, but it may also occur with a chromosomal abnormality, and the incidence can vary with the different associated genetic syndromes. For example, classic congenital central hypoventilation syndrome is associated with Hirschsprung disease in 16% to 20% of affected individuals. Twelve percent of Down syndrome patients have Hirschsprung disease. In Bardet-Biedl syndrome, Hirschsprung disease is found in 2% of affected individuals. In cartilage-hair hypoplasia, it is present in 9%. Among different racial groups, the incidence for whites, blacks, and Asians is 0.75, 1.05, and 1.4 per 5000 live births, respectively.

Hirschsprung disease is a multigenic disease and is associated with mutations in at least 9 to 11 genes (Table 10-4). In addition to those shown in the table, the gene for the glial cell–derived neurotrophic factor receptor (*GRFα₁*) and *PAX3*, a DNA-binding protein important in early neurogenesis, have been identified in animal models. Many of these genes control morphogenesis and differentiation of the enteric nervous system. Of particular interest among these genes is the *RET* gene.

RET is expressed in tissues of neural crest origin and is a susceptibility gene for several inherited diseases including the multiple endocrine neoplasia (MEN) syndromes and

TABLE 10-4. Genes Associated with Hirschsprung's Disease

Gene	Location	Protein Function	Frequency
RET	Chr 10q11.2	Tyrosine kinase receptor	70% to 80% long segment 50% familial 15% to 20% sporadic
GDNF	Chr 5p12-13.3	Glial cell–derived neurotrophic factor	<10%
NRTN	Chr 19q13.3	neurturin, RET ligand	<1%
EDN3	Chr 20q13	Endothelin B	<10%
EDNRB	Chr 13q22	Endothelin B receptor	<10%
ECE-1	Chr 1p36.1	Endothelin-converting enzyme	<1%
SOX10	Chr 22q13.1	Sry/HMG box transcription factor	<1%
PHOX2B	Chr 4p12	Paired-like homeobox 2b	<1%
SIP1	Chr 2q22	SMN-interacting protein	6 Cases

Data from Puri P, Shinkai T. Pathogenesis of Hirschsprung's disease and its variants: recent progress. *Semin Pediatr Surg.* 2004;13:18–24

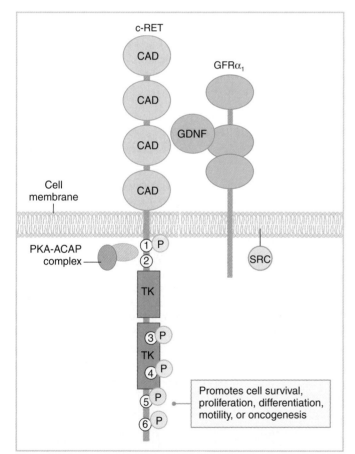

Figure 10-6. RET signaling receptor. GDNF binds preferentially to the sphingolipid-rich region of GFRα1 and activates the SRC-family of tyrosine kinases. Binding of GDNF to GFRα1 also causes recruitment of cRET and dimerization, resulting in activation of tyrosine kinases and phosphorylation of six tyrosines in the cytoplasmic domain. Four of the tyrosines are binding sites for signaling proteins important in a variety of cellular functions. CAD, cadherin-like domains that bind Ca^{++}; GDNF, glial cell–derived neurotrophic factor; GFRα1, GDNF receptor α; TK, tyrosine kinase.

Hirschsprung disease. This gene was originally identified as a proto-oncogene, encoding a receptor tyrosine kinase (Fig. 10-6). The transmembrane protein is composed of a signal peptide, a cysteine-rich region, a transmembrane region, a conserved intracellular tyrosine kinase domain, and an extracellular cadherin-related binding domain. This transmembrane receptor is the signaling component of receptor complexes with four ligands: glial-derived neurotrophic factor (GDNF), neurturin (NRTN), artemin (ARTN), and persephin (PSP). Members of the GFRα family bind to RET, permitting the binding of a specific ligand. RET/GFRα$_1$ binds GDNF, RET/GFRα$_2$ binds NRTN, RET/GFRα$_3$ binds ARTN, and RET/GFRα$_4$ binds PSP. The enteric nervous system fails to develop in the absence of RET-GFRα$_1$/GDNF signaling. Less dramatic effects are seen in the absence of RET-GFRα$_2$/NRTN signaling.

Mutations in the *RET* gene are also responsible for MEN type II cancer syndromes: MENIIA, MENIIB, and familial medullary thyroid carcinoma (FMTC). Each of these has an autosomal dominant mechanism of inheritance. *RET* mutations in Hirschsprung disease tend to be inactivating, or loss-of-function, mutations whereas those for MENII are activating. As seen in Table 10-4, other mutations compromising the developmental expression or activity of the RET pathway also cause Hirschsprung disease. However, the co-occurrence of MENII and Hirschsprung disease in some families with the same mutations suggests a common mechanism for both disorders.

●●● HEPATIC DISORDERS

There are three primary genetically determined diseases that target the liver with acute, subacute, or chronic manifestations. One of these, α$_1$-antitrypsin (AAT) deficiency, is discussed in Chapter 9. Here, hereditary hemochromatosis and Wilson disease will be discussed along with Menkes syndrome, which demonstrates several similarities to Wilson disease. As is the case for AAT deficiency, disorders of the liver are not necessarily restricted to the liver and in fact may not be a chief complaint at presentation. Hemochromatosis and Wilson disease can have devastating effects on the liver owing to iron and copper overload; however, they also have serious consequences in other systems. Menkes syndrome is due to a mutation in a gene quite homologous to the gene causing Wilson disease. However, the effects are more pronounced in neurologic manifestations and catabolism because of copper deficiency. These examples emphasize the power of genetics in complex metabolic disorders involving the liver.

Hemochromatosis

The function of iron is controlled by the need for hemoglobin synthesis. Most of the iron in the body is recycled repeatedly, as transferrin bound iron is transported to marrow precursors that become erythrocytes, which are then ingested by macrophages in the reticuloendothelial system after a life span of about 120 days. Iron is removed from hemoglobin by heme oxygenase, and most is returned to the plasma, where it is bound to transferrin again. Only a small quantity of iron leaves this cycle and enters the liver and other tissues, where it participates in the synthesis of other hemoproteins such as cytochromes and myoglobin.

Iron overload occurs by two basic mechanisms: too much is absorbed or too many erythrocytes are destroyed. In the first case, iron in excess of the iron-binding capacity of transferrin is deposited in parenchymal cells of the liver, heart, and some endocrine tissues. In the second case, iron accumulates in the reticuloendothelial macrophages. If this capacity is exceeded, iron is then stored in the parenchyma. It should be apparent that the first situation is far more serious and can lead to tissue damage and fibrosis if not corrected. Both types of overload can be dangerous and lead to damage, but macrophages function to protect organs as long as possible.

Several genes play an important role in the regulation of iron absorption (Table 10-5). Mutations in *HFE* are associated with the most common form of iron-overload disorder, known as hemochromatosis. Mutations in the transferrin receptor 2 gene (*TFR2*) are much less common than *HFE* mutations but present a clinical picture very similar to HFE-associated hemochromatosis. A third gene is hemojuvelin, *HJV*, which is mutated in most cases of juvenile hemochromatosis. Juvenile hemochromatosis is rare but is associated with more severe iron overload than with mutations in either *HFE* or *TFR2* genes. Each of these genes is expressed in the liver, and it is now becoming clearer that the liver plays a critical role in the regulation of iron absorption through an iron regulatory hormone known as hepcidin. Specifically, hepcidin is central in determining the amounts of iron that must be mobilized from macrophages, enterocytes, and hepatocytes.

Iron absorption is influenced by a variety of factors that affect the expression of enterocyte iron transport molecules (Table 10-6). A brush border ferric reductase, *DCYTB*, reduces dietary iron to the ferrous state (Fe^{++}). The brush border iron transporter divalent metal transporter 1 (*DMT1*) mediates the actual uptake of iron from the intestinal lumen across the apical membrane and into the enterocyte. Iron that is not needed by the body is stored in the enterocyte as ferritin and eventually lost by ultimate cell turnover. Iron is transferred across the basolateral membrane and into the circulation by the iron transport protein ferroportin 1, *SLCA401* (also known as IREG1) and hephaestin, a ferroxidase with homology to ceruloplasmin. Hepcidin expression regulates these activities.

BIOCHEMISTRY

Ferritin

The ferritin concentration in blood is related to the amount of iron in stored in tissues and therefore is used as a marker of iron load. It is an iron-containing protein complex that is found principally in the intestinal mucosa, spleen, bone marrow, and liver.

Translation is regulated by the iron regulator protein (IRP). In low concentrations of iron, IRP binds to the iron response element (IRE) located in the 5′ UTR of ferritin mRNA and thus inhibits translation. Conversely, at high concentrations of iron, iron binds to IRP and changes its conformation, releasing it from IRE; ferritin mRNA is then translated.

TABLE 10-5. Classification of Types of Hemochromatosis (HFE)

Type	Gene	Location	Protein	Inheritance
Classical HFE or HFE-1	*HFE*	Chr 6p21.3		Recessive
HFE-2				
HFE-2A	*HJV*	Chr 1q21	Hemojuvelin	Recessive
HFE-2B	*HAMP*	Chr 19q13	Hepcidin	Recessive
HFE-3	TFR2	Chr 7q22	Transferrin receptor-2	Recessive
HFE-4	SLC40A1	Chr 2q32	Ferroportin	Dominant

TABLE 10-6. Factors influencing Iron Absorption

Factors Increasing Iron Absorption	Factors Decreasing Iron Absorption
Inadequate diet	Regular blood transfusions
Impaired absorption	High-iron diet
Achlorhydria	Iron-loading vitamins
Gastric surgery	
Celiac disease	
Pica	
Increased iron loss	
GI bleeding	
Duodenal and gastric ulcers	
Hiatal hernia	
Gastritis from drugs or toxins	
Diverticulosis	
Hookworm	
Meckel's diverticulum	
Anemias, decreased erythropoiesis	
Hypoxia	
Inflammation	
Pregnancy	

Hepcidin expression in the liver is up-regulated when iron stores are increased and down-regulated when iron stores are decreased. Once expressed, hepcidin interacts directly with ferroportin 1 at the basement membrane, resulting in internalization and degradation of this transmembrane protein; hence, the iron associated with ferroportin is then released into the cell. A decrease in ferroportin 1 decreases iron transfer to the body. Since it is known that the expression of DMT1 and DCYTB is affected by cellular iron concentrations, this suggests that signals of excess iron from the body affect the ferroportin 1 protein before expression of DMT1 and DCYTB expression is affected. Stated differently, if iron is not transported across the basolateral membrane, the iron concentration within the enterocyte increases, which leads to decreased ferric reduction at the apical surface and decreased iron transport into the enterocyte (Fig. 10-7). This interaction replaces the previously held hypothesis that the crypt cells of the duodenum regulate iron absorption.

Iron is transported in the body by transferrin, which binds two iron molecules. Transferrin and HFE compete for binding sites at the transferrin receptor, TFR1, found on hepatocytes and other cells. It is proposed that transferrin has a higher binding affinity for TFR1 than HFE does and that higher transferrin levels lead to increased free HFE on the cell surface. It is further proposed that increased HFE stimulates increased hepcidin. During iron overload, TFR2 receptors are expressed more than TFR1 receptors. With a lower affinity for transferrin, TFR2 receptors will bind more transferrin, resulting in increased hepcidin expression. Thus, increased HFE availability and TFR2 expression can lead to decreased absorption at the basolateral surface of the enterocyte by increased expression of hepcidin.

Mutations in either HFE or TFR2 produce iron overload. Hepcidin levels are lower but detectable with these mutations, and therefore iron absorption can still be regulated minimally; however, regulation is insufficient to decrease the high rate of absorption or reduce the iron stored. Mutations in hemojuvelin, on the other hand, are more severe, and no hepcidin is present. As might be expected, a double mutation in HFE and TFR2 produces a severe phenotype.

Hereditary hemochromatosis (HH) is an autosomal recessive, late-onset disease featuring altered iron metabolism. Specifically, increased iron absorption in the gastrointestinal tract leads to excessive iron deposits in the primary storage targets, namely, the liver, pancreas, heart, and endocrine organs (Fig. 10-8), resulting in a toxic situation for the organ. There is no major mechanism for iron excretion. The hereditary form of the disease differs from secondary hemochromatosis due to acquired iron excess, as might be seen with repeated transfusions.

Clinically, symptoms for the classical hereditary form of hemochromatosis generally do not manifest until the fifth or sixth decade of life. Early symptoms are generally nonspecific and can include fatigue, arthralgia, erectile dysfunction, and increased skin pigmentation. With progression, hepatosplenomegaly and tenderness occur and lead to liver fibrosis and cirrhosis. The incidence of hepatocellular carcinoma increases after liver damage. Iron deposition in the heart causes cardiomyopathy. The accumulation of iron also initiates endocrinopathies including diabetes mellitus, hypopituitarism, hypogonadism, and hypoparathyroidism. In addition, affected individuals experience increased infections owing to decreased hepcidin, which has antimicrobial properties.

Expression of hemochromatosis in women occurs later than in men, presumably owing to loss of iron during menses and pregnancy. As a result, onset of a full phenotypic clinical expression for hemochromatosis generally occurs after menopause. Unlike men who initially have cirrhosis or diabetes, women at the outset have vague symptoms of fatigue, arthralgia, and pigmentation. The differences in these presentations may contribute to more men being diagnosed than women until progressive hepatic involvement becomes significant in women.

Nearly 90% of all HH patients are homozygous for an HFE missense mutation that changes cysteine at amino acid residue 282 to tyrosine (C282Y). A second HFE variant that substitutes aspartate for histidine at amino acid 63 (H63D) also is associated with HH and typically occurs in the homozygous state or as a compound heterozygote with C282Y. HFE heterozygotes may also accumulate iron but rarely, if ever, demonstrate clinical signs.

The frequency of C282Y homozygotes in individuals of northern European ancestry is as high as 1 in 250, indicative of a high allele frequency and characteristic of a very common disease. However, HFE-associated hemochromatosis serves as a classical example of incomplete penetrance in that roughly half of C282Y homozygotes demonstrate some degree of iron overload and only 10% develop pathologic indicators of iron overload. For the majority of clinically

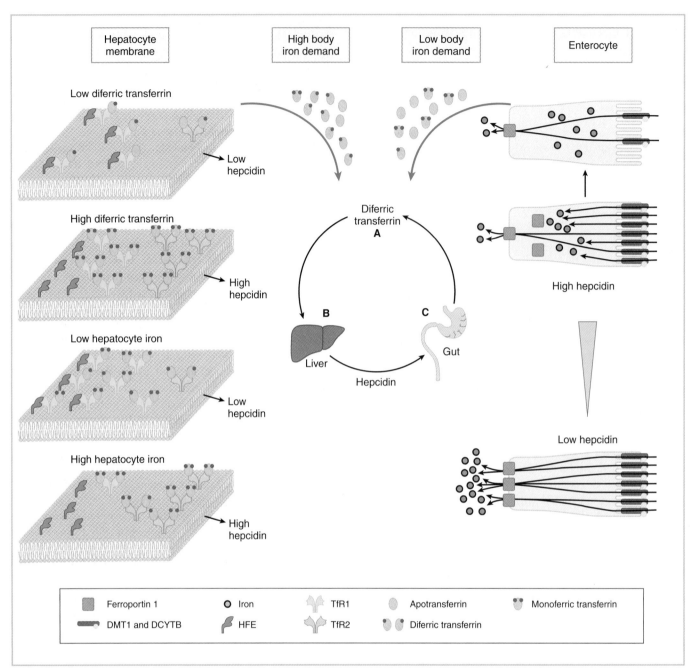

Figure 10-7. Model for the regulation of intestinal iron absorption. Changes in body iron usage alter the amount of diferric transferrin in the circulation (A). This molecule is preferentially taken up by cells requiring iron. The change in diferric transferrin concentration is detected by transferrin receptor (TFR) 2 and the hemochromatosis protein (HFE)/TFR1 on the plasma membrane of hepatocytes and leads to changes in the expression of hepcidin (B). Hepatocyte iron stores also affect hepcidin production by altering the amount of TFR1 on the plasma membrane. Circulating hepcidin interacts with ferroportin 1 at the basolateral membrane of the villus enterocytes of the small intestine, causing the iron transporter to be internalized and degraded and reducing iron export (C). The accumulation of iron within the cell decreases the expression of divalent metal transporter 1 (DMT1) and DCYTB at the brush border. Any changes in iron absorption affect diferric transferrin levels, thereby completing a negative feedback loop that regulates body iron homeostasis. (Redrawn with permission from Frazer DM, Anderson GJ. Iron imports. I. Intestinal iron absorption and its regulation. *Am J Physiol Gastrointest Liver Physiol.* 2005; 289:G631–G635.)

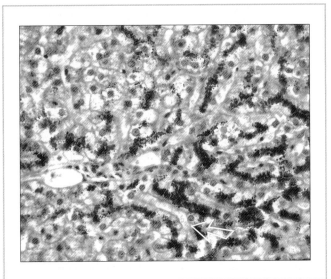

Figure 10-8. Hereditary hemochromatosis. Hepatocellular iron deposition (blue) is stained with Prussian blue stain in an early stage of the disease. Parenchymal architecture is normal. (From Kumar V, Abbas A, Fausto N. *Robbins & Cotran Pathologic Basis of Disease*, 7th ed. Philadelphia, WB Saunders, 2005.)

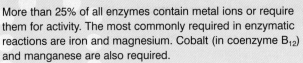

BIOCHEMISTRY

Metal Ions

More than 25% of all enzymes contain metal ions or require them for activity. The most commonly required in enzymatic reactions are iron and magnesium. Cobalt (in coenzyme B_{12}) and manganese are also required.

Most are divalent ions. Iron and manganese change oxidation states during reactions.

identified HH patients, it is clear that HFE mutations serve as predisposing entities and may be necessary but not sufficient for disease expression.

Among the many populations that have been studied, mutations in C282Y have not been found in individuals from Africa, Asia, Southeast Asia, or Micronesia. A few alleles have been identified in Australian aborigines, Melanesians, and Polynesians, but these are linked to HLA haplotypes commonly observed in Europeans, thus suggesting admixture. Hemochromatosis is occasionally recognized in blacks with C282Y alleles with a frequency of 1 in 6000, significantly less than in individuals of European ancestry. Non-HFE-associated hemochromatosis among blacks apparently results from an unidentified gene.

Menkes Syndrome

Copper is required in trace amounts for several reactions (Box 10-4). It is absorbed in the stomach and duodenum and bound to albumin for transport to the liver. Two highly homologous genes are involved in copper homeostasis: *ATP7A* expressed in most cells and *ATP7B* expressed in hepatocytes, brain, kidney, and placenta. The liver has a high affinity for copper-bound albumin, and in hepatocytes the ATP7B protein facilitates copper incorporation in apoceruloplasmin, followed by release of copper-rich ceruloplasmin in the circulation; thus, copper is a rate-limiting element for ceruloplasmin formation.

PHYSIOLOGY & BIOCHEMISTRY

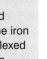

Iron Absorption

Dietary iron is absorbed in the duodenum from heme and nonheme sources but by different mechanisms. Nonheme iron is usually in the ferric (Fe^{+++}) form, which is easily complexed with anions, thereby reducing its solubility and absorption. Absorption is increased by glucose, fructose, some amino acids, and vitamin C. Vitamin C complexes with iron, reducing it to the ferrous (Fe^{++}) form, thereby enhancing its absorption.

Heme iron, derived from myoglobin and hemoglobin, is more readily absorbed than nonheme iron. Iron absorption is decreased in the presence of PO_4, HCO_3^-, and bile acids.

PHYSIOLOGY & PATHOLOGY

Transferrin

Transferrin is produced predominantly in the liver but also in the testes and central nervous system; it carries iron from the intestine, reticuloendothelial system, and liver parenchymal cells to all proliferating cells in the body. Owing to the mildly alkaline pH of the extracellular fluid, the iron-transferrin complex binds to membrane-bound transferrin receptors with high affinity. During endocytosis, iron is released from transferrin because of the decreased pH in the endosome. The apotransferrin (transferrin without iron) and transferrin receptor are then recycled to the cell membrane surface, where the change in pH (more alkaline) causes dissociation of the apotransferrin from the receptor.

PATHOLOGY

Iron Overload Among Africans

Iron overload in Africans results from a predisposition to iron loading. This condition was formerly called Bantu siderosis. It occurs among Africans who drink beer from nongalvanized steel drums and differs from HFE-associated hemochromatosis. Iron loading occurs in Kupffer cells as well as hepatocytes. However, cardiomyopathy and diabetes are less frequent. Serum ferritin levels are elevated, but transferrin levels may not reflect the extent of overload.

There is a concern that affected individuals may be more susceptible to infections and tuberculosis than individuals with HFE-associated hemochromatosis.

Box 10-4.   ENZYMES REQUIRING COPPER AS A COFACTOR

Lysyl oxidase—connective tissue formation
Superoxide dismutase—free radical scavenging
Cytochrome-*c* oxidase—electron transfer
Tyrosinase—electron transfer
Monoamine oxidase—neurotransmitter formation
Dopamine β-hydroxylase—conversion of dopamine to
    noradrenalin

Ceruloplasmin, a ferroxidase, is important also for iron transport. By oxidizing ferrous iron to the ferric form, ceruloplasmin promotes iron loading onto transferrin, which binds only the ferric form of the metal. Oxidizing ferrous to ferric iron also serves an antioxidant function and thus helps prevent or reduce oxidative damage to proteins, lipids, and DNA. Aceruloplasminemia shares features with other neurodegenerative diseases.

Both ATP7A and ATP7B proteins provide copper to copper-dependent enzymes as they migrate through the trans-Golgi, the final portion of the Golgi network. However, under conditions of elevated extracellular copper, ATP7A proteins relocate to the plasma membrane and ATP7B relocates to an intracellular vesicle to assist in copper efflux.

Two genes are implicated in copper transport in the brush border of intestinal cells: *CRT1* and *DMT1*. The latter has been discussed with iron transport and may transport as many as eight metals, has four or more isoforms, and carries out transport for multiple purposes. CRT1 (copper transporter 1, also known as SLC31A1) is located on the basolateral surface as well as the apical surface, since copper can enter enterocytes from the blood. The mechanism of copper absorption is not as well understood as that for iron. However, it is known that once in the enterocyte, most copper is bound to metallothionein or other proteins having a high affinity for copper.

BIOCHEMISTRY & PATHOLOGY

Ceruloplasmin

Ceruloplasmin is an α-globulin. Ninety percent of copper is bound to ceruloplasmin; each molecule binds six copper atoms, and albumin carries the remaining 10% with less avidity (i.e., albumin donates copper more readily).

Ceruloplasmin concentration is decreased with liver disease. Its absence, however, does not produce marked changes in copper metabolism although it will cause a gradual accumulation of iron in the liver and other tissues. This occurs because the ferroxidase activity of ceruloplasmin is important for oxidizing ferrous iron to ferric iron. Without oxidation, iron is not bound to transferrin. Copper deficiency is accompanied by a hypochromic, microcytic anemia similar to that produced by iron deficiency.

Both ATP7A and ATP7B proteins are localized predominantly in the trans-Golgi network, where they facilitate the addition of copper to certain enzymes. However, when cells are exposed to excessive copper, the copper-transporting protein is rapidly relocated to the plasma membrane, where it functions in copper efflux to decrease the concentration of copper in the cytoplasm. The normal function of ATP7A is to move copper from the intestinal mucosa into the bloodstream, where it is bound to albumin proteins and transported to tissues. If the ATP7A protein is nonfunctional, the uptake of copper from the intestines is impaired and a state of copper deficiency results. Mutations in this gene result in Menkes syndrome, which is sometimes referred to as kinky hair disease. It is an X-linked disorder characterized by early retardation in growth, peculiar hair, and focal cerebral and cerebellar degeneration. Severe neurologic impairment begins within a month or two of birth and progresses rapidly to decerebration.

These manifestations underscore the critical function of copper for the proper function of several enzymes. Lysyl oxidase is important for the cross-linking of collagen and elastin, and deficiencies lead to problems in connective tissue, such as bone. The enzyme dopamine-β-hydroxylase (or dopamine-β-monooxygenase) requires copper to catalyze the conversion of dopamine to noradrenalin. Individuals with Menkes syndrome have a reduced activity of this enzyme with high levels of dopamine and low levels of noradrenalin and its neuronal metabolite dihydroxyphenylglycol. Cytochrome oxidase is part of complex IV of the electron transport chain in mitochondria; it contains bound copper atoms. Since copper is insufficient, the activity of the enzyme is reduced and less ATP is produced, leading to lipid catabolism in the body to provide adequate energy for essential biochemical reactions. In addition, lower cytochrome oxidase activity leads to neuromuscular disorders and progressive brain degeneration.

Wilson Disease

There are only two routes for copper excretion. Excess copper intake induces metallothionein production in enterocytes that capture it for storage followed by normal shedding. The physiologic route for balancing copper is through incorporation into ceruloplasmin and compartmentalization into a vesicular membrane compartment in preparation for excretion into bile (Fig. 10-9). Mutations in the *ATP7B* gene, located on chromosome 13q14.3-q21.1, prevent release of copper from hepatocytes and cause an inability to use or excrete the metal. As an additional consequence, apoceruloplasmin is degraded and ceruloplasmin levels decrease (Table 10-7). This can be a significant event because ceruloplasmin is required for iron homeostasis and neuronal maintenance in the central nervous system. Ceruloplasmin also serves an acute-phase reactant with increased levels during inflammation, infection, and trauma. Without copper incorporation, only apoceruloplasmin is produced.

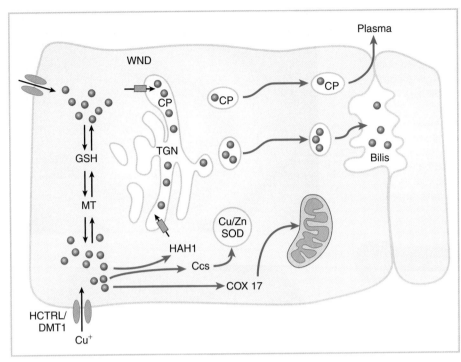

Figure 10-9. Model of Cu$^+$ uptake and metabolism in hepatocytes. Crossing the plasma membrane through either CTRL1 or DMT1, most of the Cu$^+$ is shuttled to the trans-Golgi network (TGN) by the chaperone HAH1/Atox1, which delivers Cu$^+$ to the P-type ATPase located in the trans-Golgi network. In the case of hepatocytes, it is ATP7B, the protein defective in Wilson disease. In enterocytes, it is ATP7A, the protein defective in Menkes syndrome. The chaperone protein, CCS, delivers Cu$^+$ to cytosolic Cu/Zn superoxide dismutase (SOD), which dismutates superoxide into hydrogen peroxide. COX 17 delivers Cu$^+$ to the mitochondria, where it is required for cytochrome C oxidase. Glutathione (GSH) may also be a chaperone by binding Cu$^+$ and delivering it to metallothionein (MT) and to some Cu$^+$-dependent apoenzymes, such as SOD.

Wilson disease was first described in 1912 as progressive lenticular degeneration characterized by bilateral softening of the lenticular nucleus and by liver cirrhosis. The original characterizations of this disease focused more on its neurologic aspects than the liver aspects. However, it has since become clear that the disease is the result of copper accumulation in the liver, and only after liver disease has initiated does neurologic involvement begin.

Wilson disease is an autosomal recessive disease resulting from mutations in the adenosine triphosphatase gene, *ATP7B*, located on chromosome 13q14.3-q21.1. More than 200 mutations have been described that affect the transport of copper across the trans-Golgi and into vesicles. These mutations specifically cause diminished copper excretion, leading to its accumulation in the liver, brain, and eye. Onset of the disease may be as early as age 3 years in families with affected members and range to age 50 years before diagnosis.

The heterozygote frequency of Wilson disease mutations is 1 in 90 in the general population, with the disease occurring in 1 in 30,000 individuals. Expression of the disease varies in different populations. For examples, the prevalence is 1 in 10,000 individuals in China, Japan, and Sardinia. As this suggests, mutations are panethnic, but the frequency of certain mutations is ancestry dependent. The H1069Q mutation accounts for 35% to 45% of mutated alleles in individuals with European ancestry. Mutations in exons 8, 14, and 18 account for 60% of the mutations detected in British populations. The R778L mutation accounts for about 57% of the Wilson disease alleles in persons of Asian ancestry. Mutations in exons 8 and 12 account for 57% of Wilson disease alleles in the Chinese population. Wilson disease alleles H714Q and delC2337 are identified in up to 45% of individuals with Russian ancestry. These data underscore the importance of family history in determining the correct mutation through specific laboratory instructions for screening.

Clinically, Wilson disease is variable but characterized by recurrent jaundice, fatigue, malaise, arthropathy, and rashes. Fulminant hepatic failure may occur with severe coagulation

TABLE 10-7. Comparison Between Menkes Syndrome and Wilson Disease

	Gene	Location	Defect	Laboratory Findings	Treatment
Menkes syndrome	*ATP7A*	Chr Xq12-q13	Intestinal absorption of copper	Increased serum copper levels Decreaed liver copper levels Increased intestinal/kidney copper levels	Daily copper histidine injections
Wilson disease	*ATP7B*	Chr 13q14.3-q21.1	Biliary excretion of copper	Decreased serum copper levels Increased liver copper levels Increased urinary copper levels	Copper chelation

NEUROSCIENCE & ANATOMY

Basal Nuclei (Ganglia) and Lenticular Nucleus

The basal nuclei (ganglia) consist of five interconnected nuclei: the caudate nucleus, putamen, subthalamic nucleus, globus pallidus, and substantia nigra. The lenticular nucleus is composed of the globus pallidus and putamen.

The organization of the basal nuclei (ganglia) leads to an order of connections. Specific cells in the putamen or caudate project to the globus pallidus or substantia nigra and allow cortex to motor neuron transmission. It is located between the caudate nucleus and the Island of Reil, or insula, with its anterior portion attached to the head of the caudate nucleus.

MICROBIOLOGY

Coombs Test

Two Coombs tests are used to detect and characterize antibodies: the direct and indirect. The indirect is almost never needed routinely.

The direct Coombs test is conducted to investigate the cause of hemolytic anemia whether it is to diagnose hemolytic disease of the newborn or hemolytic anemia in adults or to investigate hemolytic transfusion reactions. A positive Coombs test supports autoimmune hemolysis (IgG, complement, or both are on the surface of erythrocytes).

Many diseases can initiate autoantibody formation leading to hemolysis. Drugs can also initiate autoantibody formation (e.g., quinidine, methyldopa, and procainamide).

PHARMACOLOGY

Chelating Properties

Chelating agents are heavy-metal antagonists with the ability to complex with metals to prevent or reverse their binding to ligands. Ideally, a chelator

- Is water soluble.
- Is resistant to biotransformation.
- Can reach sites of metal storage.
- Can form nontoxic complexes with toxic metals.
- Is active at physiologic pH.
- Can be excreted.

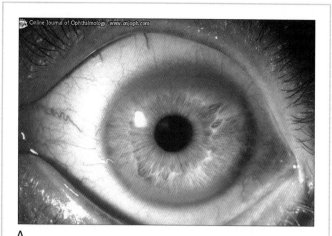

A

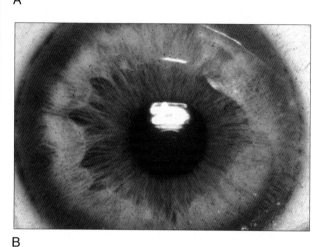

B

Figure 10-10. Kayser-Fleischer rings. Yellow-brown discoloration of the Descemet membrane surrounding the cornea resulting from copper deposition. (Reproduced with permission of the Verlag Online Journals of Ophthalmology. Available at: http://www.atlasophthalmology.com.)

problems, encephalopathy, acute Coombs' negative hemolysis, and renal failure. Chronic liver disease poses additional issues with separate consequences including portal hypertension, hepatosplenomegaly, ascites, and low serum albumin.

As the disease progresses, neurologic manifestations of Wilson disease increase as hepatic manifestations begin to decline. After the age of 18 years, 70% of clinical features are neurologic and about 20% are liver-associated, classified as acute and chronic hepatitis, cirrhosis, and fulminant hepatic failure. Lenticular degeneration is associated with dystonia, its most common feature. Additional features include dysarthria, tremors, dysphagia, and psychiatric disturbances. Ninety-eight percent of individuals with neurologic disease and 80% of all individuals with Wilson disease have *Kayser-Fleischer rings*, seen as discoloration of Descemet's membrane of the corneal endothelium (Fig. 10-10). Although common in affected individuals, they are not pathognomonic, since they may be associated with other causes of liver disease such as autoimmune hepatitis and cholestasis.

The first line of treatment is copper chelation. Dysarthria and tremors are more amenable to chelation therapy than dystonia. Renal tubule disease is usually improved with chelation therapy. In severe disease, however, individuals may not respond to chelation and may require liver transplantation.

Disorders of Gender Differentiation and Sexual Development

11

CONTENTS

Historically, the area of genetics that perhaps engenders the most enthusiasm among students of all ages involves disorders adversely affecting gender and normal sexual development. The best known are those caused by nondisjunction of the sex chromosomes. Unlike the outcome for a fetus or newborn that is monosomic or trisomic for an autosome, the same mechanism affecting sex chromosomes results in viable individuals with normal or near-normal life expectancy.

This chapter provides highlights of genes involved in gender differentiation in the developing embryo and fetus along with examples of how certain mutations change the expected outcome. In addition to specific genes involved, the best known chromosomal anomalies—Turner syndrome and Klinefelter syndrome in particular—are discussed followed by the effects of mixed genotypes, or mosaicism, in an individual. These examples demonstrate a primary effect on sexual development.

Finally, attention is given to disorders having a primary effect on the adrenocortical pathway and a secondary effect on sexual development. These outcomes revisit the underlying biochemical dogma of accumulating substrate with the inability of enzymes to produce product. In these cases, the accumulating substrates can also be used in the production of sex steroids and thus secondarily affect sexual development and function.

●●● GONADAL DIFFERENTIATION AND DISORDERS OF GENDER DEVELOPMENT

Gonadal development begins during the fifth week of gestation as a thickened ridge on the medioventral border of the urogenital ridge. During the sixth week, the primordial germ cells, which migrated into the yolk sac during gastrulation, increase mitotically and migrate back through the dorsal mesentery of the hindgut to the gonadal ridge, where they become incorporated into the primary sex cords. The primary sex cords begin developing to define the outer cortex and inner medulla. Before the sixth week of gestation, gender is indistinguishable; primordial germ cells are undifferentiated epiblast cells specified during gastrulation to become germ cells. Germ cells not arriving in the gonad prior to gender differentiation usually degenerate, but occasionally they may persist and later develop into extragonadal germ cell tumors. The difference in gender differentiation is a reflection of gene expression from the X and Y chromosomes. Under the influence of Y chromosome genes, testis organization begins in the sixth and seventh week. Ovary differentiation begins at about the twelfth week.

Early cytogenetic evidence indicated that the Y chromosome possessed a gene or genes controlling the destiny of a bipotential gonad to become an ovary or testis. Several candidate genes were investigated. The hypothetical gene sought was called the *testis determining factor* (TDF). The location of the gene producing this factor was localized to the short arm on the Y chromosome through a study of patients with translocations and deletions of the Y chromosome. The discovery of 46,XX males with a translocation of the Yp terminus to the Xp led to the discovery that the terminal region of Yp was essential for testicular differentiation.

At the termini of Y chromosomes are pseudoautosomal pairing regions (PARs). The few genes within these regions are the same on the X and Y chromosomes and are inherited in an autosomal manner, as the name implies. Males have two copies of these genes, one allele on the Y chromosome and one on the X chromosome, just as females have one allele on each of the X chromosomes. During meiosis I, Xp and Yp align at the PAR and recombination may occur. In translocations involving genes adjacent to the pseudoautosomal region, molecular analyses revealed a 1.1-kb transcript expressed only in testes, and this gene was designated as the sex-determining region of the Y chromosome (*SRY*) (Fig. 11-1). In the case of 46,XX males, recombination between Xp and Yp translocated the *SRY* gene to the Xp chromosome along with genes in the pseudoautosomal region; some of these PAR genes are also expressed specifically in testes. The *SRY* gene is the gene encoding the TDF and has become the general designation for the gene product, which may also be referred to as the SRY protein.

The *SRY* gene contains only one exon and no introns. The 5′ flanking promoter region of *SRY* differs from the vast majority of genes. It contains no TATA or CCAAT boxes, is GC rich, and contains two zinc finger recognition sites for the SP1 transcription factor. The single exon produces an 841-bp transcript that produces a 204-amino-acid protein. Within the SRY protein is a centrally located high mobility group (HMG) octamer that binds to the minor groove of the DNA helix, inducing a large conformational change. This explains the observation that almost all *SRY* mutations in 46,XY females have been localized to the HMG region: mutant SRY proteins may not effectively bind to the DNA to cause the conformational change needed for other genes to be transcribed.

The *SRY* gene was identified first because of the interest in gender differentiation. However, within the developmental pathway, steroidogenesis factor (*SF-1*) gene expression is necessary for *SRY* transcription (Fig. 11-2). If *SRY* is expressed, another gene, *SOX9,* is up-regulated and SRY expression remains high throughout Sertoli cell development. SOX proteins are related to SRY and have HMG boxes that are 71% homologous to those of SRY.

SOX9 expression is required not only for proper gender differentiation but also for chrondrogenesis. Mutations in the *SOX9* gene result in a severe dwarfism syndrome, *camptomelic dysplasia,* characterized by bowing of long bones and skeletal dysplasia including hypoplastic scapulae, unmineralized thoracic pedicles, and narrowed iliac bones (Fig. 11-3). As seen in Figure 11-2, mutations in *SOX9,* which can be in both the regulatory and the coding region, also lead to XY female sex reversal owing to gonadal dysgenesis in about 75% of the cases. Inherited as an autosomal dominant disorder, normal development does not occur in a heterozygote. Consequently, among the variable phenotypical expressions, Sertoli cells will either not initiate differentiation or not be maintained. An important target for SOX9 in sex determination is antimüllerian hormone (AMH), also called müllerian inhibitory factor (MIF).

Development of both male and female gonads and adrenal glands requires the expression of the *SF-1* gene that also regulates the steroid hydroxylase enzyme system. Failure of *SF-1* expression to occur in adrenals causes a cascade of events in which insufficient corticosterone produces significant

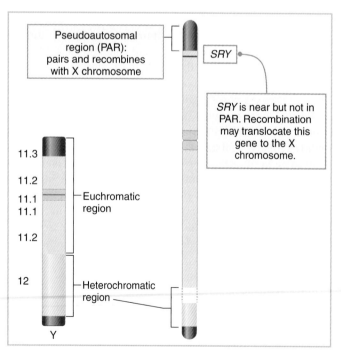

Figure 11-1. Anatomy of the Y chromosome. The pseudoautosomal region of the Y chromosome contains genes also found on the X chromosome.

BIOCHEMISTRY

Zinc Finger Proteins

Several amino acid motifs are commonly found in transcription factors. In a helix-turn-helix motif, which includes homeodomain proteins (proteins with a recurring 60-amino-acid motif, important in controlling development), a recognition helix binds in the major groove of DNA and is stabilized by the turn and the other helix.

The zinc finger motif includes general transcription factors such as TFIIIA, and SP1. This motif binds in the major groove of DNA and uses a repeating Zn^{++} motif to create the final structure.

In the helix-loop-helix motif, including the transcription factors MYOD, MYC, and MAX, two helices are separated by a loop that acts as a sequence-specific DNA binding domain.

The leucine zipper motif, including FOS, JUN, and CREB, does not directly interact with DNA. It contains leucine repeats on two protein α-helices that interdigitate in a zipper-like fashion to stabilize the protein.

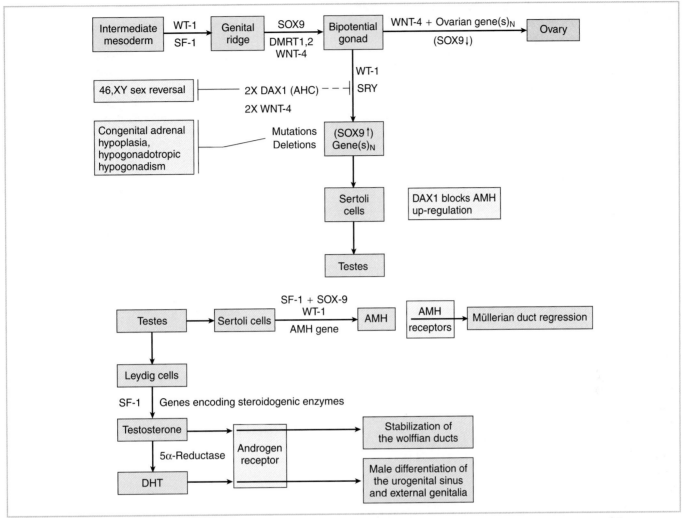

Figure 11-2. Diagrammatic representation of genes involved in sex differentiation. WT-1, Wilms' tumor suppressor; SF-1, steroidogenic factor-1; DAX1 (AHC), critical region on the X chromosome gene 1; AHC, adrenal hypoplasia congenita, hypogonadotropic hypogonadism; AMH, antimüllerian hormone. (From Larsen PR, Knonenberg HM, Melmed S, et al., *Williams Textbook of Endocrinology*, 10th ed. Philadelphia, WB Saunders, 2003, p 864.)

consequences. *SF-1* is expressed in the Sertoli cells after initiation of gonad development when mitosis is suppressed and inhibin is produced. SF-1 acts synergistically with WT to up-regulate AMH. AMH diffuses from Sertoli cells to the paired müllerian duct primordia and effects apoptosis through serine-threonine protein kinase surface receptors. Further internal and external male differentiation is regulated by testosterone synthesis in the Leydig cells, beginning at about 9 weeks, and by dihydrotestosterone. Testosterone synthesis may be stimulated by placenta-derived human chorionic gonadotropin (hCG) prior to fetal pituitary luteinizing hormone (LH) expression, since hCG and LH share regions of high homology and can interact with the same receptors on Leydig cells.

ANATOMY & EMBRYOLOGY

Adrenal Development

The adrenal cortex and medulla have different origins. The cortex is a mesoderm derivative. It first appears in week 6 as a mesenchyme aggregation between the root of the dorsal mesentery and the gonad. Cells are derived from the mesothelium of the posterior abdominal wall.

The medulla is a neural crest cell derivative. Cells of the medulla are innervated by presynaptic sympathetic fibers, similar to sympathetic ganglia.

ANATOMY

Bowlegs

Bowleg is the outward curvature of the lower limbs with medial concavity. It includes genu varum and tibia vara. Normal physiologic bowing is observed in newborns and infants and, like idiopathic bowing, generally self-corrects. In camptomelic dysplasia, femoral and tibial shafts are bowed. This may be secondary to generalized bone softening. Examples of disorders in which bowing occurs are rickets, osteogenesis imperfecta, secondary hyperparathyroidism, and hypo- or hyperphosphatasia.

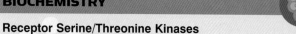

BIOCHEMISTRY

Receptor Serine/Threonine Kinases

Receptor serine/threonine kinases are one of five classes of catalytic receptors. They phosphorylate serine and/or threonine residues on proteins. An example of these is the transforming growth factor-β (TGF-β) superfamily. This large family includes members important during embryogenesis and control of cellular differentiation in adults: antimüllerian hormone (AMH), inhibins, activins, bone morphogenic proteins, and other glycoproteins.

The receptors are single membrane-spanning glycoproteins and consist of two types, RI and RII. Ligands bind to RII but RI, which recognizes ligand is bound to RII but cannot itself bind ligand, transmits signals downstream. Formation of a stable RII-ligand/RI complex results in phosphorylation of RI at serines and threonines. This activates the kinase activity of RI to downstream effectors.

Substrates of activated RI include the SMAD family of transcription factors. When phosphorylated by the TGF-complex, the activated factor translocates to the nucleus, binds to DNA, and effects transcription.

PHYSIOLOGY

Human Chorionic Gonadotropin (hCG)

hCG shares structural homology with LH, FSH, and TSH. It functions after binding to a G-protein receptor on target cells, and it may also interact with receptors for LH, FSH, and TSH because of shared homologies.

The syncytiotrophoblast, which forms the placenta, produces hCG beginning in the second week after fertilization. Production begins to decline during the eighth week and thereafter occurs from the chorion, the outer embryonic membrane. Its major function is to maintain the corpus luteum during the first trimester of pregnancy via LH/hCG membrane receptors. This function is important because the corpus luteum secretes progesterone and estrogen to maintain pregnancy. Excess hCG is excreted in urine and is the basis of most pregnancy tests. During the second trimester, the placenta begins secreting progesterone, which plays a critical role in supporting the endometrium of pregnancy and hence the survival of the fetus.

Duplication of a region on the X chromosome can result in sex reversal. This region, called DSS (*dosage-sensitive sex reversal*), is regulated by *SF-1* through feedback inhibition. DSS contains a gene designated as *DAX1* for *d*osage-sensitive reversal-*a*drenal hypoplasia on the *X* chromosome. Prior to testis determination, DAX1 is expressed in both gonads. As SRY expression increases from the Y chromosome, *DAX1* expression declines in testes. DAX1 is present normally in the ovary, where *SRY* expression is not normal or expected in 46,XX females. DAX1 also normally blocks the synergistic activity of SF-1 and WT-1 to up-regulate *AMH* expression.

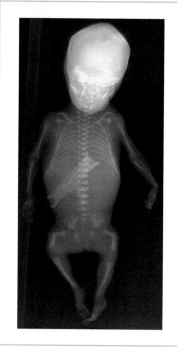

Figure 11-3. Camptomelic dysplasia is caused by mutations in the *SOX9* gene. This gene plays an essential role in sex determination as well as in chrondrogenesis. In the latter, SOX9 protein binds to sequences in the collagen gene, COL2A1, to regulate its expression. (Used with permission of GE Healthcare: http://www.medcyclopaedia.com.)

When *SRY* expression increases, *DAX1* expression is repressed. Then accordingly *DAX1* expression does not occur in testes, where SRY expression is high, and thus prevents ovary formation. An interesting situation occurs when the *DAX1* gene is duplicated on the X chromosome. Here, the amount of SRY is insufficient to antagonize the increased DAX1 activity. *DAX1* remains active and continues to prevent testis formation, resulting in a 46,XY female.

DAX1 is expressed in all tissues of the steroidogenic axis: hypothalamus, pituitary, adrenal cortex, and gonads. As might be expected, mutations in *DAX1* can affect these tissues. The X-linked form of *adrenal hypoplasia congenita* (AHC) is caused by loss of function mutations in *DAX1*, resulting in hypogonadotropic hypogonadism in males. In the severest clinical presentation, infants have primary adrenal insufficiency characterized by hyponatremia, hyperkalemia, acidosis, and hypoglycemia—a life-threatening situation if untreated. Less severe mutations may present with hypogonadotropic hypogonadism at adolescence. Mutations resulting in this presentation are due to decreased *DAX1* expression rather than to absence of expression in the hypothalamus and pituitary.

Understanding the generalities of gender development and several disorders that can occur with mutations allows a better appreciation of the survival of individuals missing an X chromosome or having additional sex chromosomes.

Turner Syndrome

Turner syndrome with a 45,X karyotype, which results from loss of an X chromosome through nondisjunction, characterizes approximately 60% of the individuals with the classical features of Turner syndrome (Box 11-1). The remaining 40% encompasses a wide range of structural abnormalities of one of the X chromosomes, including Xp and Xq deletions (Box 11-2). Many patients with Turner syndrome have a mosaic pattern comprising two or more cell lines and have a milder phenotype.

Women with Turner syndrome have rudimentary ovaries, also called streak ovaries. Germ cells in the primitive gonad begin to differentiate but then undergo degeneration, sometimes referred to as dysgenesis, and oocytes are lost during fetal development. By birth, the number of oocytes is severely diminished, and by adolescence ovarian tissue has regressed to ridges of white streaks devoid of both germ cells and hormone-producing cells and consisting of fibrous connective tissue. The degeneration of ovaries has secondary consequences, notably, an inhibition of breast development and the presence of infantile external genitalia. The decreased secretion of sex hormones is largely responsible for the immaturity of the external genitalia.

Turner syndrome is often diagnosed at birth by the presence of webbed neck, edema of the hands and feet, and a very low birth weight (below the third percentile) (Fig. 11-4).

PHYSIOLOGY

Secondary Sexual Characteristics

Secondary sexual characteristics are generally those changes that occur at puberty. For females, breast and associated apocrine gland development follow stimulation by estrogens secreted by ovaries. Estrogen also causes the pelvis to widen, and deposition of fat in the hips, buttocks, and thighs. It also induces uterine growth, proliferation of the endometrium, and menses. Pubic and axillary hair also grow, controlled by androgens secreted by adrenals and ovaries.

Through testosterone and dihydrotestosterone (DHT), males experience growth of the penis, testes, and pubic hair. Testosterone directly increases muscle mass and size as well as the mass of vocal cords, which leads to deepening of the voice, and the mass of bones, leading to increased strength and changes in skeletal shape.

5α-reductase converts testosterone to DHT at peripheral target tissues, such as the skin, and contributes to beard growth, acne, and temporal balding. DHT binds to the same androgen receptor as does testosterone but with greater affinity, and the DHT-receptor complex binds with greater avidity to DNA.

Box 11-1. FEATURES OF TURNER SYNDROME

45,X karyotype

Webbed neck, coarctation of aorta, high arched palate, shield-like chest with widely spaced nipples, short metatarsals, renal abnormalities; gonadal dysgenesis; may also have cubitus valgus, renal abnormalities, edema of hands and feet, micrognathia

Lack of ovarian development leading to deficient secretion of sex steroids

Increased incidence of diabetes mellitus, inflammatory bowel disease, and autoimmune disease

Box 11-2. TURNER SYNDROME GENOTYPES*

45,X
45,X/46,XX
45,X/47,XXX
45,X/46,XY
46,X,i(Xp)
46,X,i(Xq)
46,X,del(Xq)
46,X,del(Xp)
45,X,46X,i(Xq)
47,X,i(Xq),i(Xq)

*Features of Turner syndrome may occur with different genotypes.

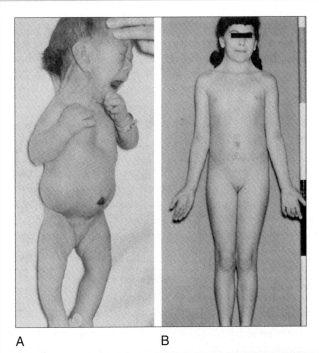

Figure 11-4. Turner syndrome. **A**, Lymphedema and webbed neck are frequent features in infants with Turner syndrome. Lymphedema in newborn females is an indication for karyotyping. **B**, A 13-year-old girl with classical Turner features, including short stature, webbed neck, delayed sexual maturation and lack of secondary sexual characteristics, cubitus valgus, and broad, shield-like chest with widely spaced nipples. (From Nussbaum RL, McInnes RR, Willard HF. *Thompson & Thompson Genetics in Medicine,* 6th ed. Philadelphia, WB Saunders, 2001, p 175.)

Short stature, the lack of secondary sex characeristics, and primary amenorrhea are significant features seen later in the development of these females. Short stature, a hallmark of the syndrome, is generally three standard deviations below the age-adjusted mean. Other features may include micrognathia, low posterior hairline, cubitus valgus, renalanomalies, and coarctation of the aorta. There is also an associated increased incidence of autoimmune disease including Hashimoto thyroiditis, Crohn disease, and diabetes mellitus.

The frequency of Turner syndrome is 1 in 2000 to 1 in 2500 live-born females. There is high intrauterine mortality, and 98% to 99% of all 45,X fetuses are spontaneously aborted—accounting for 20% of all chromosomally abnormal aborted embryos. Given the high incidence of in utero loss, one might expect 45,X fetuses that come to term to be severely affected, particularly mentally. Nevertheless, Turner syndrome is associated with normal intelligence.

Turner syndrome presumably results from *haplo-insufficiency* of certain genes on the X chromosome. Gene dosage considerations led to the prediction that the genes implicated in the Turner phenotype *escape* lyonization. This further suggests that a functional Y chromosome homolog may exist, since two copies are suggested in XX females. As discussed earlier, genes possessing these characteristics are those residing in the PAR of X and Y chromosomes. Genes in the PAR that are dosage sensitive probably contribute to the short stature observed in Turner syndrome. One such gene has been identified in the Xp22 and Yp11-3 regions containing a homeobox that is mutated in individuals with idiopathic short stature. This gene is designated *SHOX*, for short stature homeobox-containing gene. There are two forms of this gene resulting from alternative splicing. SHOXa protein is expressed in skeletal muscle, placenta, pancreas, heart, and bone marrow fibroblast. SHOXb protein expression is restricted to fetal kidney and skeletal muscle and has its greatest expression in bone marrow fibroblasts.

Turner females are short because they are missing one *SHOX* allele. *SHOX* expression is most evident in the midportion of limbs and the first and second pharyngeal arches. Expression in these sites supports the involvement of this gene in the development of other Turner stigmata beyond

short stature, such as cubitus valgus, genu varum, high-arched palate, micrognathia, and sensorineural deafness. This also provides an explanation for the greater height attained by 46,Xi(Xp) females who possess many Turner syndrome features. The Xp isochromosome contains *SHOX* alleles, and these females express 3 *SHOX* alleles.

Treatment for Turner syndrome usually includes growth hormone therapy to improve growth followed by estrogen replacement to improve development of secondary sex characteristics. Estrogen therapy is also important for reducing the risk of osteoporosis, which is common in Turner syndrome.

Turner syndrome is phenotypically mimicked in *Noonan syndrome*, which features webbed neck, short stature, pectus excavatum/carinatum, characteristic facies, cryptorchidism, and cardiac anomalies. However, whereas Turner syndrome results from an absent X chromosome, Noonan syndrome is inherited in an autosomal dominant manner and thus occurs in both males and females. At least 50% of Noonan syndrome is associated with mutations in the *PTPN11* gene, a non–receptor protein tyrosine phosphatase. Mutations affect the ability of the protein to convert from an inactive to active form. Other unidentified gene mutations are expected to explain other Noonan syndrome phenotypes. Although fertility may be reduced in Noonan syndrome, both males and females are fertile. Individuals with Noonan syndrome often have pulmonary stenosis, particularly those with *PTPN11* mutations, whereas females with Turner syndrome have coarctation of the aorta.

Klinefelter Syndrome

Klinefelter syndrome, the *most common cause of hypogonadism in the male*, occurs in males with the 47,XXY karyotype at a frequency of 1 in 1000 live-born males. Also known as seminiferous tubule dysgenesis, it is usually detected at adolescence because of the lack of sexual maturation or later because of infertility. Prepubertal suspicion of Klinefelter syndrome is generally associated with

---

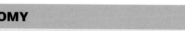

disproportionately long legs, small external genitalia, and behavioral disorders (Box 11-3).

In affected males, testes are about one-third of the normal size and gynecomastia may occur in 50% of individuals. Most patients are sterile owing to decreased testosterone production. Microscopic studies of testes show degenerative changes in the seminiferous tubules (Fig. 11-5). Studies suggest that the number of germ cells is normal or near-normal at birth but this is followed by a dramatic loss of germ cells leading to a defective testis with increasing hyalinization of the seminiferous tubules and clumping of Leydig cells.

The mechanism resulting in Klinefelter syndrome is directly related to dosage compensation. Many X chromosome genes are expressed in higher doses before and after inactivation in the Klinefelter male. Although lyonization of additional X chromosomes occurs just as in females, several characteristics of the additional X chromosomes are atypical. Recall that lyonization does not occur until the blastomere stage. Prior to this, all X chromosome alleles are active and capable of expression, which implicates an elevated level of many proteins as contributory to abnormal development. Similarly, between 15% and 20% of genes escape inactivation and are expressed from the inactive and active X chromosome, again representing a difference in dosage between males and females. For example, as previously discussed, the *SHOX* gene in the pseudoautosomal region of the X and Y chromosomes is not inactivated and the increased number of *SHOX* alleles is associated with increased height in individuals who are 47,XXY, 47,XYY, and 47,XXX.

Another gene of interest is the steroid sulfatase (*STS*) gene located on the X chromosome. This gene is expressed from the inactive X chromosome. Estrone sulfate is a major circulating plasma estrogen that is converted to the biologically active estrogen—estrone—by steroid sulfatase. This enzyme also hydrolyzes sulfate ester bonds in other steroids such as cholesterol and DHEA. The level of *STS* expression is higher in fetal tissues than in adult tissues, and thus it is not surprising that the placental syncytiotrophoblast produces large quantities of biologically active estrogens during pregnancy. Estrogens play important roles in fetal development, but excessive estrogen exposure affects development—just as seen with excessive androgen exposure.

The limbs of males with Klinefelter syndrome are longer than average and facial hair is sparse (Fig. 11-6). Although some are passive with poor self-image, most have an IQ in the normal range. Less than 1% of mentally retarded males have a 47,XXY complement. A few 47,XXY males are free of any clinical signs of Klinefelter syndrome, with the exception of infertility.

Individuals with Klinefelter syndrome have a 20-fold increased risk of developing breast cancer. The incidence of breast cancer in patients with Klinefelter syndrome is comparable to the incidence in females, suggesting an association between abnormal hormonal balance and breast cancer. Klinefelter individuals with unusually high numbers of X chromosomes have been reported, such as 48,XXXY, 49,XXXXY, and 50,XXXXXY. With more than two X chromosomes, the deleterious effect on IQ is increasingly severe. Despite numerous X chromosomes, however, the individual is male by virtue of the Y chromosome.

Testosterone replacement beginning in the early to the mid-adolescence years is recommended for Klinefelter syndrome. This therapy will not reverse gynecomastia but will support secondary sexual characteristics. Individuals with Klinefelter syndrome are at an increased risk for osteoporosis because of decreased androgens, and testosterone therapy will reduce this risk. Similarly to women with Turner syndrome, these men have an increased risk of autoimmune disorders such as diabetes, thyroid disorders, and systemic lupus erythematosis.

Another condition genotypically similar to Klinefelter syndrome is *XYY syndrome*, which affects 1 in 850 to 1 in 1000 males. Unlike Klinefelter males, these individuals have normal sexual behavior and normal secondary sexual characteristics. 47,XYY males are taller than average with low weight compared with stature and may have minor skeletal anomalies. They have larger facial features, large hands and feet, severe acne as adolescents, and possibly mild-to-moderate hyperactivity. There are reports that XYY males are more aggressive and have behavioral and learning problems.

Box 11-3. FEATURES OF KLINEFELTER SYNDROME

47,XXY and variants for karyotype
Prepubertal features: small testes, disproportionately long legs, personality and behavioral disorders
Postpubertal features: small testes, gynecomastia, and other signs of androgen deficiency (e.g., diminished facial and body hair, small phallus, poor muscular development, eunuchoid habitus, taller than average height)
Increased risk of osteoporosis if untreated
Increased risk of breast cancer and extragonadal germ cell tumors

---

PHARMACOLOGY

Androgen Replacement

Various drugs and routes of administration can treat androgen deficiency. Methyltestosterone, oxymetholone, and fluoxymesterone may be given sublingually or orally, but have disadvantages such as erratic absorption and potential for cholestatic jaundice and are less effective than intramuscular preparations. Testosterone propionate is a short-acting treatment. Testosterone enanthate and cyclopentylpropionate are given intramuscularly and can cause virilization. Transdermal patches mimic normal diurnal testosterone fluctuation.

Therapy is contraindicated in adolescents prior to epiphyseal fusion and in patients with prostate cancer.

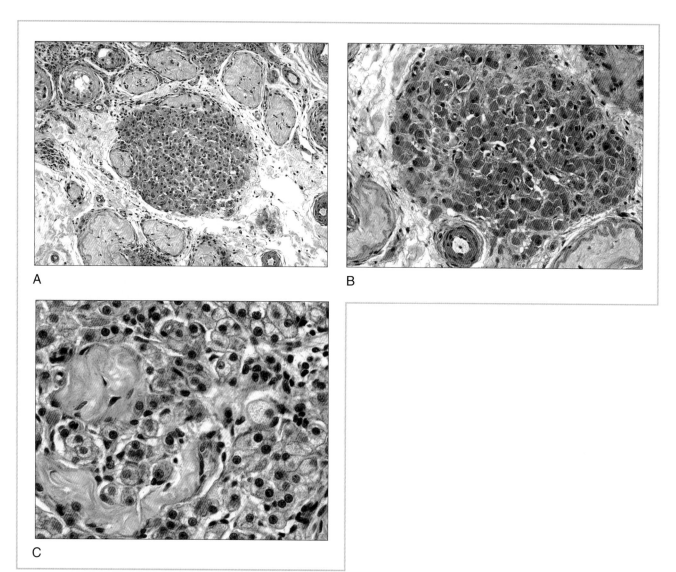

Figure 11-5. Leydig cells in Klinefelter syndrome. **A,** Testicular biopsy shows small, hyalinized seminiferous tubules and pseudoadenomatous clusters of Leydig cells. Patient had normal semen volume and severe oligospermia. **B,** Atrophy of seminiferous tubules and reduced testicular volume gives a false impression of Leydig cell hyperplasia in Klinefelter syndrome. Studies have shown that the total number of Leydig cells is actually reduced. **C,** A few hyalinized seminiferous tubules surrounded by Leydig cells contain abundant microvacuolated cytoplasm. Even though Leydig cells may appear morphologically normal in Klinefelter syndrome, they are often functionally deficient and androgen levels are often reduced, accompanied by elevated FSH and LH levels. (Used with permission of Dr. Dharam Ramnani at Webpathology.com.)

Chromosomal Mosaicism

Clinical records include many mosaic forms of Klinefelter and Turner syndromes, including 46XX/45X, 46,XY/45X, 46,XX/47XXY, 46,XY/47,XXY, and others. The actual phenotypical manifestation of mosaicism depends on the relative proportion and distribution of the two types of cells in the body. As a consequence of the many bizarre mosaic combinations, a graded series of clinical Turner and Klinefelter syndrome features has been found in individuals ranging from a severe presentation to a nearly normal physical presentation. In all cases of fertility in individuals with

Klinefelter or Turner syndrome, mosaicism is suspected even if not proved. As previously described, individual cells with multiple X chromosomes undergo X inactivation for all but one X chromosome per cell, but all are active until inactivation occurs. As in nonmosaic males, increasing numbers of Barr bodies are correlated with decreasing IQ.

Mitotic nondisjunction explains the following self-contradictory finding. Individuals affected with Klinefelter syndrome are born more often to older women, yet a maternal-age effect cannot be demonstrated for Turner syndrome. If both disorders were to stem from a meiotic nondisjunction event during the formation of the mother's

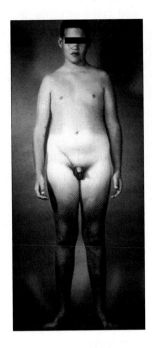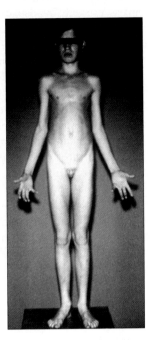

Figure 11-6. Klinefelter syndrome. Physical characteristics are variable as shown in these two patients. Puberty generally occurs at the normal time, but the testes remain small. As hyalinization of the seminiferous tubules increases, androgen production does not increase for proper pubertal development, leading to abnormal body proportions; sparse or absent facial, axillary, pubic, and body hair; female distribution of adipose, gynecomastia, decreased libido, decreased muscle mass and strength, and osteoporosis. The pituitary-gonadal system appears to function well until puberty when testosterone production diminishes and gonadotropins increase. Hyalinization leads to a decrease in inhibin B levels and follicle-stimulating and luteinizing hormone levels become greatly increased. (Courtesy of Dr. Mark Stephen, Madigan General Hospital.)

gametes, then both disorders should be subject to the same strong influence of the mother's age. This has led to the conclusion that the vast majority of Turner cases arise from chromosomal errors that occur in a cell of the early embryo by mitotic nondisjunction rather than in a maternal or paternal germ cell by meiotic nondisjunction. If this is the case, it is likely that most, if not all, live-born 45,X individuals are mosaics. This implies that the extraordinarily high in utero lethality of the 45,X condition reflects that those 45,X conceptuses lack a second cell line. In support of this view, the extent of mosaicism is exceedingly high in females with Turner syndrome—as high as 75%.

It is important to determine the genotype in females with Turner syndrome to distinguish 45,X and 45,X/46,XX individuals from mosaic individuals with any cells containing a Y chromosome, such as 45X/46,XY. The presence of any Y chromosome material increases the risk of gonadoblastoma to greater than 95%. This can be avoided through correct identification of mosaicism and subsequent removal of the streak ovary and gonadal remnants.

Triple-X Female

The 47,XXX constitution occurs once in every 1000 newborn females and accounts for about 50% of all females with more than two X chromosomes. Similar to 47,XYY males, most 47,XXX females have no apparent physical abnormalities and many are fertile. Evidently, the presence of an additional X chromosome does not impair fertility, and its presence is far less hazardous to the developing oocyte than is the absence of an X chromosome in 45,X females. There is evidence that the developing oocytes of the 47,XXX female actually discard the additional X chromosomes by a mechanism known as selective disjunction. Thus, no XXY or XXX offspring can be born to 47,XXX females. Children born to 47,XXX females are either normal males or normal females.

Clinically, triple-X females may appear as quiet infants who later have delayed motor, verbal, and emotional development. However, very few of these females are distinguished by the features in adulthood. Social problems may occur at puberty, since these girls are tall for their age. As in Klinefelter males, the extremities of these females are longer than normal, giving a greater lower body to upper body ratio. As a result of vertical growth, back problems and scoliosis may develop. Intellectually, there may be learning disabilities and intelligence may be slightly lower than that of siblings or a control group, but overall intelligence is within the normal range. Several studies have highlighted the importance of environment and social interaction for the normal development of these females.

⬤⬤⬤ DISORDERS OF SEX STEROIDOGENESIS

In addition to several similarities in the genes required for their development, steroidogenesis occurs in both the adrenal gland and the reproductive system. Beyond the impact of chromosomal anomalies and gene mutations affecting the establishment of gender, steroidogenesis is critical for proper development and function of gonads. Many disorders in this pathway result from specific gene mutations that affect gender—as either a primary or a secondary consequence—through development of abnormal gonads and adrenals.

Steroid hormones, with the exception of retinoic acid, are synthesized from cholesterol in the gonads, the adrenal cortex, and peripherally in such sites as skin, fat, brain, and placenta. Sex steroids include androgens, estrogens, and progestins. Mineralocorticoids, such as aldosterone, and glucocorticoids, such as cortisol, also are steroids and require some of the same enzymes as sex steroid synthesis. The effects of mutations in these latter pathways may have broad and complex ramifications due to mineralcorticoid insufficiency. A few examples of genetic disorders of sex steroidogenesis

BIOCHEMISTRY

Cholesterol

There are three sources of cholesterol for its many functions in the body, such as the need for membranes and steroidogenesis. The liver is the major organ controlling cholesterol metabolism. Cholesterol may be made extrahepatically and de novo in the liver from acetate, or it may be received by the liver in the form of cholesterol-enriched remnant chylomicrons from the intestine. It can also be taken up by the liver as plasma lipoprotein, primarily in the form of low-density lipoprotein (LDL). Once cholesterol is synthesized or taken up by liver cells, it is exported by two mechanisms. Cholesterol is used to synthesize bile acids or it is included in bile as cholesterol and cholesteryl esters. It is also exported to the blood in the form of very low density lipoprotein (VLDL).

ANATOMY & PHYSIOLOGY

Gonads and Steroidogenesis

The ovarian follicle is composed of theca cells, granulosa cells, and the primary oocyte. 3β-Hydroxysteroid dehydrogenase (HSD3B) is stimulated by gonadotrophs. Theca cells lack aromatase and produce androgens. Granulosa cells lack 17α-hydroxylase and produce estrogen—primarily estradiol in the proliferative phase and progesterone in the luteal phase.

The primary male steroids are testosterone, dihydroxytestosterone, and estradiol. DHT and estradiol are produced by the testes and by peripheral conversion (80% is from peripheral conversion). Leydig cells produce more than 95% of testosterone and secrete estradiol, estrone, pregnenolone, progesterone, 17α-hydroxypregnenolone, and 17α-hydroxyprogesterone. Target cells convert testosterone to DHT with 5α-reductase.

that result in anomalies of sexual determination and differentiation are discussed below.

True Hermaphroditism

A true hermaphrodite possesses both ovarian and testicular tissue. The most common karyotype is 46,XX, but 46,XX/46,XY and 46,XY may also occur. The most common presentation of gonadal tissues is in an *ovotestis*, a gonad containing both tissues. Other presentations include a testis that may be present on one side and an ovary on the other side, ovarian and testicular tissue on one side and an ovary or testis on the other side, and an ovotestis or testis on one side along with an ovary in its normal position.

Genital ducts generally reflect the gonad that is present. In individuals with an ovary on one side and a testis on the other, müllerian derivatives develop on one side and wolffian derivatives on the other. In the presence of an ovotestis, genital ducts are usually müllerian derivatives. External

genitalia may be ambiguous, male, or female (Fig. 11-7). If a penis is present, hypospadias and cryptorchidism are not uncommon, but generally gonads or an ovotestis are palpable in the labioscrotal fold (see Fig. 11-7). Breast development and menses may occur at puberty. For 46,XX individuals, pregnancy has been reported, but there is only one report of a 46,XY individual fathering a child (Box 11-4).

From earlier discussions, it is plausible to consider that translocation of an *SRY* allele, or another mutation in a gender determination, might result in 46,XX true hermaphrodites. While most true hermaphrodites are SRY negative, 10% of those individuals studied demonstrated *SRY* expression in the ovotestis. Other genes have not been identified; however, it is not difficult to hypothesize that mutations in other differentiation genes might perturb development. The 46,XX/46,XY individual is usually a chimera resulting from double fertilization. These individuals have two populations of cells.

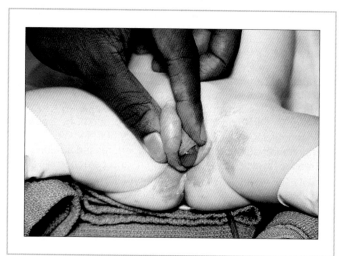

Figure 11-7. 46,XX/46,XY infant with palpable gonad. (Courtesy of Tarek Bisat, MD, Mercer University School of Medicine.)

ANATOMY & EMBRYOLOGY

Genital Ducts

Mesonephric and paramesonephric ducts are important for establishing male and female reproductive systems. Mesonephric ducts establish the male reproductive system. The proximal portion becomes convoluted to form the epididymis, and the remainder forms the ductus deferens and ejaculatory duct.

The paramesonephric ducts establish the female reproductive system. These ducts develop lateral to the gonads and mesonephric ducts. The mesonephric ducts degenerate due to lack of testosterone. The cranial portions of the paramesonephric ducts form the uterine tubes and the caudal portions fuse to form the uterovaginal primordium, which forms the uterus and vagina.

Box 11-4. CLINICAL FEATURES OF A TRUE HERMAPHRODITE

Genitalia are ambiguous.
Cryptorchidism is frequent.
Ovotestis may be located in labioscrotal fold.
Testis, ovary, or ovotestis is present.
Menses may occur.
Spermatogenesis is rare.
Breast development and virilization occur at puberty.

ANATOMY

Hypospadias

Hypospadias can occur anywhere along the urethral groove when fusion of the urethral fold stops proximal to the tip of the glans penis. It occurs in 1 in 100 to 1 in 200 boys. Conditions known to result in hypospadias are the following:

- Inadequate testosterone produced by testes—enlargement and development of genital tubercle and scrotal swellings does not occur properly
- Lack of androgen receptors
- Lack of 5α-reductase
- Congenital adrenal hyperplasia

Male Pseudohermaphroditism

Enzyme Deficiencies

Testosterone, like other steroids, is synthesized from cholesterol in a series of steps requiring the steroidogenic enzymes P450scc (cholesterol side chain cleavage enzyme), HSD3β2 (3β-hydroxysteroid dehydrogenase), CYP17 (17α-hydroxylase/c17,20-lyase), and 17β-hydroxysteroid dehydrogenase (17β-HSD). Male and female embryos have the same androgen receptors; differences between males and females result from differences in levels of androgens.

17β-HSD plays an important role in the balance of gonadal steroids. It maintains a balance between active 17β-hydroxysteroids and relatively inactive 17-ketosteroids. Reducing the 17-ketosteroids is the last step leading to testosterone in Leydig cells and estradiol in granulosa cells. Oxidation of 17-ketosteroids occurs predominantly in the periphery and is the balancing force.

There are at least six isozymes of 17β-HSD in humans. Type 3 17β-HSD is the most frequent cause of male pseudohermaphroditism due to defective testosterone biosynthesis (Fig. 11-8). At birth, 46,XY males with a 17β-HSD mutation generally appear female or have mildly ambiguous genitalia resulting from testosterone deficiency during differentiation. Although having female external genitalia, these males have testes and typical male derivatives of the wolffian ducts: epididymes, vas deferens, seminal vesicles, and ejaculatory

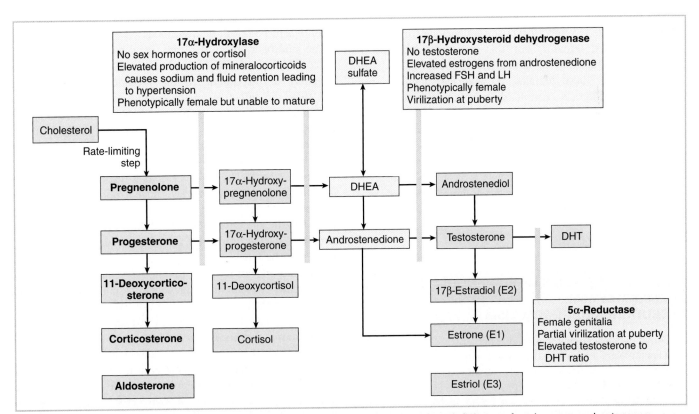

Figure 11-8. Synthesis of androgens and estrogens. Enzyme mutations lead to a deficiency of androgens and estrogens. Deficiency of 17α-hydroxylase (P450c17) shunts precursors into the aldosterone pathway. Deficiency of 17β-hydroxysteroid dehydrogenase will shunt precursors to estrogens primarily as will a deficiency of 5α-reductase.

ANATOMY & EMBRYOLOGY

Chimera

A chimera, or a person with two genetically distinct cell types, may occur by one of three mechanisms:

- There is anastomosis of placental vessels.
- A cell line is artificially introduced, such as with a transfusion or transplant.
- Two zygotes, which normally would form twins, fuse.

ducts. As testosterone levels increase at puberty, these males experience marked virilization with clitoral hypertrophy and breast enlargement.

5α-Reductase is required for the conversion of testosterone to dihydroxytestosterone (DHT) (see Fig. 11-8). There are two isozymes of this gene. Type 1 is expressed postnatally, primarily in the liver and skin. Type 2 is expressed pre- and postnatally, predominantly in prostate, internal genital structures derived from wolffian ducts, genital skin, and liver. 46,XY individuals with mutations in this gene look like other male pseudohermaphrodites with female or ambiguous genitalia along with testes and male genital ducts. Classical features include a clitoris-like, hypospadiac phallus bound down in chorde, a bifid scrotum, a urogenital sinus opening onto the perineum, and a blind vaginal pouch opening into the urogenital sinus or the perineum (Box 11-5). At puberty, virilization occurs owing to the increased testosterone even though there is an inability to convert it to DHT.

As an X-linked gene, 5α-reductase deficiency may also occur in 46,XX females, but this primarily requires a homozygous condition, or mutations in both alleles, for presentation. In these females, the external genitalia are normal because female genitalia do not require testosterone or DHT to develop normally. Postpubertal development is normal. Menarche is delayed, but fertility is normal. The effects of this mutation in females are seen at the sites particularly sensitive to DHT; development of axillary and pubic hair is decreased and body hair is absent. Not surprisingly, type 2 5α-reductase is the predominant form of 5α-reductase found in hair follicles.

Box 11-5. FEATURES OF 5α-REDUCTASE DEFICIENCY MALE PSEUDOHERMAPHRODITISM

External genitalia appear female at birth.
Testes are extra-abdominal, usually inguinal.
Hypospadiac microphallus with bifid scrotum is present.
There is a blind vaginal pouch.
Is sometimes referred to as "penis at twelve syndrome."
Is strongly suspected with normal blood testosterone level but elevated T:DHT ratio.

17α-Hydroxylase (P450c17) is a bifunctional enzyme. Unlike 17β-HSD and 5α-reductase, mutations in this gene have consequences beyond those of androgens and estrogen. Mutations affect P450c17 and c17,20-lyase activities by reducing the production of cortisol, androgen, and estrogen and thus cause a corresponding increase in the production of certain mineralocorticoids (see Fig. 11-8). A severe deficiency impairs androgen synthesis, causing the appearance of female external genitalia in XY males. No uterus is present because Sertoli cells produce AMH. Sexual infantilism is observed in XX females at puberty. In this case, the uterus is hypoplastic. ACTH levels are elevated owing to the decrease in cortisol production, further exacerbating excess mineralocorticoid production. This leads to hypertension and hypokalemia. Less severe mutations have less effect on the presenting phenotype. Adrenal hyperplasia can occur with severe deficiency.

Androgen-Insensitivity Syndrome

Androgens require a receptor to mediate function. Generally speaking, testosterone enters target cells and is converted to dihydrotestosterone by 5α-reductase (see Fig. 11-8). DHT binds to the intracellular androgen receptor, also known as the DHT receptor, and a cascade of events is initiated that leads to the binding of specific hormone response elements to DNA and ultimately causes the androgen action. Disorders may occur if a mutation affects any step leading up to DHT binding to the appropriate receptor (i.e., leading up to the production of DHT, or at any point affecting binding or affecting androgen action after binding occurs). Examples of both will be described.

The androgen receptor itself may have mutations that affect binding of DHT. In these cases, target cells are incapable of responding to the presence of testosterone, and thus the effect is an appearance of no testosterone. Previously known as testicular feminization, *androgen insensitivity syndrome* (AIS) is an X-linked disorder occurring 1 in 20,000 births and in which more than 300 mutations have been described. Over 200 of these occur in exons 2 to 8. These 46,XY males respond to androgen variably, and phenotypes may range from a normal male phenotype with a small phallus to a female phenotype with female or ambiguous genitalia. Clinically, AIS has complete, partial, and mild forms. In milder presentations, males may be fertile.

In the absence of receptor function, resistance to androgens during early development prevents masculinization of the external genitalia and development of wolffian ducts. Sertoli cells secrete AMH, and müllerian structures degenerate. In this scenario, newborns have female genitalia and a blind vaginal pouch. Testes are present either in the abdomen or in the inguinal canal. At puberty, breasts develop in response to increased LH and subsequent increases in testosterone and androstenediol that is converted peripherally to estradiol. LH is increased as a result of the ineffective response of the hypothalamus to testosterone at mutated surface receptors.

BIOCHEMISTRY

Androgen Receptor

The androgen receptor is a nuclear hormone receptor produced from a gene consisting of eight exons and organized like other steroid hormone receptors. The gene produces two mRNAs via differential splicing. The function of this hormone receptor is to bind testosterone and regulate expression of genes involved in the development of male secondary sex characteristics. The receptor has ligand-binding domains that regulate the receptor's DNA binding and transcription activating functions. The major transcription activation function of the receptor is located in the NH$_2$-terminal domain, which is the hormone-binding domain. The DNA binding domain has two Zn^{++} clusters.

Mutations in this gene produce receptors that fail to bind androgen or fail to bind DNA effectively. The most severe mutations in this gene present clinically as *androgen-insensitivity syndrome*, characterized in 46,XY males by a lack of male secondary sex characteristics and the presence of female secondary sex characteristics. Testosterone is present, but cells cannot respond to it. Another type of mutation of the androgen receptor is present in Kennedy disease, a neuromuscular disease causing spinal and bulbar muscular atrophy and characterized by proximal limb and facial muscle wasting. It is caused by expansions of a CAG repeat.

ANATOMY & PHYSIOLOGY

Adrenal Cortex

The adrenal cortex comprises three zones having different roles in steroidogenesis: zona glomerulosa, zona fasciculata, and zona reticularis. The zona glomerulosa produces aldosterone, the main mineralocorticoid, but lacks 17α-hydroxylase and 17,20-lyase and thus cannot synthesize cortisol and androgens. Cortisol, the main glucocorticoid, is produced in the zona fasciculata and zona reticularis. The zona reticularis also produces androgens and small amounts of estrogens. The latter two zones (fasciculata and reticularis) cannot produce aldosterone because they lack the 11β-hydroxylase enzyme.

Cortisol is considered a glucocorticoid because it was originally recognized that it could increase plasma glucose levels. Aldosterone promotes salt and water retention by the kidney and is therefore a mineralocorticoid. There is great similarity in the structures of cortisol and aldosterone, but aldosterone has no glucocorticoid activity. Glucocorticoids have many actions beyond glucose regulation, including immunosuppressant and anti-inflammatory actions, effects on protein and fat metabolism, behavioral effects on the central nervous system, and effects on calcium and bone metabolism.

Female Pseudohermaphroditism with Maternal Virilization

Aromatase Deficiency

Cytochrome P-450 aromatase catalyzes the aromatization of androgens to their respective estrogenic derivative. In addition to the testis and ovary, aromatase is found in skin, fat, brain, and placenta. Its expression is dependent on tissue-specific promoters. In ovarian granulosa cells, FSH and cAMP induce aromatase. In fibroblasts, it is induced by glucocorticoids and certain lymphokines. Mutations in the coding part of the gene will alter the activity of aromatase, whereas those in the 5′ regulatory region will affect expression in a tissue-specific manner.

Pathogenesis of a mutation in aromatase may result from an accumulation behind the block or from estrogen depletion. Androgen excess can masculinize the external female genitalia or prematurely virilize the male external genitalia during fetal development. Similarly an affected fetus can cause virilization of the mother during pregnancy.

Female pseudohermaphroditism may also occur from defects in adrenocortical pathway enzymes, as discussed below. In these females, virilization occurs at birth even in the presence of ovaries.

●●● DISORDERS OF COMBINED ADRENOCORTICAL AND SEX STEROIDOGENESIS

Deficiencies in enzymes of adrenocortical steroidogenesis may have severe consequences reflecting the absolute requirement for these end products. While agenesis or dysgenesis of gonads has certain undesired outcomes for individuals, adrenal dysgenesis is a far more critical and potentially life-threatening event. In these cases, sex steroidogenesis is

PHYSIOLOGY

Evaluating the Adrenal Cortex

There are three major tests to consider when evaluating the function of the adrenal cortex. Abnormalities in the cortex are reflected by overproduction or underproduction of hormones, and therefore these tests are designed to stimulate or suppress production.

- The ACTH stimulation test is the most reliable screening test for decreased adrenal production. Synthetic ACTH (250 μg) is administered, and serum steroids are measured 45 and 60 minutes later. The normal cortisol response by the adrenal gland to this challenge is 20 μg/dL.
- Corticotropin-releasing hormone (CRH) challenge is useful to distinguish between ACTH-dependent and ACTH-independent hypercortisolism. For this procedure, 1 μg/kg ACTH is administered, and ACTH levels are measured between 3 and 30 minutes.
- The dexamethasone suppression test is used to test for hyperfunction of the adrenal cortex but is plagued by false negatives and false positives. However, it has some value for evaluating mineralocorticoid excess. One procedure provides for the administration of 0.5 mg of dexamethasone by mouth every 6 hours for 2 days.

To distinguish the various forms of congenital adrenal hyperplasia, specific steroid substrates that accumulate in response to decreased enzyme activity are measured.

secondarily affected. These defects comprise a group known as *congenital adrenal hyperplasias* (Fig. 11-9).

Adrenal hyperplasia occurs owing to the feedback control of the hypothalamus and pituitary. In the absence of sufficient products, such as cortisol and sex steroids, ACTH and gonadotropins stimulate the adrenals to produce more products, and thus cellular hyperplasia occurs. An important consideration for each of the following enzymes is the mutation itself. Recall that the location and extent of change in the DNA can be demonstrated as either a negligible or mild effect or as a serious effect due to little or no enzyme production.

glands and gonads. As expected, a mutation in the type II gene will interfere with mineralocorticoid, glucocorticoid, progesterone, androgen, and estrogen synthesis (see Fig. 11-9). If a mutation is severe, salt-losing crises, hypomasculinized external genitalia in males, and clitoromegaly at birth in females may occur along with adrenal hyperplasia. Obviously, milder mutations, characterized by the type and position of the mutation affecting the protein's function, may not display the broad spectrum of phenotypes. Type I mutations are less problematic but may explain masculinization or virilization of some affected 46,XX females.

3β-Hydroxysteroid Dehydrogenase Deficiency

3β-Hydroxysteroid dehydrogenase (*HSD3B*) is expressed as two highly homologous genes and identified as type I and type II. Type I gene expression is found predominantly in the placenta and the peripheral tissues of skin and mammary gland. Type II gene expression occurs mainly in the adrenal

21α-Hydroxylase Deficiency

21α-Hydroxylase (P450c21) is responsible for conversion of progesterone to deoxycorticosterone (DOC) in the aldosterone biosynthetic pathway (see Fig. 11-9). The precursors and substrates that accumulate behind these blocks are directed into the androgen biosynthesis pathway. Deficiency of this enzyme is the *most common cause of congenital adrenal*

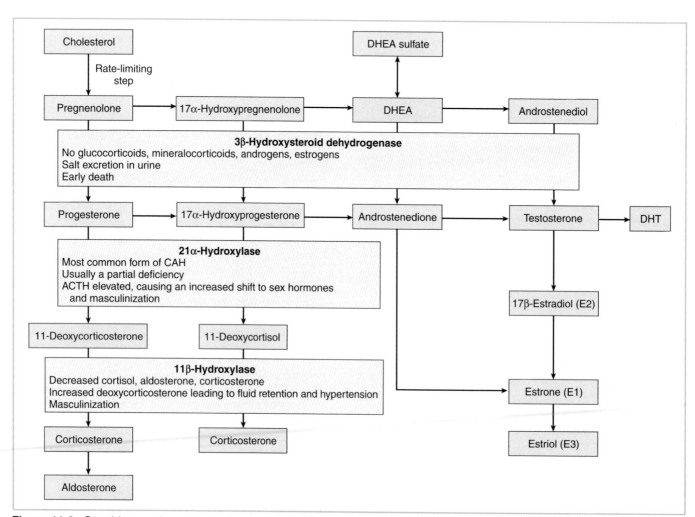

Figure 11-9. Steroidogenesis pathway. Mutations affecting enzymes primarily responsible for the production of mineralocorticoids and cortisol can have secondary effects on sex steroid production. Substrates that accumulate are shunted to the right.

PHYSIOLOGY

Salt Wasting

Salt wasting can accompany two forms of congenital adrenal hyperplasia: 21α-hydroxylase deficiency and 3-β-hydroxysteroid dehydrogenase deficiency. Since the former is more common, salt wasting is seen most often with this form. Severe salt wasting will occur in about 75% of infants with severe 21α-hydroxylase deficiency. This deficiency leads to decreased cortisol and aldosterone synthesis. Reduced aldosterone, which functions normally to stimulate the kidney to reabsorb Na^+ and water and enhance K^+ secretion, will cause electrolyte and fluid loss due to hyponatremia and hyperkalemia, which lead to acidosis, dehydration, and vascular collapse if not corrected.

The decrease in circulating volume also causes an increase in renin, which activates the renin angiotensin system through stimulation of the baroreceptor reflex and a decrease in renal arteriole pressure. Angiotensinogen is cleaved into angiotensin I, which is then converted to angiotensin II. This octapeptide is unable to stimulate the adrenal cortex directly or indirectly through stimulation of the anterior pituitary and release of ACTH to effect aldosterone production. Therefore, the net result is life threatening unless reversed.

The situation is different with 11β-hydroxylase deficiency (CYP11B1 deficiency). In these infants, the lack of cortisol causes an increase in ACTH resulting in increased aldosterone. This increases Na^+ reabsorption and K^+ secretion by the kidney, leading to "salt retention" rather than "salt wasting." Directly related to the enzyme deficiency is an increase in 11-deoxycortisol. This and the excess 11-deoxycorticosterone contribute to hypertension.

TABLE 11-1. Incidence of Congenital Adrenal Hyperplasia

Location	Frequency
Alaska, Yupik Eskimo population	1 in 280
France and Italy	1 in 11,000
La Reunion, France	1 in 2,100
Scotland	1 in 17,000
New Zealand	1 in 14,500
Japan	1 in 15,800
China	1 in 28,000

Data from *Pediatrics* 1988;81:866-874.

with a milder mutation; however, the incidence is significantly increased among Hispanics and Ashkenazic Jews.

Mild CAH is much more common than the classical form. Men and women with mild CAH may have normal height compared with the general population, yet shortened when compared with their parents. Glucocorticoid precursors accumulate and are converted to androgenic steroids, causing shortened stature, early puberty, severe acne, and virilization and infertility in females. Mineralocorticoid synthesis can also be affected, resulting in electrolyte disturbances, hypotension, and syncope. Some people with mild CAH can mount limited glucocorticoid stress responses and are thus never recognized as having the disorder. Others, however,

hyperplasia (CAH) and is responsible for *at least 90% to 95% of cases.* Depending on the population, the incidence of this disorder ranges from 1 in 280 among the Yupik Alaska natives to 1 in 28,000 among Chinese (Table 11-1) About two-thirds of affected patients have the "salt-wasting" form resulting from seriously deficient aldosterone as well as cortisol. If untreated, these infants die in early infancy of hyponatremia, hyperkalemia, hypovolemia, and acidosis. Females are more likely to be diagnosed and treated early because they have ambiguous genitalia or masculinization of genitalia (Fig. 11-10). They may have clitoromegaly and labioscrotal fusion with a phallic urethra. Ultrasonograms will demonstrate a uterus.

Impaired cortisol synthesis due to 21α-hydroxylase deficiency leads to increased ACTH levels and increased levels of adrenal androgen precursors and androgen secretion. Elevated androgen levels before 12 weeks of gestation lead to labioscrotal fusion and clitoral enlargement, whereas after 12 weeks of gestation only clitoromegaly is induced. Virilization continues after birth, resulting in rapid bone growth and maturation (Fig. 11-11).

The hallmark of CAH is inadequate production of glucocorticoids. Patients with mild CAH are frequently unable to mount sufficient stress responses to trauma and infection. One in 100 persons of all ethnic backgrounds are affected

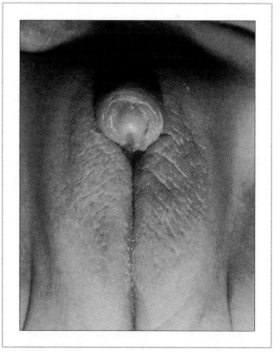

Figure 11-10. Congenital adrenal hyperplasia. This 46,XY child was raised as a female. (Courtesy of Roberta Sonnino, MD, Creighton University School of Medicine.)

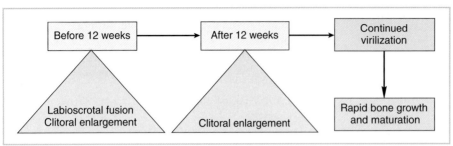

Figure 11-11. Elevated androgens and development. Exposure to high levels of androgens during fetal development affects fetal development in a time-dependent manner.

have frequent illnesses and decompensate when challenged by common infections or minor trauma.

11β-Hydroxylase Deficiency

11β-Hydroxylase (*CYP11B1*) converts deoxycorticosterone (DOC) to corticosterone and 11-deoxycortisol to cortisol (see Fig. 11-9). A deficiency of this enzyme is the *second most common cause of congenital adrenal hyperplasia*. Most mutations completely abolish the enzyme activity although the clinical presentation may be variable. The resulting cortisol deficiency leads to an increase in ACTH and a subsequent increase in precursors that are diverted to the androgen synthesis pathway. Females may have ambiguous or masculinized external genitalia at birth and become virilized in early childhood. In cases of ambiguity, there is clitoral enlargement and labial fusion (Fig. 11-12). Virilization varies from mild to severe. Male infants have normal external genitalia, as with 21α-hydroxylase deficiency, but virilize prematurely. Both DOC and 11β-deoxycortisol are increased in blood, but 11-deoxycortisol has little activity; it is the action of DOC that provides the mineralocorticoid actions. Should an individual have a late onset of *CYP11B1* deficiency, it is most likely the result of a less pronounced mutation that allowed adequate expression during earlier years.

It is interesting to note that a related gene, *CYP11B2*, representing a duplication of *CYP11B1*, is located adjacent to *CYP11B1*. These genes are 95% homologous in exons and 90% homologous in introns. The function of this gene is the conversion of corticosterone to aldosterone, and therefore a mutation would cause an aldosterone crisis but not the cortisol crisis that can occur with *CYP11B1* deficiency.

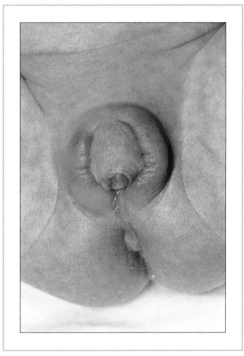

Figure 11-12. Ambiguous genitalia. (Courtesy of Tarek Bisat, MD, Mercer University School of Medicine.)

CYP11B1 deficiency occurs in 1 in 100,000 live births. However, in some populations the incidence is higher. For example, in Israel, the incidence is 1 in 5000 births among Sephardic Jews. While uncommon in European women, this deficiency is reportedly responsible for 15% of congenital adrenal hyperplasia in Muslim and Jewish women.

Population Genetics and Medicine

Prior chapters have focused on variations within DNA molecules that lead to disease. Oftentimes, specific variations are identified within particular populations at a greater frequency than in other populations. Many examples have been given in which groups such as the Ashkenazi Jews, whites of northern European ancestry, or black populations have a propensity for specific disorders. Understanding DNA variations by combining the study of populations with the advancing molecular diagnostics is leading to a better understanding of gene action and the development of disease.

●●● HISTORICAL PERSPECTIVE

At the turn of the 20th century, an intriguing question was posed to the English geneticist R. C. Punnett. He was asked to explain the prevalence of blue eyes in humans in view of the acknowledged fact that the blue-eyed condition was a recessive characteristic. Would the dominant brown-eyed trait in time supplant the blue-eyed state in the human population? The answer was not self-evident, and Punnett sought out his colleague Godfrey H. Hardy, an astute mathematician at Cambridge University. Hardy had only a passing interest in genetics, but the problem fascinated him as a mathematical one. The solution ranks as one of the most fundamental theorems in population genetics. As fate would have it, Hardy's formula was arrived at independently in the same

year (1908) by a physician, Wilhelm Weinberg, and the well-known equation bears both their names.

●●● HARDY-WEINBERG EQUILIBRIUM

Basic Algebraic Formula

Assume there are only two possible alleles, A and a, at a particular locus on an autosome. In addition, assume the frequency of the A allele in the population is designated "p," and "q" is the frequency of the a allele. Under these conditions, $p + q = 1$, since this is the totality of these alleles in an individual within a population. The probability of bringing two gametes bearing the A allele together is simply $p \times p = p^2$. The chance of obtaining the aa genotype is q^2, and the chance of obtaining Aa is $2pq$. The "2" in $2pq$ derives from the fact that there are two ways of forming the heterozygote, since each allele can be contributed to the zygote either through the egg or through the sperm.

The simplest case for understanding gene expression is the gene with only two alleles; however, as discussed in great detail in prior chapters, any change in DNA at a locus results in a new allele, making the possibilities seemingly endless. Though Hardy and Weinberg developed this formula prior to a proper appreciation of alleles, only two alleles are considered at a time and the formula still has applicability.

An important factor that influences the genetic composition of a population is the system of mating among individuals. The simplest scheme of breeding activity in a population is referred to as *random mating* (or *panmixia*) wherein any one individual has an equal chance of pairing with any other individual. Random mating does not imply promiscuity; it simply means that those who choose each other as mating partners do not do so on the basis of similarity or dissimilarity in a given trait or gene.

The absence of preferential mating in a population has interesting consequences. The gametes in a panmictic population are mixed at random. Each gamete carries either A or a. To predict the outcome of the random mixing of gametes, the "Punnett square" is used (Fig. 12-1). This matrix essentially brings into play the multiplication rule of probability: *the chance that two independent events will occur together is the product of their chances of occurring*

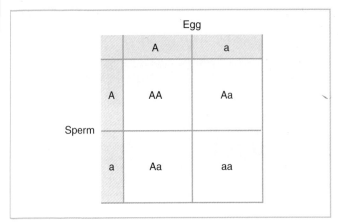

Figure 12-1. The distribution of genotypes in the next generation: p^2:AA 2pq:Aa q^2:aa.

separately. The Punnett square checkerboard displayed in Figure 12-1 reveals the outcome of all possible combinations.

The distribution of genotypes in the next generation of a randomly breeding population is p^2AA: $2pqAa$: q^2 *aa*. The algebraic expansion of the binomial equation $(p + q)^2$ is reflected in this distribution, p^2:$2pq$:q^2. The Hardy-Weinberg theorem states that the proportions of *AA*, *Aa*, and *aa* genotypes, as well as the proportions of *A* and *a* alleles, will remain constant from generation to generation, provided that the bearers of the three genotypes have equal opportunities of producing offspring in a large, randomly mating population. If blue-eyed persons are equally as fertile as brown-eyed individuals and leave equal numbers of offspring each generation, then blue-eyed persons as well as brown-eyed individuals will persist in the population with the same frequency from one generation to the next.

Application of Hardy-Weinberg Theorem

It may seem ironic that the Hardy-Weinberg theorem is entirely theoretical. The following set of underlying assumptions can scarcely be fulfilled in any natural population. It is implicitly assumed that there is the absence of recurring mutations, the absence of any degree of preferential mating, the absence of differential mortality or fertility, the absence of immigration or emigration of individuals, and the absence of fluctuations in gene frequencies due to sheer chance. But therein lies the significance of the Hardy-Weinberg theorem. In revealing the conditions under which changes in gene frequencies cannot occur, it brings to light the possible forces that could cause a change in the genetic composition of a population (Box 12-1).

A population is a group of individuals living within a defined geographic area. Historically, it may have been easier to define a population because of the tendency for groups of individuals to remain in a location for long periods of time, represented by centuries in some cases. As groups within a population became segregated or separated from the larger population, subpopulations developed. Just as different populations may have developed unique mutations, subpopulations

may have developed a specific genetic complement due to unique mutations that differ from other subpopulations or the population as a whole. In both cases, the gene pool is limited by the DNA variation contributed by individuals through mating. These differences among gene pools, which are directly affected by the DNA sequences available, develop through variations in meiotic reassortment and mutations (Box 12-2). These changes may confer a *selective advantage* or *disadvantage* to the gene and the individual or have a neutral affect. Of course, only those changes that are neutral or that confer a selective advantage are important for the survival of the population.

An understanding of Hardy-Weinberg equilibrium provides a basis for recognizing the forces that permit a change in gene frequencies. A few of the more obvious factors that prevent a natural population from attaining stationary equilibrium are (1) mutation, (2) natural selection, (3) chance events in a small population (genetic drift), and (4) migration. In any population, the more individuals contributing to the gene pool, i.e., the larger the population, the more stable the allele frequencies within the population and the more difficult it will be for frequencies to change. Conversely, small populations may have fluctuations in frequencies often; in some cases this can even occur between generations. The factors or forces affecting gene pools can profoundly modify the gene frequencies in natural populations. In essence, the Hardy-Weinberg theorem represents the cornerstone of population studies, since deviations from Hardy-Weinberg expectations direct attention to the forces that disturb, or upset, the theoretical equilibrium. The Hardy-Weinberg theorem is exceedingly useful in enabling us to estimate (1) the

---

Box 12-1. FORCES THAT CAN CHANGE THE EQUILIBRIUM OF ALLELES

Mutations
Preferential matings
Mortality
Infertility
Immigration and emigration
Chance fluctuations

Box 12-2. DIFFERENCES THAT DEVELOP WITHIN AND BETWEEN GENE POOLS

Meiotic assortment of DNA to gametes
  Random assortment
  Recombination
Development and persistence of mutations
  Failure of repair mechanisms
  Development of a selective advantage—mutation favors survival
  Development of a selective disadvantage—mutation does not favor survival of gene function

frequencies of heterozygous carriers of deleterious recessive alleles and (2) the risk of bearing offspring with detrimental recessive disorders in various marriages (Table 12-1).

Estimating the Frequency of Heterozygotes

Contrary to popular opinion, heterozygotes of a rare recessive abnormality are rather common instead of comparatively rare. Recessive albinism may be used as an illustration. The frequency of albinos is about 1 in 20,000 in human populations. When the frequency of the homozygous recessive (q^2) trait is known, the frequency of the recessive allele (q) can be calculated, as follows:

$$q^2 = \frac{1}{20,000} = 0.00005$$

$$q = \sqrt{0.00005} = 0.007$$

$$= \text{about } 1/140 \text{ or 1 in 40 (frequency of recessive allele)}$$

The heterozygotes are represented by 2pq in the Hardy-Weinberg formula. Accordingly, the frequency of heterozygous carriers of albinism can be calculated as follows:

$$q = 0.007$$

$$p + q = 1$$

$$p = 1 - 0.007 = 0.993$$

Therefore:

$$2pq = 2(0.993 \times 0.007) = 0.014$$
$$= \text{about } 1/70 \text{ (frequency of heterozygous carrier)}$$

Thus, although 1 person in 20,000 is an albino (recessive homozygote), about 1 person in 70 is a heterozygous carrier—or, there are 280 times as many carriers as affected individuals. The rarity of a recessive disorder does not signify a comparable rarity of heterozygous carriers. In fact, when the frequency of the recessive gene is extremely low, nearly all the recessive genes are in the heterozygous state.

Significance of the Heterozygote

When the frequency of a detrimental recessive allele becomes very low, most affected offspring (aa) will come from mating of two heterozygous carriers (Aa). For example, in the human population, the vast majority (> 99%) of newly arising albino individuals (aa) in a given generation will come from normally pigmented heterozygous parents.

Detrimental recessive alleles in a population are unquestionably harbored mostly in the heterozygous state. As shown in Table 12-1, the frequency of heterozygous carriers is many times greater than the frequency of homozygous individuals afflicted with a trait. Thus, an extremely rare disorder such as *alkaptonuria* (blackening of urine) occurs in 1 in 1 million

BIOCHEMISTRY

Natural Selection for a Heterozygote: Sickle Cell Trait

Sickle cell trait (HbS) is a heterozygous condition for a specific mutation in hemoglobin that is called hemoglobin S. The occurrence of this mutation overlaps the distribution of malaria in Africa and is an example of a heterozygous condition that conveys a survival advantage in areas where malaria is endemic. Sickle trait cells, those with only one mutant allele, generally undergo little sickling at normal O_2 tension. Though some sickling will occur as O_2 tension lowers, it is not as much as in sickle cell anemia with two mutant alleles and twice as much mutant hemoglobin. *Plasmodium falciparum* requires normal intracellular K^+ concentration. With lower O_2 tension in the cell, potassium diffuses out. *P. falciparum* grows poorly in the lower than normal O_2 tension occurring in HbS cells and dies because of the inadequate oxygen and reduced potassium.

TABLE 12-1. Frequencies of Homozygotes and Heterozygous Carriers

Disease	Frequency of Homozygotes	Frequency of Heterozygous Carriers (Aa)	Ratio of Carriers to Homozygotes
Sickle cell anemia	1 in 500	1 in 10	50:1
Cystic fibrosis	1 in 2500	1 in 25	100:1
Tay-Sachs disease	1 in 60000	1 in 40	150:1
Albinism	1 in 20,000	1 in 70	286:1
Phenylketonuria	1 in 25,000	1 in 80	313:1
Acatalasia	1 in 50,000	1 in 110	455:1
Alkaptonuria	1 in 1,000,000	1 in 500	2000:1

persons. One in 500 persons, however, carries this detrimental allele in the hidden state. There are 2000 times as many genetic carriers of alkaptonuria as there are individuals affected with this defect. For another recessive trait, cystic fibrosis, 1 in 2500 individuals is affected with this homozygous trait. One in 25 persons is a carrier of cystic fibrosis. In modern genetic counseling programs, an important consideration has been the development of simple, inexpensive means of detecting heterozygous carriers of inherited disorders. Molecular diagnostic techniques have increased the number of carrier screening programs available for at-risk populations.

X-Linked Loci

In the above discussions, the genes and alleles considered were autosomal genes with two possible alleles, *A* and *a*. For those loci located on the X chromosome, the principles are similar but the male gamete may or may not carry an X chromosome (Fig. 12-2). Since there is only one X chromosome in males, the genotype frequency of any allele on that X chromosome is equal to the allele frequency. In females, alleles may be distributed as p^2AA: $2pqAa$: $q2aa$, and thus a heterozygous carrier is determined just as with an autosomal trait. For example, if the frequencies of two X-linked alleles are 0.3 (A) and 0.7 (a), then for a female offspring, the probability of carrying both alleles (Aa) is

$$2pq = 2 (0.3 \times 0.7) = 0.42$$

whereas the probability that a male offspring will carry either allele is 0.3 or 0.7 for the *A* allele or *a* allele, respectively.

	Egg	
	A	a
Sperm a	Aa	aa

A

	Egg	
	A	a
Sperm A	AA	Aa

B

Figure 12-2. X-linked loci. **A**, The sperm carries the *a* allele on the X chromosome, and two female offspring have an equal chance of being Aa or aa from an Aa mother. **B**, The sperm carries the A allele on the X chromosome, and two offspring have an equal chance of being AA or Aa from an Aa mother.

For recently arising mutations on the X chromosome, there may be a difference in *allele frequencies* between males and females. However, with each successive generation, differences in frequencies between males and females becomes less until equilibrium is approached. Allele frequencies will approach equilibrium or be in equilibrium for those alleles that have been in the gene pool for many generations. The *expression* of a recessive allele will occur at a higher frequency in males than in females just as implied above. In females, the frequency of expression is q^2. The X-linked form of color blindness affects 1 in 20 white males, so q = 0.05. The expected frequency in females is $q^2 = (0.05)^2 = 0.0025$ or 1 in 400 females.

CONSANGUINITY AND RECESSIVE INHERITANCE

Offspring afflicted with a recessive disorder tend to arise more often from consanguineous unions than from marriages of unrelated persons. Close relatives share more of the same alleles than would individuals chosen at random from the general population (Table 12-2). If a recessive trait is extremely rare, the chance is very small that unrelated mating partners would both harbor the same defective allele. The mating of close relatives, however, increases the risk that both partners have received the same defective allele through some common ancestor. Therefore, the frequency of occurrence of a recessive disorder increases at the expense of the frequency of heterozygotes in the population.

With increasing rarity of a recessive gene, it becomes more and more unlikely that unrelated parents will carry the same recessive allele. With an exceedingly rare recessive disorder, the expectation is that most affected children will come from cousin marriages. Human geneticists often infer that a recessive allele transmits a rare disorder when the incidence of consanguineous marriages is high. Thus, the finding that Toulouse-Lautrec's parents were first cousins is the basis for the current view that the French painter was afflicted with *pycnodysostosis*, characterized by short stature and a narrow

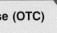

BIOCHEMISTRY

Lyonization of Ornithine Transcarbamylase (OTC) Deficiency in Females

Another example of X chromosome genes and the role of lyonization is ornithine transcarbamylase (OTC) deficiency, the most common disorder of the urea cycle. This enzyme, part of a mitochondrial matrix, catalyzes the conversion of ornithine and carbamyl phosphate to citrulline. It is the second step in the urea cycle.

As an X-linked disorder, OTC deficiency can be fatal in newborn males owing to hyperammonemia. In females, however, expression is variable because of lyonization. As might be surmised, penetrance is 100% in males (with a severity index of 50), whereas it is only 20% in females and the severity is low.

TABLE 12-2. Alleles Shared by Consanguineous Matings

Mating	Proportion of Shared Alleles
Parent-offspring	1/2
Brother-sister	1/2
Half-sibs	1/4
Uncle-niece, aunt-nephew	1/4
First cousins	1/8
Double first cousins	1/4
Half first cousins	1/16
First cousins once removed	1/16
Second cousins	1/32
Second cousins once removed	1/64
Third cousins	1/128

One of the first indications that phenylketonuria (PKU) in humans is controlled by a recessive allele was the relatively high percentage of first-cousin marriages among parents of affected children. Data from the United States, England, and Norway indicate that, for this trait, the parents are often close relatives. Individuals suffering from phenylketonuria have peculiarities of posture and make jerky, or convulsive, movements. Untreated phenylketonuric patients are mentally retarded, usually so severely that they are institutionalized (see Chapter 4).

The number of heterozygous carriers of a detrimental recessive PKU allele is about 1 in 80. Thus, the probability that two carriers from the general population will marry is 1 in 6400 (80 × 80). If both marriage partners are carriers, then theoretically 1 of every 4 children will be afflicted with PKU. The first probability figure (1 in 6400) multiplied by the second probability figure (1 in 4) gives the total chance of 1 in 25,600 for affected children from two normal persons who marry at random from the general population. This probability is increased enormously if two normal individuals marry, both of whom had heterozygous carrier parents. The marital partners would each have a two-thirds chance of being carriers themselves, and the risk of affected children from such a marriage would be 1 in 9. Calculations of the risk of PKU in offspring from different types of marriages are shown in Table 12-3.

The offspring of consanguineous marriages are said to be "inbred." Thus, the expectation is that more genetic disorders

lower jaw, which is governed by a rare recessive gene, rather than as had been formerly thought, with *achondroplasia*, which is determined by a dominant gene. Both demonstrate similar phenotypes, but in the absence of laboratory data and with the knowledge that the parents were related, the choice of an autosomal recessive disorder is a better probable diagnosis.

TABLE 12-3. Risk of PKU Offspring in Various Mating Relationships

Mating Partners				Theoretical Frequency of Affected Children If Both Parents Were Carriers	Chances of Affected Children from Such a Mating
A		B			
Carrier Status	Chances of Carrying Allele	Carrier Status	Chances of Carrying Allele		
Unknown	1 in 80	Unknown	1 in 80	1 in 4	1 in 25,600
Unknown	1 in 18	Normal sibling of phenylketonuric	2 in 3	1 in 4	1 in 480
Unknown	1 in 80	Parent of phenylketonuric	1	1 in 4	1 in 320
Unknown	1 in 80	Phenylketonuric	1	1 in 2	1 in 160
Normal sibling of phenylketonuric	2 in 3	Normal sibling of phenylketonuric	2 in 3	1 in 4	1 in 9
Normal sibling of phenylketonuric	2 in 3	Parent of phenylketonuric	1	1 in 4	1 in 6
Normal sibling of phenylketonuric	2 in 3	Phenylketonuric	1	1 in 2	1 in 3
Parent of phenylketonuric	1	Parent of phenylketonuric	1	1 in 2	1 in 2
Parent of phenylketonuric	1	Phenylketonuric	1	1	1
Phenylketonuric	1	Phenylketonuric	1	1	1

resulting from recessive traits will occur in these individuals. However, many recessive genetic disorders occur within the general population that are not the result of consanguinity. In fact, most result from the chance event of heterozygous carriers mating and unknowingly passing an affected allele to an offspring.

General Aspects of Consanguinity

One way to show the effects of consanguinity is to consider a situation in which a widow marries her late husband's brother. As Figure 12-3 shows, a child with phenylketonuria (III-1) was born in the first marriage of the man (II-1) and the woman (II-2). The man dies, and his brother (II-3) feels obliged, as required by certain religious laws, to marry the widow and assume responsibility for the family. The couple may ask the question: what are the chances that the second marriage will produce a child with PKU? Alternatively, what would be the chances of a phenylketonuric offspring if the widow were to marry instead an unrelated man (II-4) with no family history of PKU?

As Figure 12-3 reveals, the widow (II-2) and the late husband (II-2) are each heterozygous. The late husband's brother (II-3) is phenotypically normal, but the probability is 1/2 that he harbors the recessive allele for phenylketonuria. This recessive allele was transmitted by one of his parents, either I-1 or I-2. Both parents might have been heterozygous, but since the trait is rare, it is more probable that only one parent was a carrier.

Individual probabilities may be categorized as follows:
- Chance that the widow (II-2) is a carrier = 1
- Chance that the late husband's brother (II-3) is a carrier = 1/2
- Chance for a homozygous recessive child = 1/4

Thus, the total chance that a child of this marriage will be afflicted with PKU is

$$1 \times 1/2 \times 1/4 = 1/8$$

If the widow marries someone other than her late husband's brother, the probability that the unrelated man (II-4) is a carrier is equal to the frequency with which carriers occur in the general population. As noted earlier, 1 in 80 persons is a carrier of the recessive allele for phenylketonuria. Hence, the chance that a man picked at random from the general population happens to be heterozygous for PKU is 1 in 80. In this circumstance, the individual events are as follows:
- Chance that the widow (II-2) is a carrier = 1
- Chance that the unrelated man (II-4) is a carrier = 1/80
- Chance for a homozygous recessive child = 1/4

Thus, the total chance that the child will be afflicted with PKU is

$$1 \times 1/80 \times 1/4 = 1/320$$

It should be evident that if the widow marries her late husband's brother, the likelihood of having a homozygous recessive child is increased 40-fold from 1 in 320 to 1 in 8. Clearly, two siblings (in this case, two brothers) have a greater chance of inheriting the same recessive gene from a common ancestor (in this case, one of their parents) than do any two individuals selected at random in a general population. As a generalization, the farther removed two individuals are from a common ancestor, the smaller the likelihood that both individuals will receive the same alleles from that ancestor.

●●● ASSORTATIVE MATING AND INBREEDING

In some circumstances, mates are selected for characteristics shared or not shared in common. These situations are referred to as *positive assortative mating* and *negative assortative mating*, respectively. For those characteristics that are genetically determined, an increase in homozygosity will be observed. This is not the same as inbreeding. Inbreeding involves all loci on all chromosomes with a resulting increase in homozygosity at many loci; assortative mating affects only those characteristics that are similar. Examples are matings that occur between individuals with similar clinical conditions such as dwarfism or congenital deafness.

●●● DNA TECHNOLOGY AND CLINICAL DIAGNOSIS

Prior to the development of DNA technology and applied diagnostic capabilities, physicians were limited in their capacity to determine whether an expectant mother might deliver a child with a serious birth defect, such as Tay-Sachs disease. This fatal disease takes its lethal toll by the age of 3 to 4 years. There are no known survivors, and there is no cure. For the most part, physicians in the past referred prospective parents with a family history of a severe congenital disorder to specialists in genetic counseling. Even then, the prospective parents could be informed only of the statistical probability that they would have a child with a particular genetic disorder. Using statistical information comparable to that shown in Table 12-3, the parents could be given no assurance that the actual outcome of the pregnancy would not be unfavorable. Many high-risk couples in the past avoided pregnancy rather than

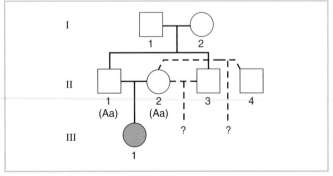

Figure 12-3. An example of the effects of consanguinity.

NEUROSCIENCE

Positive Assertive Mating

Positive assertive mating examples include selection of mates for the following:

- Intellectual ability
- Athletic talent
- Physical characteristics
- Parental income
- Place of birth
- Home town

hazard the birth of an affected child. Today, this situation has been altered dramatically by the availability of molecular techniques that reveal a disorder in the fetus or in preimplantation embryos. This approach to detecting genetic disorders, referred to as *prenatal* or *preimplantation diagnosis*, is now available to prospective parents for many single gene disorders (see Chapter 13).

Similarly, suspected genetic disorders at most stages of development and detection can be evaluated with development of proper diagnostic tools for gene evaluation. The Human Genome Project has provided copious amounts of DNA sequence information about genes of interest. Most importantly to the application of this information to clinical evaluation are those disorders resulting from single genes. For complex multifactorial disease, DNA diagnostics is not recommended.

Limitations to the use of DNA diagnostics for single gene disorders occur when there are many alleles for a particular gene. The larger the gene, the more opportunities for mutations to occur and the less likely an individual can be tested for all alleles. An example is cystic fibrosis, for which over 1000 mutations have been described (see Chapter 9). About 80% of cystic fibrosis results from a single mutation in the *CFTR* gene. Different allele frequencies vary with different populations. Using a panel to screen for the most common mutations in a single population may not adequately identify

BIOCHEMISTRY

Diagnosis of Sickle Cell Disease

A single nucleotide change in the normal β-globin allele produces a change in the amino acid conformation.

- A to T mutation in the sixth codon results in a glutamic acid to valine substitution.
- A to T mutation changes the CTGAGG recognition site, and a diagnostic test can be designed with this information.
- Mutation replaces a charged glutamic acid with an uncharged valine that affects structure.
- Testing may be done prenatally by amniocentesis or chorionic villus sampling.

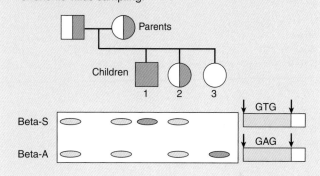

TABLE 12-4. Mutation Detection Rates Using a Panel of 25 Alleles*

Population	Detection Frequency
Askenazi Jewish	95%
North American	80–85%
Spanish	75%
Blacks	64%
Mexican	58%
Colombian	46%
Venezuelan	33%
Other groups	Variable

*Recommended by the American College of Medical Genetics for routine screening and carrier testing.

NEUROSCIENCE

Tay-Sachs Disease

Tay-Sachs disease is an autosomal recessive metabolic disease distinguished by a deficiency of hexosaminidase A resulting in the accumulaion of gangliosides in neurons, axons, and glial cells. Neuropathy occurs in these individuals because of demyelination, gliosis, and neuronal loss. In the early phase of the disease, changes are seen by magnetic resonance spectroscopy in the basal ganglia and thalamus. In the later phase of the disease, changes are demonstrated by advanced brain atrophy and diffuse white matter lesions of the basal ganglia, thalamus, and cortical layer of the cerebrum.

cystic fibrosis in other populations (Table 12-4). However, this same information may provide better diagnostic screening within specific populations because of the propensity of specific mutations to occur within a population. It may not remove all doubt about a result and false negatives may still occur, but increased confidence occurs when specific mutations are known to occur. Likewise, for disorders with a high incidence of spontaneous mutations, identifying the molecular defect with molecular techniques provides a tool for testing of the proband's offspring. Even with the advent and increased reliance on molecular DNA techniques, the Hardy-Weinberg theorem remains a powerful component of risk analysis and family counseling.

Modern Molecular Medicine 13

CONTENTS

Over the last 15 years, the relationship between genetics and the physician has undergone a radical change. Today, "molecular medicine" is recognized as the "cutting edge" of modern medicine. Whereas genetics was once an explanation for inheritance patterns, it is now recognized that essentially all disease has a genetic basis. The completion of the Human Genome Project in 2003 coupled with an explosion of technological advances has permitted elucidation of genetic mechanisms for common and rare disorders that range from simple single-gene etiologies to complex polygenic or multifactorial disease susceptibilities. Because a genetic signature typifies disease, individualized genetic profiles can be obtained and the age of "personalized medicine" becomes possible. Such a concept recognizes that each individual has a certain biology that is dictated by a unique set of alleles. As more is revealed about how these alleles interact with each other and the environment, specific treatments will be customized following genetic diagnosis. In this chapter, modern medicine in its appropriate molecular context is

discussed with a focus on three essential areas: (1) the tools of molecular medicine; (2) the role of genetics in diagnosis, screening, and counseling; and (3) molecular genetic approaches to treatment.

●●● TOOLS OF MOLECULAR MEDICINE

Determining the complete DNA sequence of *Homo sapiens* has provided a template for understanding molecular defects that underlie human infirmities. By elucidating the 25,000 to 30,000 genes that make up each person, the ability to see pathologic states as integrated entireties rather than snapshots of a single altered biochemical pathway is unfolding. In other words, modern biomedical scientists can take a "systems-based" approach to the molecular basis of disease. From a genetics point of view, this underscores a transition for medical genetics, from focusing on single-gene etiologies with biological and clinical manifestations toward medical genomics and an understanding of how multiple genes simultaneously interact to precipitate disease.

Today, physicians and biomedical scientists are using data extrapolated, or "mined," from the Human Genome Project as the foundation for furthering the understanding of molecular and cellular processes. For example, considerable effort has been invested in characterizing the function of proteins expressed from the human genome and how these gene products interact with each other, a study known as proteomics. Likewise, since many diseases result from the dysregulation of gene expression, transcriptomics, or the integrated study of global gene expression and regulation, has been vitalized. Other integrated areas of study such as pharmacogenomics, metabolomics, and nutrigenomics have emerged; all feature the current ability to see the larger picture regarding genes and proteins including expression and interaction.

The knowledge base of molecular genetics has grown hand-in-hand with the technologies that created the rapidly expanding knowledge base. The challenge for the modern physician and medical geneticist is to apply the evolving genetic paradigms and investigative and diagnostic methodologies to clinical practice. To do so requires an understanding of the tools and approaches used in molecular medicine. These include the diagnostic paradigm, molecular genetic techniques used for diagnosis and prognosis, and an understanding of the relevance of medical genetics to the modern health care system.

Revised Diagnostic Paradigm

For many years, a typical generalized paradigm for initial patient-physician interaction has consisted of three central elements. First, the physician interviews the patient, paying special attention to the initial complaint. Questions generally focus on signs and symptoms and quality-of-life issues. A physical examination ensues, followed by the third element, laboratory testing, to assess either the functionality of organ systems or biochemical parameters in bodily fluids; typically these include tests of blood, urine, and cerebrospinal fluid. Such inputs lead to a clinical diagnosis and an appropriate standard of care.

In the current age of molecular medicine, however, additional steps are added to this paradigm (Fig. 13-1). The first part of the revised paradigm remains as described with one important special emphasis. Given the genetic basis of most disease and the recent progress made in understanding genetic predisposition, it is essential that physicians pay close attention to family history and perform detailed pedigree analyses. Observations made here can provide important diagnostic clues.

The remainder of the diagnostic algorithm requires additional input. Following the family history/patient interview, physical examination, and supportive laboratory tests, a diagnosis can typically be made. In the post–Human Genome Project era, however, the diagnosis may be considered preliminary in some cases, with confirmation based on DNA-

based analysis or genetic testing. The association of a known mutational or chromosomal variant with a disease phenotype confirms the diagnosis and may even provide prognostic value if significant genotype-phenotype correlations are documented. The importance of this portion of the modern diagnostic paradigm is evidenced by the dramatic increase in genetic testing laboratories over the last 10 to 15 years, accompanied by the acceptance of insurance companies that molecular genetic diagnostics provides a high degree of accuracy and specificity.

In the absence of a known pathogenic genetic variant, a physician may feel unsure of a clinical diagnosis. In this case, it may be that the patient harbors a new, previously uncharacterized mutation. Such patients and families are the foundation for the discovery aspects of modern biomedicine. Hence, it is important that today's physician realize the vital role of public and private research efforts to the biomedical enterprise. By means of appropriate dialogue and approved *informed consent*, the physician-patient axis can collaborate with medical geneticists and biochemists to discover new disease-causing mutations (Box 13-1). This, in turn, promotes robust genetic databases, new diagnostic capacity, and the possibility of novel or enhanced genotype-phenotype associations of interest to patient care.

Finally, with the explosion of genetic information available to the physician comes a responsibility to accurately convey the implications of genetic findings to the patient. This indicates that genetic counseling should be added to the paradigm. Whether done by the physician or by professional genetic counselors, this medical service conveys an essential service to the patient because it can describe confirmation of

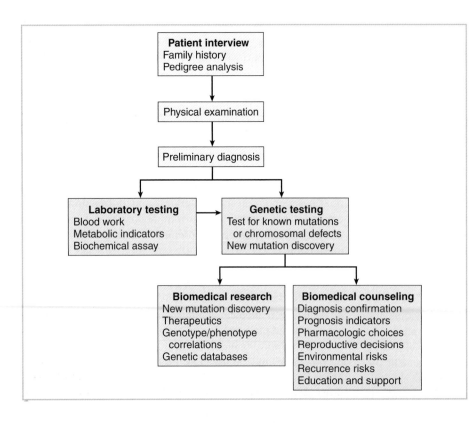

Figure 13-1. Diagnostic algorithm. Molecular diagnostics is changing the approach to diagnosis and treatment of disease. Beyond standard laboratory tests, genetic testing is providing unique patient information leading to personalized treatment regimens as well as family and patient information that until recently was limited.

Box 13-1. INFORMED CONSENT FOR HUMAN SUBJECTS RESEARCH*

Components of Informed Consent

Risks to subjects are minimized.

Procedures are used that are consistent with sound research design and that do not unnecessarily expose subjects to risk.

Whenever appropriate, procedures are used that are already being performed on the subjects for diagnostic or treatment purposes.

Risks to subjects are reasonable in relation to anticipated benefits.

Only those risks and benefits that may result from the research (as distinguished from risks and benefits of therapies subjects would receive even if not participating in the research) are considered.

Long-range effects of applying knowledge gained in the research are not considered.

Selection of subjects is equitable.

There may be special problems with vulnerable populations: children, prisoners, pregnant women, mentally disabled persons, or economically or educationally disadvantaged persons.

Informed consent will be sought from each prospective subject or the subject's legally authorized representative.

Informed consent will be appropriately documented.

When appropriate, the research plan makes adequate provision for monitoring the data collected to ensure the safety of subjects.

When appropriate, there are adequate provisions to protect the privacy of subjects and to maintain the confidentiality of data.

*Requires approval of an Institutional Review Board to provide certain safeguards to the participants. (Data from U.S. Department of Health and Human Services, Office for Human Research Protections, 45 CFR §46.111.)

---

diagnosis (refer to Table 7-4), prognostic indicators, risk assessment for patient and relatives, information critical for reproductive decisions and prenatal genetic testing, and even direct disease management (Box 13-2). New essentials in the generalized diagnostic paradigm are added to the core essentials of patient interview and family history, physical examination, and laboratory testing. These include molecular genetic diagnostics, collaboration with biomedical scientists, and genetic counseling.

Molecular Genetic Techniques

Physicians should be able to interpret fundamental genetic data just as they interpret biochemical data, ECGs, or respirometry results. To do so, an understanding of basic molecular genetic methodologies is necessary. Below, these fundamental approaches and applications to molecular diagnostics are described.

Nucleic Acid Visualization

Patient cells are necessary to initiate molecular genetic analysis. Typically, patient material is a blood sample, biopsy specimen, and amniotic fluid or chorionic villus sample. Using blood as an example, total genomic DNA is extracted and the DNA is visualized or prepared for subsequent analysis by a number of techniques including restriction fragment length polymorphism (RFLP) and Southern blotting, DNA amplification using the polymerase chain reaction (PCR), and DNA sequence analysis.

RFLP and Southern Blot Analysis

Southern blotting is a method to visualize DNA of interest. There are three fundamental elements to the Southern blot procedure: (1) fragmentation of the DNA, (2) separation of the DNA on the basis of fragment size, and (3) identification and visualization of informative fragments using a probe. Fragmentation typically occurs through the use of restriction endonucleases, which are also referred to as restriction enzymes. Restriction endonucleases are enzymes of bacterial origin that bind to the DNA at specific sites and cleave both strands of the DNA. The DNA recognition sites for restriction enzymes are typically palindromic sequences 4 to 8 bases in length, and the double-stranded breaks occur within or adjacent to the recognition sites. For example, the restriction enzyme *Eco*RI recognizes and binds to the six nucleotide sequence of 5′-GAATTC-3′. In this case, the enzyme nicks the phosphodiester bond between the G and the A on both strands, generating two DNA fragments with so-called sticky ends (Table 13-1). Because a six-base-pair sequence such as GAATTC is encountered frequently in the human genome, treatment of genomic DNA with the *Eco*RI enzyme generates roughly 1 million DNA fragments. A single-base change in a restriction enzyme recognition site prevents an endonuclease from binding to the DNA, resulting in no cleavage of the DNA. Conversely, a single-base change may create a new recognition site where none existed prior to the base change. Different individuals in the population harbor a variety of benign point mutations that alter restriction enzyme recognition sites, thus resulting in a different collection of fragments. Such variation in the sizes of DNA fragments obtained by restriction endonuclease digestion is visualized by gel electrophoresis and Southern blotting; this procedure is termed restriction fragment length polymorphism, or RFLP, analysis (Fig. 13-2).

For gel electrophoresis, DNA fragments are loaded onto a porous, gelatinous material to which an electrical field is applied. By virtue of the inherent negative charge of DNA molecules, fragments migrate to the positive pole. Smaller

Box 13-2. THE HEALTH INSURANCE PORTABILITY AND ACCOUNTABILITY ACT (HIPAA) PRIVACY RULE*

Elements of an Authorization

Core Elements

The name(s) or other specific identification of person(s) or class of persons authorized to make the requested use or disclosure.

The name(s) or other specific identification of the person(s) or class of persons who may use the PHI or to whom the covered entity may make the requested disclosure.

Description of each purpose of the requested use or disclosure. Researchers should note that this element must be research study specific, not for future unspecified research.

Authorization expiration date or event that relates to the individual or to the purpose of the use or disclosure (the terms "end of the research study" or "none" may be used for research, including for the creation and maintenance of a research database or repository).

Signature of the individual and date. If the Authorization is signed by an individual's personal representative, a description of the representative's authority to act for the individual.

Required Elements

The individual's right to revoke his/her Authorization in writing and either (1) the exceptions to the right to revoke and a description of how the individual may revoke Authorization or (2) reference to the corresponding section(s) of the covered entity's Notice of Privacy Practices.

Notice of the covered entity's ability or inability to condition treatment, payment, enrollment, or eligibility for benefits on the Authorization, including research-related treatment, and, if applicable, consequences of refusing to sign the Authorization.

The potential for the PHI to be re-disclosed by the recipient and no longer protected by the Privacy Rule. This statement does not require an analysis of risk for re-disclosure but may be a general statement that the Privacy Rule may no longer protect health information.

Optional Elements: Examples that may be relevant to the recipient of protected health information.

Your health information will be used or disclosed when required by law.

Your health information may be shared with a public health authority that is authorized by law to collect or receive such information for the purpose of preventing or controlling disease, injury, or disability, and conducting public health surveillance, investigations or interventions.

No publication or public presentation about the research described above will reveal your identity without another authorization from you.

If all information that does or can identify you is removed from your health information, the remaining information will no longer be subject to this authorization and may be used or disclosed for other purposes.

If you revoke this Authorization, you may no longer be allowed to participate in the research described in this Authorization.

*Provides comprehensive Federal protection for the privacy of personal health information. Research organizations and researchers may or may not be covered by the HIPAA Privacy Rule. (Data from U.S. Department of Health and Human Services, Office for Human Research Protections, 45 CFR §164.508.)

---

fragments migrate faster than larger fragments, thereby resolving in the gel on the basis of size. The fragments are visualized by the addition of a dye molecule, such as ethidium bromide, that intercalates between the DNA base pairs and fluoresces upon illumination with UV light. Other fluorescent dyes with greater sensitivity for staining small quantities of DNA and of less toxicity are also used. Often however, a particular fragment of diagnostic value is of interest, but it is impossible to identify an individual fragment with many fragments resolved in the gel. The ability to visualize single DNA fragments requires the addition of a DNA probe that hybridizes specifically to the fragment of interest. A DNA probe is typically single stranded and complementary to the gene or region of DNA interest. It is labeled with a fluorescent or radioactive tag so that the probe-target complex can be detected. Probes can be DNA

fragments purified from restriction endonuclease digestion or small, synthetic DNA oligonucleotides.

A gene-specific probe is not hybridized to its complement in an agarose gel owing to the difficulty of working with the gel matrix itself and to any radioactive background that could occur with this type of labeling. Instead, the fragmented DNA is transferred to a dry filter and the probe is added. This is the essence of the Southern blot procedure (see Fig. 13-2). Specifically, following gel electrophoresis, the DNA strands are denatured with a strong base while still in the gel. The single-stranded DNA is then transferred to a nylon or nitro-cellulose membrane support by capillary action; sometimes application of a vacuum facilitates transfer. At this point, the denatured DNA is "fixed" to the membrane and a probe is applied under conditions that favor the reestablishment of DNA duplexes. As suggested above, it is the Watson-Crick

TABLE 13-1. Examples of Commonly Used Restriction Endonucleases

Enzyme	Source	Type of Product	Recognition Sequence*	Fragment Ends	
AluI	Arthrobacter luteus	Blunt ends	AG↓CT TC↑GA	5′ AG 3′ TC	CT 3′ GA 5′
EcoRI	Escherichia coli strain R	5′ Overhang	G↓AATTC CTTAA↑G	5′ G 3′ CTTAT	AATTC 3′ G 5′
PstI	Providencia stuatii	3′ Overhang	CTGCA↓G G↑ACGTC	5′ CTGCA 3′ G	G 3′ ACGTC 5′
MnlI	Moraxella nonliquefaciens	Nonpalindromic sequence	CCTCNNNNNNN↓ GGAGNNNNNN↑N	5′ CCTC(N_7) 3′ GGAG(N_6)	3′ N 5′

*Arrows show recognition sites of sequence; N, any nucleic acid.

hydrogen bond base-pairing between the single-strand probe and its single-stranded complement restriction fragment that enables the probe to specifically anneal only to its complement. Visualization of a DNA fragment of interest is performed by laser-facilitated detection of the fluorescent probe or by exposure of the filter to x-ray film in the case of a radioactive probe. Thus, by means of a combination of restriction endonuclease digestion, gel electrophoresis, and Southern blotting, visualizing a DNA fragment of interest is accomplished.

Polymerase Chain Reaction

The introduction of polymerase chain reaction (PCR) has revolutionized DNA-based diagnostics. The rapid, inexpensive amplification of specific DNA sequences made possible with PCR has tremendously enabled both preparative and analytic procedures. PCR is the in vitro enzymatic amplification of a short (up to 5–6 kb) and specific DNA sequence. Amplification can be initiated with even a single DNA molecule and produces millions of copies in a period of a few hours. There are four essential components to PCR: two deoxyoligonucleotide primers, a thermostable DNA polymerase, target DNA, and nucleotides. The primers add specificity to the amplification by defining the flanking regions of DNA sequences to be amplified. Primers are "designed" to reflect the complementary nucleotide sequence of the target. These are usually 15 to 30 nucleotides in length and synthesized by an automated process. Primers bind to targets in a 5′-3′ direction on each strand, and amplification occurs between them.

Amplification occurs during a series of denaturing, heating, and cooling phases that are repeated numerous times. These serve to dissociate double-stranded DNA, allow primers to anneal, and facilitate new strand extension. The polymerase used in this procedure must be thermostable at high temperatures, a feature not characteristic of enzymes. The best known of the special thermostable polymerases was isolated from *Thermus aquaticus*. Designated DNA *taq* polymerase, it withstands repeated cycles of 95°C or greater.

During denaturation, the target DNA in the reaction is heated to 95°C, rendering the target DNA single-stranded by breaking the hydrogen bonds between the two strands. The

reaction is then cooled, typically to 45–65°C, to permit annealing of the single-stranded primers to complementary sequences in the target DNA. Finally, the temperature is increased to 70–75°C to allow extension or synthesis of the new DNA most efficiently. During the extension phase, DNA polymerase uses the free 3′-OH group on the primers to synthesize new DNA. This three-step, or three-phase, cycle is repeated with the newly synthesized DNA strands serving as templates for additional strand formation. Early in the process, the original genomic DNA is diluted out and the ends of the newly synthesized DNA strands are entirely defined by the primers. Overall, this cycle is repeated 20 to 35 times and the number of DNA copies doubles with each cycle, thus resulting in millions of copies of specific, primer-directed DNA fragments (Fig. 13-3). It should be noted that the thermostable DNA polymerase, an excess of primers, and the formation of newly synthesized DNA fragments that serve as templates for subsequent cycles permit the iterative cycles of amplification.

Later, application of the PCR in molecular genetic diagnostics will be described. It should be apparent, however, that PCR has two direct uses. First, it can provide abundant substrate for mutation detection strategies. Second, it can be a stand-alone diagnostic tool for detecting changes in DNA length, such as small insertions or deletions. In either case, PCR has greatly facilitated the era of genetic medicine by providing a rapid and inexpensive tool to biomedical scientists working on both diagnostic and research procedures (Table 13-2).

DNA Sequence Analysis

In the post–Human Genome Project era, "unknown" regions of the chromosome are no longer sequenced to find new disease-causing mutations. More typically, genes or certain regions of genes are sequenced to detect a disease-specific mutation. Because the entire sequence of the human genome is known, PCR primers can be designed to amplify specific DNA for sequencing. Since DNA sequencing is greatly facilitated by abundant target DNA, only one application of PCR amplification of a specific DNA substrate is generally needed for sequencing.

A B C

Blood samples

Digest DNA with
restriction enzyme

A B C

Separate by gel
electrophoresis

−

+

Denature DNA

Blot onto membrane

Add radioactive probe

Expose to x-ray film

A
B
C

Figure 13-2. RFLP and Southern blotting.

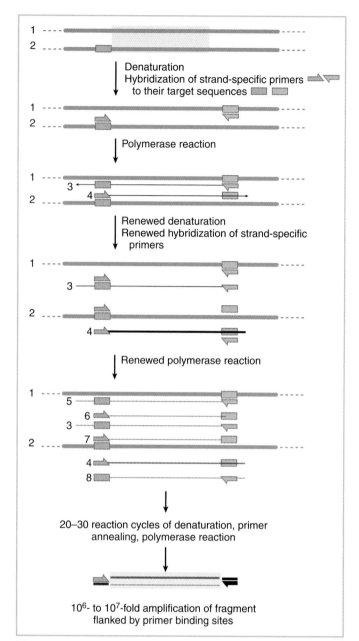

Figure 13-3. Polymerase chain reaction.

The most common method of DNA sequencing is the Sanger dideoxynucleotide chain-terminating technique (Fig. 13-4). Here, heat-denatured, single-stranded template, such as PCR products, is added to each of four tubes. Each tube contains a mixture of the four nucleotides (A, G, C, and T), which acts as a substrate for DNA polymerase. Each tube also contains *one* of the four chain-terminating dideoxyribonucleotides (ddA, ddG, ddC, or ddT). Hence the "A" tube contains a mixture of the four normal radioactively labeled

nucleotides (dA, dG, dT, and dC) plus the chain-terminating ddA; a similar mixture of dNTPs to ddNTPs is found in the "G," "C," and "T" tubes. The incorporation of any dideoxynucleotide prohibits further DNA polymerization because these lack the 3′-OH group required by DNA polymerase to add the next nucleotide. The addition of DNA polymerase and oligonucleotide primers, which are required to anneal to the target and initiate DNA polymerization via the free 3′-OH, to each reaction tube initiates DNA synthesis. However, the chains are terminated at different positions owing to the random insertion of a dideoxynucleotide instead of a normal deoxynucleotide. Stated differently, when a ddG is inserted by the DNA polymerase instead of a dG, synthesis stops at that point. In the "G" tube reaction, for example, some chains will be terminated at the initial G encountered by the DNA

TABLE 13-2. Comparison of PCR and RFLP

Characteristic	RFLP	PCR
Time requirement	Days	Hours
Amount of DNA required	Micrograms to milligrams	Picograms or less
Cost	May be high with radioactivity usage and disposal; less costly if nonradioactive probes used	Rarely needs radioactivity and therefore less expensive
Sensitivity	Less sensitive to small quantities of DNA	More sensitive to small quantities or copy numbers of DNA

BIOCHEMISTRY

Ribonucleotides

The fundamental concept of the dideoxynucleotide chain terminating technique is that some deoxyribonucleotides lack an OH at the 3′ position of the sugar. For those deoxyribonucleotides in which this occurs, called dideoxyribonucleotides, a phosphodiester bond cannot form with a 5′ H and chain elongation stops. These ddNTPs can be labeled with a radioactive or nonradioactive tag for visualization of fragments incorporating them, or rather of the fragments that terminated elongation at that point.

Ribonucleoside triphosphate (NTP)

Deoxyribonucleoside triphosphate (dNTP)

Dideoxyribonucleoside triphosphate (ddNTP)

polymerase, while other chains will be halted at other G positions of the chain. In the "G" tube, the ratio of dGTP/ddGTP is such that there will be a number of chains that have terminated at each G position along the template.

The four reactions are separated by gel electrophoresis on a polyacrylamide gel to produce a visual "ladder" of DNA fragments. Labeling either the DNA sequencing primers or the individual nucleotides with a radioactive or fluorescent tag enables this visualization. In automated sequencing, the ddNTPs are labeled with fluorescent dyes that are detected by a scanner. Because the gel lane containing "A" (from the "A" tube), "T," and so forth is known, it is a straightforward matter to read the sequencing ladder.

Most DNA sequencing was once done by polyacrylamide gel electrophoresis but more recently is being replaced by capillary electrophoresis (see Fig. 13-4B). This technique adds automation to the process while introducing several highly regarded features. DNA separation occurs in a capillary with a diameter of 25 to 100 μm, which provides a high ratio of surface area to volume that acts to dissipate heat produced. This feature allows the use of higher electric fields, which decreases time of separation and increases resolution of DNA.

Mutation Detection

The true basis of molecular diagnostics is the detection of specific disease-causing mutations. Here, the most common methods associated with genetic variation that are employed in laboratories for the detection of common diseases are discussed, including point mutations, deletions, and trinucleotide repeat expansions.

Point Mutation Detection
Mutation-specific RFLPs

In some single-gene disorders, the causal mutation is a point mutation that alters a restriction endonuclease recognition site. This type of mutation can either abolish an existing recognition site or create a novel site. When this happens, it permits a mutation-specific test that can be used for diagnostic purposes. Perhaps the best example of a mutation-specific RFLP test is found in sickle cell anemia. As described in

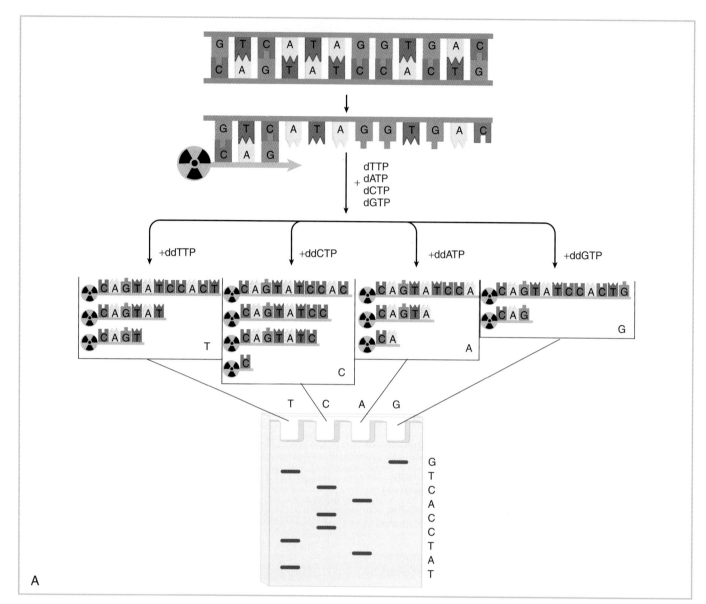

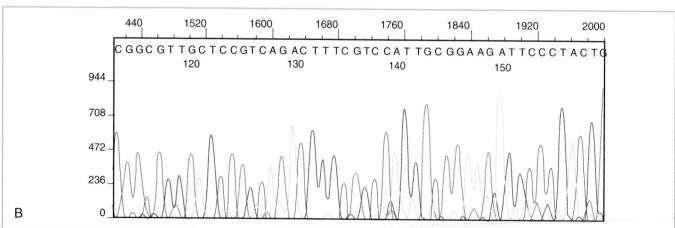

Figure 13-4. DNA sequencing. **A,** Sequencing is diagrammed using radioactively labeled deoxynucleotides. DNA fragments of varying lengths are produced by the dideoxynucleotides and separated on a polyacrylamide gel. The sequence is read from the top to the bottom of the gel. **B,** Four different fluorescent labels are used to tag the primer which is used in dideoxynucleotide sequencing reactions as shown in part **A.** The reaction products are then pooled and separated by capillary electrophoresis. A laser-induced fluorescence detector monitors the signals in four spectral channels, which are plotted as four colors corresponding to each base in the ladder. (Courtesy of NBII Program administered by the Biological Informatics Office of the U.S. Geological Survey.)

Chapter 6, sickle cell anemia results from an A to T missense mutation and the substitution of a valine for a glutamate at the sixth amino acid of the β-globin polypeptide. This base change affects the 5′-CCTNAGG-3′ (where N can be any nucleotide) recognition site for the *Mst*II restriction endonuclease because the central A is replaced by a T, rendering a similar but different 5′-CCTNTGG-3′ sequence. *Mst*II does not recognize or cleave this altered DNA sequence. Hence, sickle cell anemia patients differ from the normal population by the loss of this particular restriction site, resulting in an RFLP for sickle cell anemia. In the laboratory, this is recognized by means of agarose gel electrophoresis in which normal individuals have two smaller DNA fragments that correspond to the affected individual's single, longer DNA fragment (Fig. 13-5). While specific and sensitive, this methodology is relatively rare in practice because the majority of point mutations do not alter a restriction endonuclease recognition site. As seen in Chapter 6 and suggested earlier in this chapter, PCR can also be used to amplify a fragment of interest for restriction analysis. The fragment sizes may differ between genomic DNA versus PCR-generated DNA and a probe may be required to visualize a fragment in genomic DNA, but the results still demonstrate the effect of the mutation.

Allele-specific Oligonucleotides

Thousands of single-base changes are associated with human disease. This has necessitated the development of other methods to identify individual point mutations because mutation-specific RFLPs are relatively rare. One of these methods is allele-specific oligonucleotide (ASO) hybridization (Fig. 13-6). For this, a DNA synthesizer creates short, synthetic oligonucleotides that are an exact complement of the normal DNA sequence. These, in turn, are radioactively or fluorescently labeled and used to probe patient or control DNA in a process similar to the Southern blot probing. During the hybridization process, these short oligonucleotides bind only to a perfect sequence complement and not to any sequence with even a single mismatched base. Thus, the oligonucleotides bind only normal DNAs, making it simple to distinguish between normal DNA and mutant DNA. Conversely, a short oligonucleotide may also be synthesized that is a perfect complement to a mutant DNA sequence. For example, an ASO can be synthesized that hybridizes only to the portion of the β-globin gene that contains the sickle cell anemia mutation. Such an oligonucleotide does not bind to normal DNA because it is mismatched at the base altered in sickle cell anemia. A mutation-specific ASO, then, can be used to screen patients, family members, and even members of the general population for the presence of the sickle cell mutation.

DNA Sequencing

In special cases when a patient is clearly suffering from a particular disease but does not harbor known genetic variants associated with the disease, the candidate gene may be subjected to complete or partial automated DNA sequence

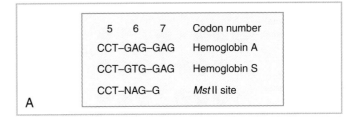

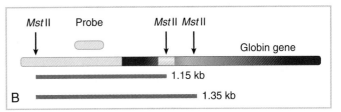

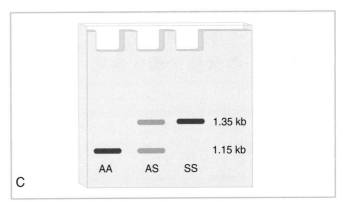

Figure 13-5. RFLP analysis of the β-globin gene and sickle cell anemia. **A**, An A-to-T point mutation occurs in codon 6. **B**, The mutation eliminates a recognition site for *Mst*II. Individuals with sickle cell trait are heterozygous and have 1.15-kb and 1.35-kb fragments. Individuals with sickle cell anemia have two longer 1.35-kb fragments. **C**, Electrophoretic gel demonstrating DNA fragments for AA, AS, and SS individuals.

analysis. DNA sequencing is much more labor intensive and time consuming than the above methods, but it is an excellent approach for the discovery of new or rare mutations. This technique is so valuable that increased technological developments are providing improvements designed to reduce the time and cost of sequencing; it is not unthinkable that samples currently referred to a research laboratory for evaluation will be sequenced in a diagnostic laboratory in the near future.

Deletion Detection

Very small deletions, typically single-base deletions that cause disease, may be screened for by means of the same methodologies employed for point mutations. Larger deletions, however, require a different approach. PCR is ideal for detecting deletions in the 100-bp to 4-kb range, since primer pairs amplify both a normal and mutated allele containing a deletion. Following PCR, DNA fragments are separated by electrophoresis and compared with molecular weight standards. Deleted alleles are obviously not so large as the nondeleted forms and hence are easily visualized.

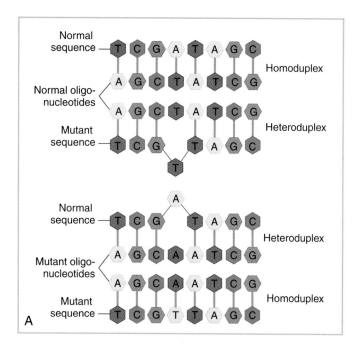

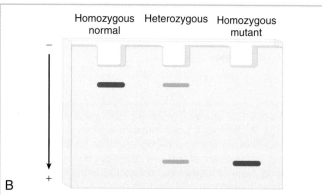

Figure 13-6. Allele-specific oligonucleotide testing. **A,** Short oligonucleotides are designed to reflect a normal sequence or a mutated sequence. These allele-specific oligonucleotides will then bind only if there is perfect complementation to either denatured normal or mutated alleles forming a homoduplex. Heteroduplexes do not form stable binding. **B,** ASOs for both the normal and mutated sequences can be used together, and the resulting homoduplexes are separated by gel electrophoresis.

Trinucleotide Repeat Expansion Detection

As described in Chapter 8, expansions of trinucleotide sequences are a relatively common genetic mechanism for neurologic disease. Fragile X syndrome, Huntington's disease, myotonic dystrophy, spinobulbar muscular atrophy, and Friedreich's ataxia are all examples of disease caused by expanding trinucleotide repeats. This class of mutation poses a special challenge for diagnostics, as illustrated by the fragile X syndrome. Fragile X is due to an expansion of a CGG trinucleotide in the 5′ untranslated region of the *FMR1* gene. Three classes of *FMR1*-associated CGG expansions are recognized in the population: normal chromosomes contain between 5 and 50 repeats; premutation chromosomes contain

between 50 and 200 repeats, and full mutation chromosomes (affected individuals) feature 200 to 2000 CGG repeats. Distinguishing between these three allelic repeats seems, intuitively, an ideal task for PCR. In practice, however, this is true for normal and premutation alleles; PCR primers flank the site of the CGG expansion and amplify the alleles. The same is not always true for the full mutation because full mutation expansions can reach 6 kb in length, exceeding the size at which accurate genotyping can be done on the basis of PCR alone. Thus, Southern blotting is typically performed when fragile X syndrome is suspected. In this case, a probe is used that hybridizes proximal to the expanded region. In this way, very large expansions can be detected. The dividing line between use of PCR and Southern blotting to size the repeat tract falls between 70 and 100 repeats. Southern blots cannot identify a precise repeat size at the normal and low premutation ranges, but PCR is unable to correctly identify repeat tracts over 70 to 100 units.

It is important to note that DNA diagnostics pervades the entirety of the health care system today. A large number of laboratories utilizing genetic techniques now exist and stand as a testament to the ubiquity of genetic defects in medicine. Even in rural or remote settings, the physician sends blood samples to a laboratory for DNA analysis. The association between medicine and molecular genetics will grow more comprehensive as additional insights are made regarding genetic predisposition to disease and the role of genetics in pharmaceutical efficacy.

●●● GENETIC TESTING AND SCREENING

Fundamentals of Genetic Testing

Currently, DNA-based tests exist for roughly 1000 diseases with about 700 in use in genetic laboratories. Clearly, genetic testing for disease mutations and predispositions will have a greater impact on medicine as more genes are identified and associated with pathology. DNA-based testing must have analytical and clinical validity and utility. Analytical (laboratory) validity, or efficiency, refers to the ability of a genetic test to accurately indicate the genetic condition or genotype. It is described by two elements—sensitivity and specificity (Table 13-3). *Sensitivity* is a measure of how effective a particular test is at identifying the mutation or genotype of interest; it is also the detection rate for true positive samples. *Specificity* indicates how often a test identifies those samples that do not have the mutation, which is the detection rate for true negative samples. To have value to the physician, gene tests must also have clinical validity *or predictive value*, defined by the ability of a particular assay to detect disease. Positive predictive value reflects the percentage of all positive tests that are true positives; the converse is true for a negative predictive value. Again, sensitivity and specificity are relevant. Here, clinical sensitivity refers to the proportion of people who have a particular disease that tested positive for a causal mutation while clinical specificity indicates the proportion of people who do not have a particular disorder and have tested negative for the associated gene mutation. Both sensitivity and specificity are measured by comparing the genetic test results with those obtained from a separate, definitive diagnostic test, such as a biochemical assay. The *clinical utility* of a DNA-based test refers to its ability to be useful to the practicing clinician. In other words, a genetic test is useful only if it clearly provides value to the diagnosis, prognosis, treatment, or prevention of a disease.

DNA-based tests have two overarching utilities: genetic testing and genetic screening. *Genetic testing* generally refers to the confirmation or establishment of a diagnosis within a patient or family that has a clear disease phenotype and family history. In this instance, a gene test is usually an effort focused on an individual or family and on a single gene. *Genetic screening*, in contrast, is a population-based approach that attempts to identify presymptomatic individuals in the population that harbor disease-associated genetic variants. Genetic screening includes such important concepts as heterozygote carrier identification, newborn screening, prenatal diagnostics, and presymptomatic testing for late-onset disorders or disease predisposition. Hence, DNA-based screens have a significant public health component, whereas genetic testing typically refers to an individual or family. Since genetic testing is a fairly straightforward concept, the following discussion centers on the principles of genetic screens.

Genetic Screening

In general, the feasibility and utility of genetic screening in a population is greatly enhanced when certain criteria are met in three general areas: disease characteristics, diagnostic test features, and the capacity of the health care system. Diseases subject to genetic screens should be reasonably common, well characterized, severe enough to warrant population screening, and treatable or preventable. The genetic test itself should have laboratory and clinical validity and be inexpensive and rapid enough to promote widespread use (see Table 4-2). Finally, the health care system itself should be prepared for the treatment of the disease including providing accessible therapeutic resources, counseling services, and educational programs.

It is important to note that not all genetic screens are tests for mutations. Biochemical tests are available that can indicate whether a particular gene is defective. Examples include the Guthrie test for hyperphenylalanine levels and creatine kinase assay for Duchenne muscular dystrophy. However, PCR-based, mutation-specific assays are being increasingly utilized, since they are typically rapid, noninvasive, inexpensive, and accurate. Examples of DNA-based genetic screening include cystic fibrosis and sickle cell anemia.

Newborn Genetic Screening

Genetic testing in the newborn represents a tremendous opportunity for disease intervention, provided the above criteria are met. In newborn screening, it is particularly relevant that a disorder be prevented or ameliorated by early and presymptomatic diagnosis and intervention. Many of the disorders identified in the newborn have been discussed elsewhere. Many do not present in the newborn with an obvious disease phenotype, and a highly specific and sensitive genetic test is ideal for early detection of disease genotypes. Certain other disorders such as sickle cell anemia and congenital adrenal hyperplasia seem to be excellent candidates for population-based newborn screening. However, because of a lowered incidence or suboptimal treatment paradigms even with early intervention, such diseases are not included in some newborn screening programs. Occasionally, newborn genetic screens are performed in certain regions of the world where they have a high incidence. For example, cystic fibrosis is one of the most common autosomal recessive diseases found in people of Northern and Western European origin. In these populations, the incidence of cystic fibrosis ranges from 1 in 2000 to 1 in 3000. Hence, several relevant countries have instituted a DNA-based newborn screening procedure to detect affected infants. Because there is no effective dietary or pharmacologic treatment for cystic fibrosis, the expectation is that early prophylactic treatment, such as physical therapy and antibiotic administration, will improve the quality of life. A similar approach and rationale are being utilized in Africa for the early detection of sickle cell anemia.

TABLE 13-3. Diagnostic Value of Tests Defined by Sensitivity, Specificity, Predictive Value, and Efficiency

Patient	Results of a Diagnostic Test	
	Test Positive	**Test Negative**
Disease present	True positive (TP)	False negative (FN)
Disease absent	False positive (FP)	True negative (TN)
Sensitivity (%)	$= \dfrac{TP}{TP + FN} \times 100$	
Specificity (%)	$= \dfrac{TN}{FP + TN} \times 100$	
Positive predictive value (%)	$= \dfrac{TP}{TP + FP} \times 100$	
Negative predictive value (%)	$= \dfrac{TN}{FN + TN} \times 100$	
Test efficiency (percentage of times the test provides a correct answer per total number)	$= \dfrac{TP + TN}{TP + TN + FP + FN} \times 100$	

Heterozygote Carrier Screening

As disease databases grow and DNA-based assays continue to be developed and optimized, the feasibility of carrier screening for autosomal recessive diseases in adults has increased. Here, the purpose is not to identify individuals at risk for disease development but rather individuals who are at risk for passing on deleterious alleles to their children. Hence, this type of genetic screen seeks to inform and educate healthy individuals regarding reproductive risks. Such screens are most effective when coupled with genetic counseling and prenatal diagnostic options.

Heterozygote screening makes the most sense when an autosomal recessive disease is present in relatively high frequency in the population. Owing to the high incidence of recessive disorders in certain subpopulations, carrier screening is therefore most effective among particular ethnic groups that harbor a high deleterious allele frequency (see Chapter 12). Tay-Sachs disease is perhaps the most striking example of this in the Ashkenazi Jewish population. Tay-Sachs disease (see Chapter 8) is a severe autosomal recessive neurologic disease that results in childhood death. It occurs commonly in the Ashkenazi Jewish population, where the frequency of heterozygotes is approximately 1 in 30, reflecting the high risk in this subpopulation and suggesting that carrier testing would be of significant value to individuals of reproductive age. In fact, genetic testing for Tay-Sachs in the Ashkenazi Jewish population has been a resounding success. Since 1970, such testing performed either by biochemical assay or direct DNA testing has resulted in an 85% decrease in the incidence of this disease in North America in this subpopulation. The majority of individuals born with Tay-Sachs disease now are of non-Ashkenazi Jewish ancestry. This decrease in incidence more accurately represents the combined effects of education, heterozygote genetic screening, and prenatal genetic diagnosis. Thus, the story of Tay-Sachs disease in the North American Ashkenazi Jewish population is a testament to the power and role of genetics in public health, presymptomatic diagnosis, and disease prevention.

Prenatal Genetic Testing and Preimplantation Genetic Diagnosis

Many methods are at the disposal of the physician to diagnose genetic maladies before birth. These include direct examination of fetal cells by chorionic villus sampling (CVS) or amniocentesis, biomarker assays such as the maternal blood serum screen (triple screen), and ultrasonography. Direct DNA-based testing and analysis is permitted by amniocentesis and CVS, and the combination of the above techniques usually permits an accurate diagnosis.

Although the above approach to prenatal testing is efficacious, it provides limited options for parents, since a diagnosis is made after implantation and fetal growth. Preimplantation genetic diagnosis (PGD) in combination with assisted reproductive technologies, such as in vitro fertilization (IVF), on the other hand, permits the implantation of only "normal" embryos. Typically, PGD is of interest to a couple at significant risk for transmitting a harmful or predisposing allele to their offspring. PGD is initiated by the biopsy of a single cell from the six- to eight-cell blastomere produced by IVF. At this point, blastomere DNA is analyzed for a particular genetic defect either by cytogenetic means or by direct mutation detection. The latter is greatly facilitated by the use of PCR, since DNA from the single cell can be exponentially amplified. Only those embryos free of the genetic defect in question are implanted, virtually guaranteeing that the fetus will not manifest the disorder of concern to the parents.

To date, PGD has been used to prevent Tay-Sachs disease, cystic fibrosis, Huntington disease, Duchenne muscular dystrophy, β-thalassemia, early-onset Alzheimer disease, and many other severe disorders. Hundreds of babies have been born using PGD coupled with IVF, and this number is sure to increase dramatically as technology improves coordinately with our understanding of the genetic basis of disease.

●●● GENETIC COUNSELING AND RECURRENCE RISK ESTIMATION

Genetic Counseling

The field of genetic counseling has emerged as an important health care resource as a result of the identification of disease-associated genes. The utility of the counselor is illustrated by considering a couple that has had a child with a certain disease. Among many questions faced by the physician and team are, "Why did this happen?" "What is the prognosis?" "Will this happen to other children that we may have?" Equally likely is the scenario in which a *consultand*, who is an individual seeking or being referred to a genetic counselor, has learned that a family member has been diagnosed with a genetic disorder and wants to know the risk for developing the abnormality or transmitting it to offspring. Other reasons for genetic counseling include infertility, teratogen exposure, prenatal diagnosis with advanced maternal age, interpretation of newborn genetic screens, or a diagnosis of genetic disease. These questions and scenarios are common and central to many patients and to the health care system in general. Thus, genetic counseling is an essential component in

---

PATHOLOGY

Prenatal Detection of Defects and Abnormalities

The triple screen has become the standard of prenatal care for detecting neural tube defects and genetic abnormalities. Maternal serum is used to analyze α-fetoprotein (AFP), human chorionic gonadotropin (hCG), and unconjugated estriol (E_3).

Anomaly	AFP	hCG	E_3
Neural tube defects	↑	Normal	Normal
Trisomy 21	↓	↑	↓↓
Trisomy 18	↓	↓	↓

the health care system and must be considered a core part of any modern medical genetic enterprise.

Genetic counseling is essentially a knowledge-based communication and educational endeavor. The counselor establishes that the patient understands the clinical diagnosis and cognate prognosis and treatment, the genetic components of the disorder including inheritance pattern and risks, treatment, reproductive risks and options, and the availability of educational information and support groups. In providing information to at-risk patients or families, consultands are not guided to a particular option, but rather provided the context, education, and information to make informed medical and reproductive decisions that are appropriate for personal and sociocultural dictates. This "nondirective" approach may actually run counter to the traditional view of medicine, where a biomedical team might suggest a course of action. Typically, a recommendation suggesting a course of action seeks the prevention of further disease or amelioration of a current disease state. However, genetic counseling seeks to provide information. The counselor communicates essential material in a manner that respects the integrity of the consultand or patient to make the decision. This communication, by the physician and the counselor, underscore the major principles of medical ethics (Table 13-4).

Recurrence Risk Assessment

An important function of the medical genetics community is estimation of the recurrence risk for a disease within a particular family. This is typically performed by a genetic counselor; the information sought is ordinarily related to risks to close family members or offspring.

Accurate risk assessment relies on the essential elements of accurate diagnosis, detailed family history and mode of inheritance determination, knowledge of DNA or biochemical tests that quantify the defect, and appropriate genetic databases that indicate carrier frequencies in the relevant population. For disorders due to a single gene, the recurrence risk to family members is often calculated by careful pedigree analysis and application of the rules of mendelian assortment of dominant, recessive, or X-linked alleles (see Chapter 12). In actuality, however, pedigree analysis can be ambiguous because of the complicating effects of incomplete penetrance, variable expressivity, unknown carrier status, late age of onset, and genetic heterogeneity. In such cases, however, modified recurrence risks are estimated using bayesian analysis.

Bayesian Analysis

Bayesian analysis is a form of probability theory that attempts to determine relative recurrence risks based on pedigree analysis, phenotype, and/or laboratory test results alone. In other words, bayesian risk analysis incorporates additional information beyond simple mendelian segregation into the risk calculation. For a given question of interest such as, "is individual A a carrier of a deleterious mutation?" bayesian analysis considers the two alternative possibilities:

TABLE 13-4. Major Principles of Medical Ethics

Principle	Description
Respect for autonomy	The patient has the right to make informed decisions without coercion. This is the basis for the practice of "informed consent."
Beneficence	Health care providers offer services that are beneficial to the patient.
Justice	Health care providers fairly distribute care to patients.
Nonmalfeasance	The health care provider is committed to protect patients from harm by providing the best standard of care.
Dignity	The patient is treated with dignity.
Integrity	Health care providers are truthful and honest to patients about conditions and treatments.

individual A is a carrier and individual A is not a carrier. This estimative approach, named after Bayes' theorem of probability first published in 1763, has four principal components:

1. A *prior probability* based on family history. This can also be considered the mendelian risk.
2. The *conditional probability*, which takes into account any additional pedigree information such as affected status in offspring. The conditional probability may also incorporate laboratory test results.
3. The *joint probability*, which is simply the product of the prior and conditional probabilities.
4. The *posterior or relative probability*, which is obtained by dividing the joint probability by the sum of all joint probabilities.

Application of bayesian probability is facilitated by an example shown in Figure 13-7. In this example, a family suffering from a sex-linked recessive disease is illustrated, and the probability that individual II-2 is a carrier is calculated. It should be noted that bayesian analysis is best understood by use of a table showing the various probabilities (Table 13-5). Calculation of prior probability is straightforward in that it is known that her (individual I-2's) mother must be an obligate carrier by virtue of the fact that she has an affected brother and son. Thus, individual II-2 has a 0.5 chance of being a carrier and a 0.5 chance of not being a carrier. This is the prior probability. How is the prior probability "conditionalized"? Here, additional ("posterior") information found in the pedigree is important. For example, individual II-2 has three sons and none are affected. If she were a carrier, the probability that she would have three healthy sons would be $1/2 \times 1/2 \times 1/2$, or $1/8$. Obviously, if she is not a carrier, the probability that she would have three healthy sons is 1.

Conditional probabilities can utilize more than family data. Particularly for autosomal dominant disorders, incomplete penetrance or delayed age of onset can complicate pedigree analysis. Empirical estimates of both can be made and included in the calculation of conditional probability. The next step asks the question, "What is the probability that individual II-2 is both a carrier and has three healthy sons?" Here, the joint probability is calculated by multiplying the prior and the conditional fractions for each of the two initial possibilities. So, under the condition that II-2 is a carrier, we would multiply $1/2 \times 1/8$ (to equal 1/16), and for the condition that she is not a carrier, we multiply $1/2 \times 1$ (to equal 1/2, or 8/16). Finally, the posterior probability is computed and turns out to be 1/16 divided by 1/16 + 1/2, or 1/9, for the condition in which II-2 is a carrier and 1/2 / 1/16 + 1/2, or 8/9, for the condition in which she is not a carrier. At this point, it has been determined that it is much more likely that individual II-2 is not a carrier for the sex-linked disease allele. In fact, the risk has been reduced from the simple 1/2, as indicated by pedigree analysis, to roughly 1/9.

Hence, bayesian analysis allows a degree of quantification for observations made in pedigree analysis. In the above example, it is inferred that individual II-2 is not a carrier because she has three unaffected sons. However, such an "educated guess" is often unsatisfying to the individual in question. In practice, bayesian analysis may be employed less today than in years past. This is due to the rise of DNA-based diagnostics. Again in the above example, the most efficient and accurate test would be to identify the mutation responsible for the disorder and directly test each interested family member for carrier status. In an appreciable number of families, however, direct mutation testing may not be economical or efficient; likewise, extreme genetic or locus heterogeneity also exists. In these cases, bayesian analysis of recurrence risk remains valuable to the family in question.

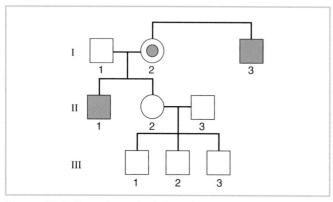

Figure 13-7. Bayesian calculations for a pedigree with X-linked recessive inheritance. (From Mueller RF, Young ID. *Emery's Elements of Medical Genetics,* 5th ed. Philadelphia, Churchill Livingstone, 2002, p 294.)

TABLE 13-5. Bayesian Calculation for Individual II-2

Probability	II-2 Is a Carrier	II-2 Is Not a Carrier
Prior conditional	$\dfrac{1}{2}$	$\dfrac{1}{2}$
Three healthy sons	$\left(\dfrac{1}{2}\right)^3 = \dfrac{1}{8}$	$(1)^3 = 1$
Joint	$\dfrac{1}{16}$	$\dfrac{1}{2}\left(=\dfrac{8}{16}\right)$
Expressed as odds	1	to	8
Posterior	$\dfrac{1}{9}$	$\dfrac{8}{9}$

From Mueller RF, Young ID *Emery's Elements of Medical Genetics*, 5th ed. Philadelphia, Churchill Livingstone, 2002, p.294.

Empirical Risk

As discussed, simple recurrence risk estimation for single-gene disorders of known inheritance patterns is based on mendelian segregation of disease alleles. However, many disorders feature multifactorial or polygenic genetic mechanisms. As discussed in earlier chapters, these diseases are characterized by a strong genetic component with relatives typically showing a higher incidence of the disease relative to the incidence in the general population. Recurrence risks for complex diseases are therefore determined empirically, since the totality of genetic and environmental factors is often unknown. In practice, empirical risks are determined by observations made in families that have the same disease. As an example, nonsyndromic cleft lip and palate has a significant genetic component and can therefore cluster in families. Theoretical probability is not used in this example because nonsyndromic cleft lip and palate is not inherited in a typical mendelian fashion. Instead, the risk to any particular relative in a pedigree is calculated based on observations from existing cleft lip and palate families.

Empirical risk calculation is valuable to the physician, genetic counselor, and patient but has limitations. For example, genetic heterogeneity may influence actual risk. In other words, a complex disease may have different genetic bases each of which might have a cognate recurrence risk. Empirical risks are typically calculated over a large population that could well encompass all of the genetic heterogeneity for a given disease. One way to potentially minimize such errors is to use families that match the patient's demographic and sociocultural characteristics. Ethnicity, geographic location, lifestyle, and socioeconomic class are all important to match, as closely as possible, with the family under consideration. In the end, an average empirical risk is provided to the physician and patient, but this risk must be interpreted carefully as an *average estimate rather than a precise probability*.

GENETIC APPROACHES TO TREATMENT

As noted in Chapter 4, genetic disease can be treated by a variety of means. In addition to some of the treatments presented in Table 4-6, gene therapy has the potential to cure a genetic disease, where "cure" is a treatment alleviating disease symptoms and restoring health. In the absence of cure, the next best option may be safe and effective drug administration. The emerging field of pharmacogenomics facilitates this option. Below, the fundamentals and medical applicability of gene therapy and pharmacogenomics are discussed.

Gene Therapy

Gene therapy is the introduction of a gene, or DNA sequence, into a cell to correct a genetic defect. Typically, it aims to correct a defective allele or to replace an absent or deficient gene product ("gene replacement") by introducing a functional allele. Such an approach, while frequently publicized as the ultimate cure for genetic disorders, is in its infancy. Nevertheless, recent advances in our understanding of the human genome have permitted significant progress in this area, and approximately 1000 gene therapy protocols for both inherited and noninherited disorders have been approved worldwide (Table 13-6).

To increase the probability of success, the disease under consideration should be amenable to genetic therapy. Most protocols involve a compensation approach for recessive disorders in which loss-of-function has occurred. In this context, many of the autosomal recessive inborn errors of metabolism (see Chapter 4) such as phenylketonuria (PKU) are good candidates for gene therapy, since restoration of as little as 10% of normal enzyme activity is sufficient to see clinical improvement. Other criteria for ideal candidates for gene therapy include diseases

1. Due to a single major gene defect.
2. With well-characterized sequence and regulatory elements.
3. With significant morbidity and mortality, i.e., there is a reasonable risk-benefit ratio.
4. Affecting cells that are experimentally accessible and otherwise represent adequate target cells.

Stem cells are ideal for many gene therapy procedures, since an introduced gene may have high replicative potential and be distributed in a large number of differentiated daughter cells. Bone marrow stem cells, in particular, provide an excellent opportunity for hematologic disease treatment because they are relatively well characterized and can be cultured. Diseases such as thalassemia and sickle cell anemia, and perhaps certain metabolic disorders, are good candidates for bone marrow therapies because marrow cells can be altered to express an appropriate gene product for delivery to relevant tissues via the circulatory system. Typically, the transfer of genes into cells relies on either a viral or nonviral vector.

Gene Transfer Procedures

Theoretically, gene therapy can either be applied to somatic or germline cells. However, because treating somatic cells yields clinical improvement in the patient and because technical and ethical concerns have limited protocols that alter the genes of gametes, the much more common somatic cell gene therapy is discussed here.

The goal of somatic cell gene therapy is to improve or cure a genetic defect within a patient's somatic cells. To do so, two general approaches may be utilized. First, an ex vivo approach involves the isolation and culturing of cells from the patient. A corrected or altered gene construct is added to these cells, and the cells are reintroduced to the patient. Second, an in vivo approach features the direct injection of a gene into a resident tissue or organ. In either case, the gene of interest requires a vector to facilitate its journey to—and entry into—the appropriate target cell.

Viral Vectors for Gene Transfer

Vectors serve as the vehicle for entry of a gene into the cell. A perfect vector is safe with no adverse reactions or harmful immunologic response, easily produced, and directable to the appropriate target cell, and it has a long half-life. Although no current vector system meets all these criteria, viral vectors are easy to manipulate and can deliver DNA to target cells and thus may be considered reasonable vectors. Three main classes of viral vectors are in use today: retroviruses, adenoviruses, and adeno-associated viruses (Table 13-7).

Retroviral vectors are derived from RNA viruses that can integrate their genomes into the host cell chromosomal DNA after making a DNA copy from their RNA genome using reverse transcriptase. This integration process is efficient and

TABLE 13-6. Examples of Diseases for Which Somatic Cell Gene Therapy Protocols are Being Tested

Disease	Target Cell	Inserted Gene
Adenosine deaminase deficiency	Lymphocytes, bone marrow stem cells	Adenosine deaminase
Cystic fibrosis	Bronchial epithelium	CFTR
Duchenne muscular dystrophy	Myoblasts	Dystrophin
Familial hypercholesterolemia	Hepatocytes	LDL receptor
Fanconi anemia	Hemopoietic stem cells	FANCC
Gaucher disease	Macrophages	Glucocerebrosidase
Hemophilia B	Hepatocytes, fibroblasts	Factor IX

stable. These vectors are genetically engineered so that they are rendered incapable of infection by removal of most of the virus's genome. For a given disease, the "corrected" gene of choice replaces the removed viral DNA, and retroviruses are capable of containing up to 8 kb of exogenous DNA. This size, while appreciable, limits the utility of retroviral vectors in that cDNAs of large genes, such as the gene responsible for Duchenne muscular dystrophy, cannot be inserted into these vectors. The inserted gene typically includes regulatory sequences such as promoter elements and polyadenylation signals. Because the vectors cannot replicate, they must be introduced into packaging cell lines. These cell lines have been infected with a retrovirus that lacks the virion packaging signals. Such cells make many viral proteins, but no virus particles can be formed. An introduced vector (sometimes termed a helper virus) contains the packaging proteins, and thus the combination of vector and packaging cell lines provides all proteins necessary for the production of infectious particles. These particles—containing the therapeutic DNA of interest yet still incapable of replication—are used to transfect the target cells. Following transfection, the introduced DNA inserts into the target cell's genome and is expressed by normal mechanisms.

Retroviral vectors have two potential drawbacks. First, they only infect replicating cells and are therefore not a viable option for certain target cell types such as neurons or skeletal muscle. Second, because retroviruses integrate into the host genome randomly, the possibility exists for random insertional mutagenesis whereby a functional allele is inactivated or an inactive allele is activated, leading to consequences of this change.

Adenoviruses are double-stranded DNA viruses that have the important advantage of being able to infect a wide spectrum of cells, including nondividing cells. They also can harbor large pieces of DNA, up to 35 kb in length, and can be purified to produce high titers of infectious particles. Adenoviruses do not integrate into the host chromosome, which means that they are unlikely to insertionally activate a proto-oncogene. On the other hand, the lack of integration renders adenovirus-mediated gene transfer unstable and transient. Finally, adenoviruses can provoke a significant immune response in the patient. This, coupled with the need for repeated introduction of the adenoviral vector owing to transient viral gene expression, hallmarks the primary disadvantage of adenovirus-mediated gene therapy.

Adeno-associated viruses (AAVs) are parvoviruses that are common in the human population and do not provoke disease or an immune response. Other advantages of this vector are that they can infect a wide range of target cell types and are capable of integrating into the host genome at a specific site (chromosome 19q13.3-qter), permitting stable gene expression without pathogenicity. However, AAVs can integrate only 5 kb of DNA.

At present, virtually all vector gene delivery systems suffer from key deficiencies limiting the promise of gene therapy. In general, these include transient or unregulated gene expression and the inability to easily access target cells or infect significant numbers of target cells. Much effort is being put forth to better understand the biology of viral vectors, target cells, and the molecular interactions of these elements to promote stable, safe, and efficient gene transfer.

Nonviral Vectors for Gene Transfer

More recently, nonviral vectors have been considered for gene transfer (Table 13-8). These vehicles are presumably less toxic and easier to produce. At least four types of nonviral vectors are being investigated, including naked DNA, DNA

TABLE 13-7. Comparison Among a Few Viral Vectors

Vector	Advantage	Disadvantage
Retrovirus	Long-term expression Integrates into DNA	7-kb insertion May inactivate or activate another gene upon insertion
Adenovirus	Does not integrate into host 30-kb insertion size	Short-term expression Immunogenic
Adeno-associated virus	Most commonly used Long-term expression Not immunogenic	Limited size inserts
Lentivirus	Infects non-proliferating cells Ex vivo delivery Integrates into DNA Not immunogenic	Requires complex expression vector systems Toxic proteins Concern that HIV will replicate Requires host DNA polymerase
Herpes simplex virus	Neurotropic 40- to 50-kb inserts	Cytotoxic Immunogenic

IMMUNOLOGY & MICROBIOLOGY

Retroviruses

Retroviruses are ssRNA viruses that bind to cell surface receptors and enter the cell. RNA is converted to DNA by reverse transcriptase and integrated into the genome with integrase. A psi sequence (packaging signal sequence) is located outside the viral genes and is required for packaging. Therefore, elimination of this sequence is preferred in order to prevent the retrovirus from repackaging itself. A cell infected with a retrovirus that has a mutated psi sequence will be able to produce viral proteins important for viral structure but will not be able to package the proteins. However, if another virus with an intact psi sequence and new genetic material in place of the structural genes (*gag, pol,* and *env*) coinfects the cell, the new genetic material can be packaged with the proteins produced from the virus with the defective psi sequence.

encapsulated in a liposome (a lipid bilayer that can fuse with cell membranes), protein-DNA conjugates that can be targeted to particular cell receptors, and artificial chromosomes (Table 13-9). Artificial chromosomes may represent the future of gene therapy vectors. They are synthetic constructs that contain the minimal functional elements of a chromosome including centromere and telomeres. These constructs can incorporate up to 10 Mb of DNA, meaning that very large pieces of exogenous DNA can be introduced to a cell by this method.

Gene Replacement Versus Gene Silencing

Gene replacement techniques are unlikely to be efficacious for diseases occurring from either a dominant negative or gain-of-function genetic mechanism. In these cases, the goal becomes to silence or reduce the expression of the pathogenic gene. Three general approaches are being developed in this context (Fig. 13-8). First, antisense oligonucleotide therapy involves the introduction of a short, synthetic DNA oligonucleotide that is complementary to the abnormal mRNA into a cell. The oligonucleotide is considered antisense relative to the mRNA, and binding of the antisense oligonucleotide to the

---

IMMUNOLOGY & MICROBIOLOGY

Adeno-Associated Viruses (AAVs)

AAVs are ssDNA nonpathogenic parvoviruses. They require a helper virus, which usually is an adenovirus, to proliferate. Adenoviruses can be inactivated by heat, thereby reducing immunogenicity associated with other viral vectors.

AAVs are composed of two genes flanked by inverted terminal repeats (ITRs). The *cap* gene produces the capsid structural proteins; *rep* is important to replication, gene expression of replication proteins, and integration (it inhibits adenovirus replication). The ITR contains the promoter region.

TABLE 13-8. Comparison Between Viral and Nonviral Gene Delivery

Feature	Viral Delivery	Nonviral Delivery
Size of insert	Limited by viral capsid	Potentially limitless
Host immune response	Potentially problematic	Minimized
Technical difficulty level	More difficult	Easier
Targetable to different cells	Possible	Possible
Gene transfer	Reasonably efficient	Inefficient
Fate of delivered gene	Transient or persistent	Transient
Stability *in vivo*	Reasonable	Not stable

TABLE 13-9. Comparison Among Several Nonviral Vectors

Vector	Advantage	Disadvantage
"Naked" DNA vaccination	Long-term protection	Limited uptake
Liposomes	Easy to vary phospholipid Inexpensive Nonpathogenic Nonimmunogenic	Less efficient than viral vectors Toxicity at high dose Not cell-specific
Polycation conjugates	Cell specific design Nonpathogenic	Targeting material to nucleus is not specific Limited expression
Artificial chromosome	Large inserts—10 kb Nonimmunogenic Does not integrate	Limited uptake Limited expression

---

target mRNA hinders or eliminates translation of that mRNA. The effect of this action is decreased expression of the disease gene.

Second, ribozyme therapy is being developed to disable target mRNAs. Ribozymes are autocatalytic RNA molecules that cleave RNA targets, including mRNA. It is possible to produce ribozymes that are specific for a particular nucleotide sequence context. This means that ribozymes can be introduced that cleave the mRNA of disease genes but not of normal copies.

Finally, RNA interference (RNAi) is an emerging technology using RNA molecules for posttranscriptional gene silencing (Fig. 13-9). Specifically, small interfering RNAs (siRNAs) may be used to block mRNAs of disease genes. In a procedure similar to the DNA-based antisense approach described above, siRNAs are short RNA oligonucleotides that are introduced into cells in the more stable form of double-stranded RNAs. The dsRNAs are processed into the single-stranded siRNAs by a multisubunit protein complex called the RNA-induced silencing complex (RISC). siRNAs can base-pair with mRNAs of a target gene and mediate either mRNA degradation or translational arrest. siRNAs as small as nine nucleotides can attain great target specificity. As with all gene therapy approaches, delivery of siRNAs to the appropriate cell and the stable, long-lasting expression of siRNAs are areas of major concern and research effort.

Pharmacogenomics and Individualized Medicine

Though most consider pharmacogenomics a recent application of genetic understanding, the concepts are not that recent. Recall that some African Americans have an acute hemolytic crisis when given primaquine (see Chapter 6). This drug sensitivity has a genetic basis that is reflected in altered

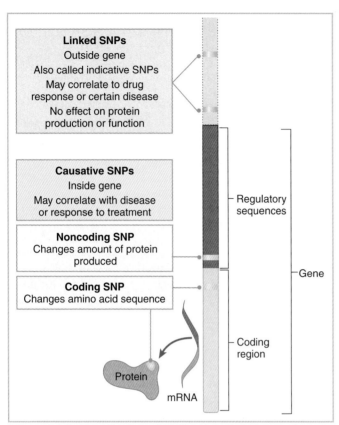

Figure 13-8. Classification of SNPs. Not all SNPs are disease causing, but they can be informative in forming genotypic signatures.

erythrocyte metabolism. Another drug, succinylcholine, is used during anesthesia to induce muscle paralysis. The extent of paralysis may last from a few minutes to a few hours in different individuals given the same dose. This difference results from the altered kinetics of pseudocholinesterase and is inherited in an autosomal recessive manner. These are only two examples demonstrating that genes determine drug effects.

To better illustrate pharmacogenomics, codeine is considered. This drug is one of many that are converted by members of the P-450 protein family to other forms. In the liver, codeine is metabolized by CYP2D6 to morphine. There are allelic variations in this gene, resulting in poor metabolism, extensive metabolism, and ultrametabolism. In about 10% of the Caucasian population, homozygosity occurs for alleles that are either nonfunctional or have very little function, and in these individuals codeine does not metabolize to morphine. There are also individuals having ultrametabolism of codeine, resulting in an increased production of morphine. These latter individuals are more likely to experience adverse effects and toxicity with any standard dose of codeine. The best scenario is those individuals who have extensive metabolism and gain pain relief without incurring risk for toxicity. Of course, once the genotype is determined for an individual, physicians will recognize which patients require

PHARMACOLOGY & PHYSIOLOGY

Uses of Succinylcholine

Succinylcholine, also known as scoline or suxamethonium chloride, is composed of two linked acetylcholine molecules. It imitates the action of acetylcholine at neuromuscular junctions but causes prolonged opening of the acetylcholinesterase receptor channels, leading to depolarization of the membrane. Initially, repetitive muscle excitation and tremors occur, followed by relaxation secondary to inactivation of Na^+ channels. Succinylcholine is degraded by pseudocholinesterase, rather than acetylcholinesterase, but at a much slower rate.

Succinylcholine is used for short-term muscle relaxation during anesthesia. It does not produce unconsciousness or anesthesia itself but is used to produce sustained muscle relaxation, or flaccid paralysis, after unconsciousness—a condition that is useful in certain types of surgery when it is important to prevent contraction and excitation of muscles.

less codeine, the ultrametabolizers, and those who require a different drug, the poor metabolizers. Since there are at least 29 morphisms for the CYP2D6 gene, this and other P-450 genes are attractive candidates for microarray analysis (see below). Determining individual genotypes for P-450 genes, responsible for clearing over half of the drugs introduced to the body, provides physicians with powerful information to anticipate and avoid potentially lethal drug interactions.

Once again, the clinical utility of the Human Genome Project is apparent with the development of a technique to identify and quantitate a high density of genetic polymorphisms, such as benign single nucleotide polymorphisms, or SNPs, that span populations and racial and ethnic groups. Not all changes in nucleotides are classified as SNPs; a SNP is defined as two or more nucleotides represented at a particular site that are present in at least 1% of the population. SNPs may not occur within a gene or have an effect on protein function, as do many point mutations. SNPs are classified as linked, causative, coding, and noncoding (see Fig. 13-8).

SNP maps are being developed in large genetic databases (Fig. 13-10). With this foundation, an individual's SNP genotype can be determined, although this can be a slow and expensive process. The advent of DNA microarrays for DNA sequencing and mutation detection, however, holds the promise to make individualized SNP surveys rapid and inexpensive. It is not inconceivable that in the near future, personal SNP profiles will be a standard part of the medical record. Once high-density SNP maps spanning the genome are completed, the next step is correlating individual or groups of SNPs with disease efficacy and adverse events. With this genetic prescreen, drugs can be prescribed that are tailored not only to the disorder but also to the individual genetic signature. In this way, medicine becomes more personalized or individualized.

Opioids

Opioids interact with receptors for three families of endogenous peptides: endorphins, enkephalins, and dynorphins. There are three major classes (with several subclasses) of opioid receptors in the central nervous system: μ, κ and δ. Opioids, in minute doses, excite neurons in the periaqueductal gray matter and nucleus reticularis paragigantocellularis. Descending pathways from the midbrain have an inhibitory effect mediated by 5-hydroxytryptamine (5-HT), enkephalins, and noradrenalin on pain transmission from the dorsal horn. Opioids can also inhibit pain directly at the dorsal horn and inhibit peripheral nociceptive afferent neurons.

Morphine is an opioid that relieves pain by interfering with the sensation of pain. It interacts with δ and κ receptors weakly but is a powerful agonist at the μ opiate receptors in the central nervous system. Manifestations of morphine and heroin include analgesia, euphoria, respiratory depression, and dependence.

The potential benefits of pharmacogenomics are not limited to individually tailored drug therapy. Others include more accurate dosing information (determined by a person's genetics rather than height and weight), rapid drug design, acceleration of drug discovery and approval, and overall decreased health care costs.

●●● NEW DIAGNOSTIC APPROACHES

A key goal for medical geneticists is the development of rapid, accurate, and inexpensive methods for genetic diagnosis, prognosis, and disease susceptibility prediction. Many such protocols, including mass spectroscopy and nanoparticle technology, are under development. However, DNA microarray analysis represents a viable diagnostic and prognostic tool that is already of clinical value and is rapidly becoming an industry standard in genetic medicine.

Microarray Analysis

DNA-based diagnostic procedures have traditionally relied on the analysis of a single gene or a small group of genes. However, a new technology permits the simultaneous measurement of thousands of gene sequences or changes in gene expression. This technology is termed DNA microarray analysis; it is also known as DNA array or gene chip analysis (Fig. 13-11). This is a hybridization-based technique that involves a nucleic acid probe hybridizing to a target nucleic acid. The targets are small pieces of DNA that are spotted in grid-like fashion on a small glass, nylon, or plastic slide, or "chip." This DNA can be gene fragments, cDNAs, or synthesized oligonucleotides. Key to this technology is that the grid contains thousands of target DNAs, each with its own position on the grid. Typical arrays contain 10 to 20 thousand

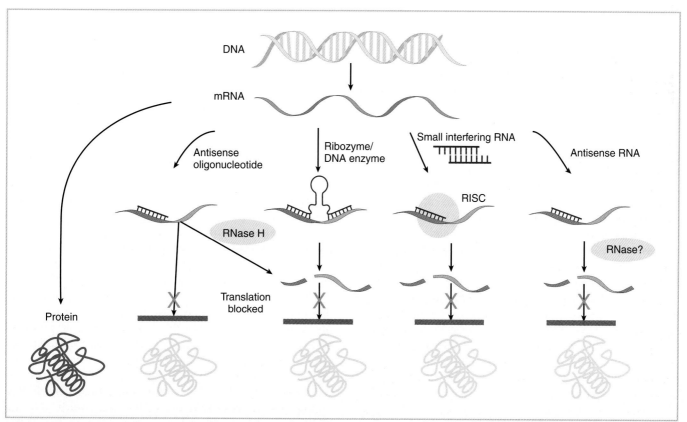

Figure 13-9. Examples of posttranscriptional gene silencing tools. Four common approaches for targeting mRNA to induce posttranscriptional gene silencing and their corresponding mechanism of action. (Modified with permission from Kukreck J. Antisense technologies. *Eur J Biochem*. 2003;270:1628–1644.)

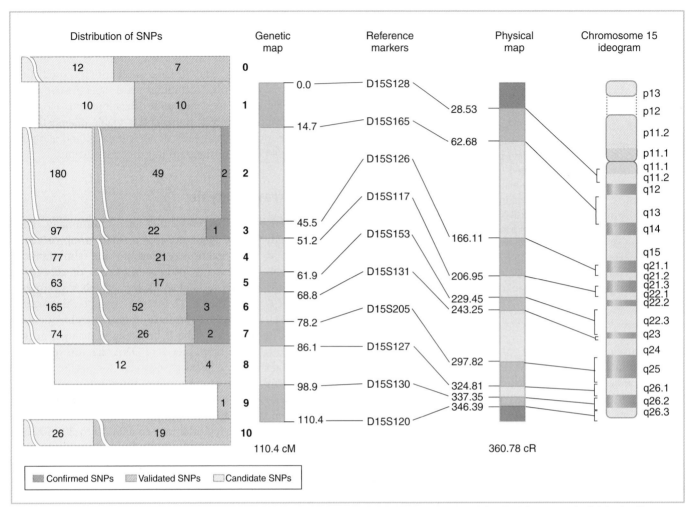

Figure 13-10. SNP map of chromosome 15. Approximately 99.9% of DNA sequences are identical between individuals. Over 80% of the remaining 0.1% of sequences differs at single nucleotide polymorphisms (SNPs). (Redrawn with permission from NCI Cancer Genome Anatomy Project. Available at: http://gai.nci.nih.gov/html-snp/imagemaps.html.)

genes per chip, and these gene targets are "spotted" using technology derived from the semiconductor microelectronics industry. To begin to see the utility of this methodology, recall that the entire human genome contains approximately 30,000 genes. The probe sequences are either DNA fragments or cDNAs derived from a control (or normal) and experimental (or disease) cell type. Probes are typically labeled with a fluorescent tag such that, following hybridization with a microarray chip, probe-target hybrids are indicated by a scanning detection system featuring lasers, cameras, and a computer that can identify precisely which spots on the grid yield a hybridization signal. The collection of positive hybridization signals on the grid results in a "molecular signature" that can be useful for the two current primary clinical uses for microarray technology: gene expression profiling and mutation detection.

Gene Expression Profiling

The use of DNA microarrays is a method to study gene expression. For example, it may be of interest to determine the gene expression profiles for a particular tissue in the normal and the diseased state. In this application, gene chips are made in which the target DNA typically consists of thousands of cDNAs. The probes may be cDNAs derived from the mRNAs from the normal and diseased tissue. Probe cDNAs from the normal tissue would be labeled with a particular fluorescent tag (red, for example), and cDNAs from diseased tissue would be labeled with a different fluorescent tag (green, for example). The "red" and "green" cDNA probes would be washed over the gene chip during the hybridization step. Encountering its complementary target, a probe forms a hybrid, and this is indicated as a "positive" hybridization by the scanner. Computer software calculates the relative amounts of the red and green signal at each address or spot on the grid. Such a ratio represents the relative amount of mRNA expression of that gene in the normal and the diseased tissue. In other words, a given address on the target grid may give a strong red signal indicating strong mRNA expression in normal tissue and weak expression in diseased tissue, a strong green signal

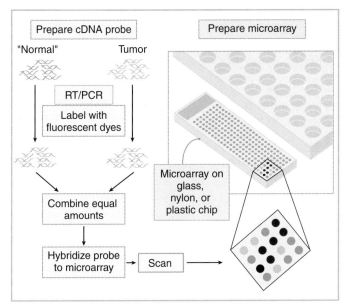

Figure 13-11. Gene expression analysis using microarray technology. Colors detected by the scanner reflect expression and level of expression in normal and tumor samples.

indicating high expression levels in the diseased tissue, a yellow signal indicating expression of the gene in both normal and diseased tissue, or a black signal indicating no expression in either tissue type. When all gene targets on the chip grid are considered, an expression signature for a given disease state is demonstrated. An illustration of this application is shown in Chapter 5 (see Fig. 5-26).

In Chapter 5, comparative genomic hybridization (CGH) was introduced as a cytogenetic technique that can be used to demonstrate changes in chromosome content, as illustrated with double minutes and heterogeneous staining regions (see Fig. 5-9). This same concept can be used with microarray analysis by placing genomic DNAs on a slide or support rather than cDNAs or DNAs as described above. The genomic DNAs are selected clones, often bacterial artificial chromosome (BAC) DNA clones, representing the physical genomic map. These microarrays are referred to as aCGH (array comparative genomic hybridization). For each gene, the ratio of red to green fluorescence corresponds to the ratio of DNA copy number of that gene in the tumor sample compared with the normal sample. Since each clone represents a known region of a chromosome and complex computer software will identify the region of chromosomes with copy number alterations, this technique provides high resolution for detecting chromosomal alterations, amplifications, deletions, and loss and gain.

Gene Chips and Mutation Detection

One of the first uses of microarray technology was the identification of point mutations. This type of array detects genetic variation among humans, as seen with SNPs. Microarrays can also detect specific disease-causing mutations, such as the spectrum of mutations that cause PKU

or cystic fibrosis. In the latter example, the DNA targets on the array grid represent pieces of DNA that contain all known or relevant variations of a gene or genes; such variations may include either benign polymorphisms or disease variants or both. This means that adjacent addresses on the grid represent the same gene but differ by as little as a single base pair. For example, a gene chip to perform genetic diagnosis for phenylalanine hydroxylase (PAH)–associated hyperphenylalaninemia contains many oligonucleotide or cDNA targets representing all known genetic variants of the *PAH* gene. Probes are generated by isolating DNA from a patient, followed by PCR amplification of the patient's *PAH* gene that also incorporates a fluorescent tag in the probe. The probe is then applied to the chip and hybridizes and fluoresces with only the grid address corresponding to the patient's PAH mutation. In this way, mutation detection is rapid and comprehensive.

There is also clinical utility in the identification of SNP patterns. As discussed above, SNPs are benign single nucleotide polymorphisms. Typically, SNPs are base changes without pathology. Several thousand SNPs have been identified in humans, and more are being added to genetic databases every week. Accordingly, and using the above method, gene chips have been produced that can test individual genomes for the presence or absence of the known SNPs. This produces an SNP signature and can indicate collections of SNPs, or haplotypes, that consistently occur together. An individual SNP or a SNP haplotype may be associated with certain disease states via genetic linkage. In this case, rapid and accurate microarray analysis reveals a haplotype or SNP signature predicting disease predisposition (Table 13-10). As discussed above, SNP profiling will also greatly enhance our ability to use genetic signatures for the determination of drug choice, as SNP genotypes will—for a given drug—predict efficacy and adverse reactions on an individual basis.

●●● SUMMARY

Within the next 15 years, most human genes will be characterized regarding location in the genome, sequence, and functional identity. At the same time, molecular genetic technology will advance to a point where it will be routine to ascertain an individual's collection of disease and disease predisposition alleles as well as benign SNPs. These data will permit a more precise form of medicine—one that is specific to an individual's unique genetic profile. Genetic predispositions will be identified, and DNA-based diagnostics will be routine. Knowledge of genetic risks will allow individual presymptomatic opportunities for disease intervention including lifestyle change. Intelligent and rational drug design will be the norm, since it will be based on integrated genetic and biochemical signatures. Gene therapy is emerging as a permanent curative approach in the treatment of both inherited and noninherited disease. Hence, it is unlikely to be an exaggeration to state that today is the dawn of the new age of molecular medicine.

TABLE 13-10. Example of an SNP-to-Haplotype-to-Phenotype Map*

Haplotype	Sequence	SNP1	SNP2	Frequency (%)	Effect
I	GGACAACC	0	0	80	None
II	AATTCGGG	0	1	10.5	Small
III	GATTAGCC	1	0	3	Small
IV	GGTCAGCC	1	1	2	Extreme

*This model demonstrates the use of four SNP haplotypes to identify informative haplotypes for a hypothetical use, whether disease severity or response to a treatment.

Case Studies

CASE STUDY 1

A 21-year-old female has sickle cell disease. She has experienced very few medical complications from the condition since diagnosis at age 4. Recently, she has become interested in having children, and she and her husband seek genetic counseling. Molecular analysis reveals that she has a T to A base change in her adult hemoglobin genes. This change causes a substitution of valine for glutamic acid in the hemoglobin proteins and is the cause of her disease. Her husband does not have the mutation.

1. What type of mutation is a T to A base change?

2. What are the consequences of this base change?

3. How are these mutations detected clinically at the molecular level?

CASE STUDY 2

The patient, a 6-month-old girl, was the second child born to a 36-year-old mother and a 47-year-old father. The patient had a round face, low hairline, hypertelorism, epicanthal folds, up-slanting palpebral fissures, long philtrum, high-arched palate, short and webbed neck, small hands and feet, clinodactyly of the fifth fingers, overlapping toes, and diastasis of the first and second toes. The facial and foot anomalies are similar to those of Down syndrome. She also had an atrial septal defect and patent ductus arteriosus. There is no family history of chromosome abnormalities.

Chromosome analyses were performed on cultured peripheral blood lymphocytes of the patient and parents. All 40 of the patient's cells analyzed had 49 chromosomes, and G-banding confirmed a karyotype of 49,XXXXX. A buccal smear revealed four Barr bodies. The chromosomes of the parents were normal without mosaicism. The child was diagnosed with penta-X syndrome with multiple congenital anomalies and congenital heart disease resulting from nondisjunction.

The patient died of heart failure at 8 months of age. Autopsy revealed a small uterus as well as dysgenesis of the ovaries.

1. How is a karyotype done?

2. How does the presence of extra X chromosomes contribute to the clinical presentation if four are inactivated as Barr bodies?

3. Explain a scenario that would result in five X chromosomes.

CASE STUDY 3

A couple, married 2 years, were both diagnosed at birth with achondroplastic dwarfism. The husband had no family history of dwarfism. The wife's brother also had achondroplasia, but both parents were normal. They are planning a family and want to discuss the possibility of dwarfism with their physician. The physician explained that they each had a mutation in the fibroblast growth factor receptor 3 gene (*FGFR3*). Since all cases reported in the literature result from the same type of mutation in the same part of the protein, it would be possible to test a fetus for the mutation or to consider in vitro fertilization with preimplantation analysis of embryos.

1. What is the significance of the two family histories?

2. How does an *FGFR3* gene mutation cause achondroplasia?

3. What is the expectation that their child will be normal or a dwarf?

CASE STUDY 4

A 29-year-old female, gravida 2, para 0, abortus 1, received a diagnosis of classical PKU as an infant but was lost to follow-up after her parents' death at age 7. Unaware of her condition, she becomes pregnant. At 22 weeks' gestation, her fetus demonstrates intrauterine growth retardation.

Microcephaly, coarctation of the aorta, and hypoplastic left ventricle syndrome are noted. She denies excessive vitamin A intake or a family history of cardiac anomalies consistent with DiGeorge syndrome. She recalls being on a special diet as a young child. Laboratory tests reveal the following:

Serum phenylalanine, 14.7 mg/dL (normal, <2 mg/dL)

Serum tyrosine, 0.85 mg/dL (normal, <2 mg/dL)

Biopterin as BH_4, normal

Biopterin as BH_2, normal

The patient was immediately started on a phenylalanine-restricted, protein-enriched diet supplemented with vitamin B_{12} and referred to a physician specializing in high-risk pregnancies. Her weight gain at term was 83% of the recommended weight gain. The baby was delivered at term. Microcephaly (5th percentile) was noted, and birth weight was 2450 g. Guthrie test was negative. The baby had maternal PKU. One week after birth, the baby's phenylalanine levels remained normal.

1. **What is the major mechanism of maternal PKU development in the baby?**

2. **Explain the baby's normal phenylalanine levels at 1 week and an expected genotype.**

3. **What outcome is expected for the baby?**

CASE STUDY 5

A 35-year-old woman visits the physician with the chief complaint of lower right abdominal cramping and pain. Past medical history and physical examination are unremarkable. Spleen is not palpable, and there is no lymphadenopathy. Laboratory values are shown.

	Patient	Normal
WBC	$50.3 \times 10^3/\mu L$	$3.07–11.77 \times 10^3/\mu L$
Hemoglobin	12.3 g/dL	11.6–15.6 g/dL
Platelets	$384 \times 10^3/\mu L$	$129–355 \times 10^3/\mu L$
Lymphocytes	6%	15%–40%
Monocytes	3%	0–10%
Blasts	3%	<1%
Promyelocytes	4%	<1%
Myelocytes	8%	<1%
Bands	10%	0–10%
PMNs	55%	40%–80%
Basophils	9%	0–2%

Laboratory values are consistent with chronic myelogenous leukemia. Cytogenetic analysis was performed on bone marrow cells and showed two populations of cells: 46,XX,t(9,22)(q34,q11),t(6;19)(q16;p13.3) in 60% of cells and 46,XX,t(9;22)(q34;q11) in the remaining 40% of cells.

The patient received a bone marrow transplant and was monitored for residual disease at 6, 9, and 12 months by RT-PCR of $p210^{BCR-ABL}$ mRNA. Residual chimera proteins were detected at each point, but additional treatment was not prescribed. The patient continued to be monitored.

1. **Explain the genetic basis of chronic myelogenous leukemia.**

2. **Explain the karyotype in the two populations of cells.**

3. **Why was RT-PCR selected to monitor the post–bone marrow transplantation course?**

CASE STUDY 6

A 26-year-old male is examined by his physician. His wife suggested the appointment because he seemed pale and easily fatigued. The patient's past medical history included a cholecystectomy 2 years previously, when he was told that he had Gilbert's syndrome, a disorder of elevated bilirubin. He has a long history of periodic anemia, and several relatives have also experienced chronic anemia or liver problems. The physician noted jaundice, scleral icterus, and a palpable spleen 4 cm below the left costal margin. Laboratory findings are shown.

	Patient	Normal
RBC	$3.95 \times 10^6/\mu L$	$4.1–4.9 \times 10^6/\mu L$
Hemoglobin	11.2 g/dL	12.7–14.7 g/dL
Hematocrit	33.3%	37.9–43.9%
MCV	84.3 fL	80–90 fL
MCH	28.4 pg	26–34 pg
MCHC	33.6 pg	31–34 pg
WBC	$5.2 \times 10^9/L$	$4000–10,000/\mu L$
Platelets	375,000/μL	150,000–450,000/μL
Reticulocytes	12.9%	1%–2%

RBC morphology: Normochromic with anisocytosis and spherocytosis.

Spherocytosis was diagnosed, and the patient was referred for splenectomy. A study of other members of the family revealed a defect in the ankyrin gene resulting in reduced ankyrin.

1. What gene mutations are implicated in spherocytosis?

2. What pertinent family history is there for this patient?

3. Why are the indices normal?

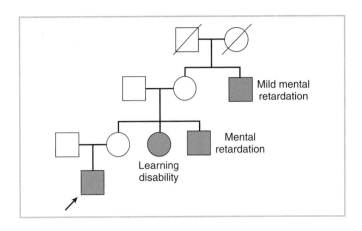

CASE STUDY 7

A 3-year-old white male has muscle weakness. His developmental milestones, particularly those involved with the lower limbs, have been delayed. He displays Gowers maneuver when standing from a sitting position. A review of the family history reveals several members who had muscular dystrophy. Laboratory tests are ordered and reveal the following:

Enzyme	Patient	Normal
AST	130 U/L	7–40 U/L
CK	1600 U/L	25–225 U/L (male)
LDH	1200 U/L	7–40 U/L
Aldolase	68 U/L	1.3–8.2 U/L

Genetic analysis of the dystrophin gene was ordered. Multiplex PCR revealed deletion of exons 45 to 48. No muscle biopsy was performed. A diagnosis of Duchenne muscular dystrophy is confirmed.

1. Explain the physical evidence that suggests Duchenne rather than Becker muscular dystrophy.

2. Explain the elevated laboratory values.

3. What is the significance of the genetic analysis?

4. Why was no biopsy performed?

CASE STUDY 8

A 3-year-old boy has delayed motor and speech development. The toddler has become very active, requiring an increasing amount of attention from adults. His parents are concerned about his language development. Family history reveals that the child's parents and maternal grandparents are normal but that a great uncle is mildly retarded. His mother's sister has a learning disability. His mother's brother is mentally retarded and lives in a group home. No mental illness or learning disabilities were noted in the child's father's family.

Physical examination reveals normal height and weight for age. Blood was drawn for chromosomal analysis and mutation analysis of the FMR1 gene. Results indicated no chromosomal abnormality; however, the child has a full mutation of the FMR1 gene with >1000 CGG repeats. Fragile X syndrome is diagnosed.

1. What is the mode of transmission demonstrated in the pedigree?

2. Explain the etiology of mental retardation and fragile X syndrome among family members.

3. Is the learning disability of the child's aunt related to fragile X syndrome?

4. What is the prognosis for the child?

CASE STUDY 9

A 5-year-old male has developed xanthomas in a bracelet pattern on both wrists and multiple xanthomas on the knees and elbows. Blood cholesterol levels are 1240 mg/dL. Both parents have previously undiagnosed elevated total cholesterol but demonstrate no xanthomas. Genetic analysis reveals that the parents are heterozygous for mutations in the LDLR gene and that the child is a compound heterozygote. One mutant allele prevents LDL binding at the cell surface, and the mutant allele from the other parent prevents endocytosis of LDL into the cell. A sibling is found to carry one mutant allele and one normal allele. Familial hypercholesterolemia (FH) is diagnosed, and the child is a compound heterozygote for two different mutations.

1. Explain the etiology of FH in the child.

2. Describe the expected progression of the disease.

3. Describe a course of action of treatment for the child.

4. What will be the outcome for the sibling?

CASE STUDY 10

At age 27 years, a man visited the physician with hepatosplenomegaly of unknown etiology. Within a few months, he developed a hand tremor and difficulty with finger dexterity. Imaging studies revealed no brain abnormalities. Over the next 2 years, the tremor worsened. Occasionally, his speech is slurred and swallowing is difficult. The patient denied use of alcohol or drugs.

Past medical history includes a father who died at age 75 after a 20-year history of Parkinson's disease. His mother died at age 79 and had a long-term tremor.

At age 31 years, the tremor has increased and balance is sometimes compromised. The patient experiences self-reported depression. New imaging studies reveal cerebellar degeneration. The liver is firm and nodular with a 14-cm span, and splenomegaly is present. Slit lamp examination of the eyes reveals Kayser-Fleischer rings. Additional laboratory tests were ordered, as follows:

	Patient	Normal
WBC	$4.0 \times 10^3/\mu L$	$3.7–11.77 \times 10^3/\mu L$
RBC	$4.7 \times 10^6/\mu L$	$3.76–5.2 \times 10^6/\mu L$
Hematocrit	40%	38.7–49.1%
Hemoglobin	13.2 g/dL	12.9–16.9 g/dL
Prothrombin	11.4	10.4
Bleeding time	10.5	2–9.5
Bilirubin	1.2 mg/dL	0.1–1.3 mg/dL
AST/GOT	18 U/mL	15–38 U/L
Alkaline phosphatase	54 U/mL	30–95 U/L
Albumin	3.8 g/dL	3.5–5.0 g/L
Urinary copper (24 h)	703 μg	1–100 μg
Ceruloplasmin	14 mg/dL	18–45 mg/dL
Thyroid function tests	WNL	—
Vitamin B_{12}	WNL	—
Hepatitis B antigens/antibodies	Negative	—
Autoantibodies	Negative	—
MCV	85	81.1–98.4
MCH	28	27.2–34
MCHC	33	32.2–35.9% Hb/cell

Genetic analysis for Wilson disease in the patient and three children was performed. The H1069Q mutation was identified in the patient. One child was heterozygous for the same mutation; she had low ceruloplasmin levels and normal levels of urinary copper.

The patient was started on penicillamine, and urinary excretion of copper increased. Within 2 months, the symptoms improved. The tremor was present only with extension of arms. Balance was nearly normal.

1. What is the significance of the patient's past medical history?

2. Explain the low value for ceruloplasmin.

3. What other disorders could have been considered in the differential?

4. How does penicillamine work?

CASE STUDY 11

A 4-year-old girl from rural Canada had a bilateral inguinal hernia. Physical examination revealed no genital abnormality or ambiguity. There was no family history of intersex disorders or consanguinity. Because of the unusual presentation, an hCG stimulation test was administered with the following results:

	2000 IU hCG for 5 days		
	Baseline	Stimulated	Normal*
Testosterone (mol/L)	<0.1	8.0	0.06 to 0.86
DHEA-S (μmol/L)	0.08	.5	0.03 to 1.0
Androstenedione (nmol/L)	0.002	0.01	0.17 to 1.78
DHT (nmol/L)	<0.1	1.78	<0.1
T:DHT	—	4	0.6 to 8.6

* For age.

During surgery to repair the hernias, bilateral gonads resembling testes were removed. Pathologic study confirmed that the gonads contained immature testicular tissue.

Additional Tests

Karyotype: 46,XY

Mutational analysis of the androgen receptor gene using PCR and sequence analysis: A G to A mutation was detected, resulting in an arginine to histidine replacement in the protein. The mother, maternal aunt, and sister of the child were also tested. The mother was heterozygous for the mutation.

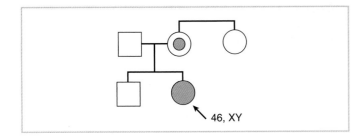

46, XY

East since birth. Her parents report that she has never been well. The child eats poorly and is plagued with infections. Her weight is at the 22nd percentile for her age. The parents have two sons who show no signs of illness, but they report that two other girls died in infancy from infections. Tests are ordered, and a diagnosis of cystic fibrosis (CF) is made. The child is treated for a pulmonary infection and pancreatic deficiency. She is referred to the nutritionist, who prescribes a diet high in protein, calories, and vitamins. She is scheduled for follow-up monitoring.

1. What is the best diagnosis for this child's disorder?

2. Explain the female appearance of the child.

3. Why does the mother have no symptoms?

4. Explain the stimulated test values.

5. Why does the child not have müllerian derivatives?

1. Describe the family pedigree.

2. What is the probability that the sons are heterozygous carriers for cystic fibrosis?

3. Further laboratory analysis revealed the specific mutation shared by both parents and determined that the frequency of this allele is 0.025 in the white population. What is the frequency of individuals affected with CF with this mutation, and who are carriers?

CASE STUDY 12

A 3-year-old white female is seen at the Saturday morning clinic for chronic diarrhea and malabsorption. Though born in the United States, she has lived with her parents in the Middle

Case Study Answers

CASE STUDY 1

1. This type of point mutation is a transversion: a pyrimidine is changed to a purine.

2. In this case, the change creates a different coding triplet that specifies a new amino acid. Not all changes will do this. Some may be silent and result in no change in amino acid even with a base change. Others may create a stop codon or cause a change in the reading frame that creates inaccurate amino acid information from that point on. Among changes with a triplet, those affecting the 3rd position are less likely to cause a change in the amino acid; this is known as the "wobble effect." More critical changes occur at positions 1 and 2 of the triplet.

3. Unlike large mutations that may be observed by merely staining the chromosomes, small mutations require newer molecular techniques. The identity of single-base-pair changes can be detected by polymorphism analysis after the polymerase chain reaction (PCR) is employed to amplify the region of interest. Amplified DNAs may be further characterized with the use of restriction enzymes to identify a loss or creation of a specific recognition site for a particular restriction enzyme. Combining the power of PCR with direct sequencing technology can also identify a mutation.

CASE STUDY 2

1. A karyotype can theoretically be done with any cell with a nucleus that can be induced to undergo mitosis. This of course eliminates red blood cells. Typically, a karyotype is done with lymphocytes that are placed in short-term culture and stimulated to divide with a lectin, phytohemagglutinin. Within a few days, large numbers of dividing cells are present. Colchicine, which inhibits the development of the mitotic spindle, blocks cell division at metaphase. To prepare chromosomes on slides, a hypotonic solution is added to make the cells swell, allowing chromosomes to spread. Chromosomes can then be stained and analyzed in many ways. Typically, this begins with organizing the homologous pairs in descending order of size, with the sex chromosomes at the end.

2. The presence of four Barr bodies indicates there are five X chromosomes in this patient, or at least in buccal cells. This confirms the finding of G-banding, which also provides additional information about any rearrangements that may exist or about these chromosomes. However, the issue with this patient is not the possibility of X chromosome rearrangements but that five X chromosomes were present early in development and actively transcribed prior to inactivation through lyonization. The five-fold increase in gene product leads to abnormal development. To a lesser extent it can be argued that genes not silenced on the inactive X chromosomes are also in excess and continue to be contributory.

3. It should be apparent that the presence of additional X chromosomes results from meiotic nondisjunction. It should also be clear that more than one nondisjunction event occurred for there to be more than one additional X chromosome. Looking at male gametogenesis first, nondisjunction in meiosis I would yield a gamete with both an X and a Y chromosome. If, however, meiosis I was normal and nondisjunction occurred during meiosis II in the cell with the X chromosome, a gamete with 24 chromosomes would be produced having two X chromosomes.

   In the female, nondisjunction can occur in either meiosis I or II as well. In meiosis I nondisjunction, both homologous chromosomes would segregate to the same cell; normal meiosis II would yield gametes with 24 chromosomes and two X chromosomes. The same result would occur if nondisjunction occurred in meiosis II alone. Nondisjunction in meiosis I and II produces gametes with 4 X chromosomes. This gamete fertilized by a normal sperm would yield 49,XXXXX, as seen in this patient. However, it is also possible that nondisjunction in meiosis I followed by normal segregation in meiosis II would yield a 25,XXX gamete. If the male gamete had also undergone nondisjunction yielding a 24,XX gamete, a zygote from both of these gametes would also be 49,XXXXX. Additional testing using polymerase chain reaction or restriction fragment length polymorphism (an older, less used technique today) to identify allelic variation in the parents would clarify the parent of origin and inheritance scenario of the additional chromosomes.

CASE STUDY 3

1. Achondroplasia, the most common form of dwarfism, has an autosomal dominant mode of inheritance with 100% penetrance. In the absence of a family history of achondroplasia, the husband's achondroplasia is consistent with a spontaneous (de novo) mutation. In the wife's case, there is also no family history, but a sibling also displays achondroplasia. Both cases are suggestive of germline mutations. However, de novo spontaneous mutations in this allele have been shown to be inherited exclusively from the father and represent de novo mutations during spermatogenesis rather than mosaicism; they are also associated with advanced paternal age.

2. Mutations in the *FGFR3* gene cause achondroplasia. All individuals studied have a transition mutation causing the substitution of arginine for glycine in the protein. Substituting arginine for glycine (G380R) is a gain-of-function mutation that causes the FGFR3 protein to inhibit endochondral bone growth by down-regulating chondrocyte proliferation and differentiation. The couple is likely to be heterozygous for a mutated allele, since the family history suggests de novo mutations and since a homozygous condition is lethal. Obviously, the presence of one normal allele is sufficient to overcome the lethal effects of two mutated alleles.

3. With the expectation that both parents are heterozygous for the mutant allele, there is a 75% chance that a child will have achondroplasia and 25% chance the child will be normal. Since most infants with two mutant alleles (a lethal condition) will not survive, the expectations are that 67% of offspring born to these parents will carry a mutant allele and 33% of the offspring will be normal. The difference in interpreting these two different probabilities is that the first is the probability of mutated alleles coming together at fertilization through independent assortment and the second reflects the probability of a child being born with a particular genotype.

CASE STUDY 4

1. The baby has been exposed to high levels of phenylalanine owing to the mother's mutations in phenylalanine hydroxylase. These mutated alleles prevent appropriate catabolism of phenylalanine to tyrosine with the accumulation of serum phenylalanine. Phenylalanine then acts as a teratogen to the developing fetus with particular affinity for brain development. Phenylalanine may compete with leucine for the transporters that decrease the amount of leucine available for myelin.

2. The baby's phenylalanine levels are normal after birth for two reasons. First, the mother was placed on a phenylalanine-restricted diet. Since phenylalanine crosses the placenta, this limits the availability of phenylalanine to the baby. Because the mother's diet was also protein enriched, the baby received tyrosine. Second, there is no evidence that the baby also has PKU, and therefore any phenylalanine would be metabolized by the baby's phenylalanine hydroxylase. Since the phenylalanine level is normal, this supports the suggestion that the baby is a PKU carrier but is not affected. The carrier status is likely, since it is more unlikely for two affected individuals to conceive a child than one affected parent and one unaffected parent. Since the mother is affected and thus possesses two recessive alleles, the baby inherits one of these alleles; a normal allele is inherited from the father.

3. The prognosis is not good. Having been exposed to high levels of phenylalanine for 22 weeks, the baby will have some developmental damage. This is observed at birth in terms of microcephaly and cardiac anomalies. Following corrective surgeries, the baby is expected to have a reduced verbal and performance IQ.

CASE STUDY 5

1. Chronic myelogenous leukemia (CML) is characterized by the juxtaposition of 3′ sequences of the *ABL* gene (Chr 9q34) to 5′ sequences of the *bcr* gene (Chr 22q11) resulting in a p210 protein with transforming capabilities. What is shown in this patient is that there are two cell lines. In one, the cells have two different translocations: t(9,22)(q34,q11) and t(6;19)(q16;p13.3). Both clones have the Philadelphia chromosome. The Philadelphia chromosome, t(9,22)(q34,q11), is represented in the first clone along with a translocation of Chr 6q16 to Chr 19p13.3. The second cell line has only one translocation, the Philadelphia chromosome.

2. The monoclonal origin of cancer is well recognized, but polyclonality originating from a simple clone is also recognized as DNA rearrangements accumulate. Translocations are frequently observed in blast formation. The crucial event in CML is apparently the chimeric *BCR-ABL* gene formation. Even in the presence of non–Philadelphia chromosome abnormalities, and even when these abnormalities represent a greater percentage, the clinical presentation may be indistinguishable from CML. It is even suggested that the mechanism causing the formation of the Philadelphia chromosome may promote additional chromosome breaks.

3. Basically, karyotyping has limited sensitivity and requires more time to complete. The use of RT-PCR provides extreme sensitivity for cells in which p210$^{BCR-ABL}$ mRNA is transcribed. These cells have either escaped chemotherapy, which is unlikely owing to the life span of the cells, or new cells are being formed with the translocation occurring. The presence of residual disease in this patient does not change during monitoring (i.e., p210$^{BCR-ABL}$ does not increase, so no new chemotherapy is initiated).

CASE STUDY 6

1. Several genes may result in hereditary spherocytosis, including ankyrin, α- and β-spectrin, band 4.2, and band 3.

2. The formation of bilirubinate gallstones is the most common complication of hereditary spherocytosis. Gilbert syndrome, along with the increased breakdown of red blood cells, may have increased the patient's risk for gallstones and may have led to the patient's cholecystectomy. The chronic anemia and liver problems within the family suggest that the patient's anemia and Gilbert syndrome may have been hereditary.

3. Like most patients (80%) with spherocytosis, this patient is probably asymptomatic most of the time. The patient is anemic with a low hematocrit; however, the size of the cells and the amount of hemoglobin per cell is normal. While these values are low, they are not a hemolytic crisis. The number of RBCs is low, but the increase in reticulocytes indicates the marrow is actively trying to replace RBCs and thus increase the hemoglobin available for oxygen binding. The large number of reticulocytes may cause the MCV to appear higher than it should, since reticulocytes are slightly larger than RBCs. In the absence of reticulocytes, the MCV would more appropriately demonstrate a smaller size of RBC owing to the rapid turnover from hemolysis. The enlarged spleen, palpated on examination, reflects the long-standing nature of the disorder.

CASE STUDY 7

1. The physician should consider several things when entertaining a diagnosis of muscular dystrophy. Age of onset and location of muscle weakness are important distinguishing factors between Duchenne muscular dystrophy (DMD) and Becker muscular dystrophy (BMD). DMD has an earlier age of onset, generally before age 5, as seen in this patient. BMD onset is generally during adolescence or early adulthood. Muscle weakness begins in the pelvic girdle and is more pronounced in the proximal muscles. This weakness leads to the Gowers maneuver that the child uses to raise himself to a standing position. Later weakness will develop in the neck and shoulder muscles in DMD, but the strength in the neck flexor muscles is spared in BMD.

2. Certain enzymes are found in relatively high amounts in normal skeletal muscle. These include aspartate aminotransferase (AST), creatine phosphokinase (CK), lactic dehydrogenase (LDH), and aldolase. These enzymes are released as muscle breaks down. AST, LDH, and aldolase can be found in other tissues and may be elevated for other reasons such as liver disease, pulmonary infarction, or myocardial infarction. CK is found in significant concentrations in the brain, heart muscle, and skeletal muscle. CK and aldolase are elevated very early in DMD, even before clinical symptoms, and continue when symptoms do begin. After muscle is replaced, the aldolase becomes normal and CK is either normal or only mildly elevated. AST and LDH values parallel CK and aldolase but with less significant change.

3. The most prevalent mutations in both DMD and BMD are deletions. These occur in 65% of DMD and 85% of BMD. The deletion itself does not identify which type of dystrophy is present. However, dystrophin is the only gene responsible for DMD and BMD, and given the physical and laboratory findings, DMD is the best diagnosis in this case.

4. A biopsy may not be informative early in the disease. Variations in dystrophin will begin as nonspecific and progressively lead to muscle degradation. Histologic studies of muscle early in the disease show nonspecific dystrophic changes. Later in the disease, fat and fibrous connective tissue replace muscle fibers, leading to the pseudohypertrophy frequently seen in calf muscles.

CASE STUDY 8

1. Fragile X syndrome does not demonstrate classical mendelian form of inheritance. Since amplification occurs during oogenesis, it can be traced in families but generally only after a family member expresses a full mutation. Premutations may not be noted because they are either asymptomatic or because the symptoms are so mild that other factors are considered.

2. As shown, the parents, grandparents, and great-grandparents all are normal. It is suggested that the first mutation, or amplification of the *FMR1* gene, occurred during oogenesis of the great-grandmother because of the "mildly" retarded son. The affected aunt and uncle demonstrate that a full mutation occurred during oogenesis in the grandmother. The fact that the mother does not show symptoms demonstrates the

independence of each amplification event and the influence of other factors, such as lyonization. PCR amplification of the region surrounding CGG repeats would show the amount of amplification in each family member.

3. Fragile X syndrome is rarely fully expressed in females, since this would imply inheriting a paternal X chromosome that already had an amplified region of the *FMR1* gene in addition to a maternal X chromosome that underwent amplification during oogenesis. A more likely scenario is to receive a maternal X chromosome that is amplified similarly to that seen in the child, but because of the presence of two X chromosomes in females, any clinical symptoms are less pronounced because of lyonization. In the case of females, learning disabilities are not uncommon in families in which males express fragile X.

4. The child will express fragile X syndrome. Phenotypic changes such as characteristic facies and macroorchidism will begin to occur at puberty.

CASE STUDY 9

1. In some compound heterozygotes, two mutant alleles may be able to compensate for each other and provide some functional protein. However, in the scenario described, one mutation in the *LRLR* gene has abolished the ability of LDL to bind to it. The other mutation allows LDL to bind to the receptor, but the receptor is unable to be internalized. This presentation is severe and equal to a homozygous condition. Since LDL transports cholesterol into the cell, this inability to bind to half the receptors and to be internalized once bound to the other half results in increased LDL cholesterol, represented by the child's value of 1240 mg/d.

2. With the inability to remove cholesterol from the circulation via the LDL receptor, there is no way to degrade cholesterol into bile acids or steroids. Therefore, atherosclerotic plaques will begin to develop; these commonly develop on the ascending aorta and cause stenosis of left and right coronary arteries, leading to severe stenosis and cardiac arrest at an early age.

3. This child's severe form of FH will be resistant to treatment, and therefore aggressive strategies should be employed. Dietary control and lipid-lowering drugs will be ineffective. Several methods of removing LDL from the blood include plasma exchange, double filtration plasmapheresis, and dextran sulfate cellulose adsorption. The first two methods are usually associated with decreasing HDL as well as LDL; this latter increases HDL concentrations.

4. The sibling, like the parents, can be treated with diet, pharmacologic intervention, and plasma exchange to decrease serum cholesterol. Xanthomas, if present, are

expected to regress, and atherosclerosis will not progress if cholesterol levels are controlled.

CASE STUDY 10

1. Wilson's disease is an autosomal recessive disease. In some disorders, the heterozygous condition is phenotypically an incomplete recessive disorder. In the case of the parents, the presentations of Parkinson's disease and tremor are suggestive of some expression of the disease. Laboratory tests may have revealed mildly elevated levels of copper and reduced ceruloplasmin. The reduced ceruloplasmin over a long period might suggest a link to the parents' conditions; aceruloplasminemia is associated with some features of neurodegenerative diseases.

2. Ceruloplasmin is a protein produced in the liver that functions as a copper transporter. It comprises six copper-binding domains. It is secreted from the liver with copper atoms attached. In this patient, some ceruloplasmin is being produced, but the levels are very low for the levels of copper being excreted. Though not provided, serum levels should be decreased because transport from the intestine to the liver is unaffected. The inability to adequately incorporate copper in ceruloplasmin causes apoceruloplasmin that is upregulated owing to copper excess to be degraded. Ceruloplasmin is also important in iron metabolism; however, there are no signs of anemia of chronic disease in this patient at this time.

3. Liver diseases presenting with abnormal liver biochemistries with or without hepatomegaly should be considered. These include chronic viral hepatitis, autoimmune hepatitis, primary sclerosing cholangitis, drug hepatotoxicity, α_1-antitrypsin deficiency, nonalcoholic steatohepatitis (NASH), alcoholic liver disease, and primary biliary cirrhosis.

4. Penicillamine is 3-mercapto-D-valine. It is the most characteristic degradation product of the penicillin antibiotics. It is used as an antirheumatic and as a chelating agent in Wilson disease, in which it forms bonds with a central metal ion. It is used to chemically remove ions from the blood and can reverse the hepatic, neurologic, and psychiatric manifestations seen in most patients.

CASE STUDY 11

1. Androgen insensitivity syndrome (AIS) is the best diagnosis. The mutation in the androgen receptor gene

and the appearance of the child suggest complete AIS rather than partial AIS.

2. The lack of androgen stimulation during fetal development failed to masculinize the male genitalia. Therefore, even though genetically male, this child appears female; the child is also a male pseudohermaphrodite.

3. The androgen receptor gene is located on the X chromosome and is inherited in an X-linked recessive manner. The mother would require two mutated alleles for expression. Although symptoms were not noted, the mother could have mild, localized symptoms depending on the tissues in which the mutated X chromosome is expressed.

4. The baseline levels of testosterone, DHEAS, androstenedione, and DHT are normal for the child, and the stimulation tests show no single enzymatic error. While appearing low, the androstenediol is most likely being converted to the testosterone that is present. The testes function normally when challenged. In the absence of an elevated T:DHT ratio, a defect in 5α-reductase is not considered. Further analysis reveals a 46,XY male. Family analysis revealed that the mother was a carrier of the mutation.

5. The testes produced normal amounts of antimüllerian factor (AMF) during development, and therefore no fallopian tubes, uterus, or proximal (upper) vagina developed.

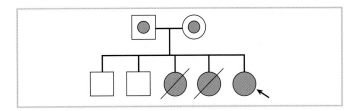

0.5. However, since it seems apparent from the history that CF does not affect the boys, the probability that they are carriers increases to 0.67 because the homozygous affected state is not a consideration.

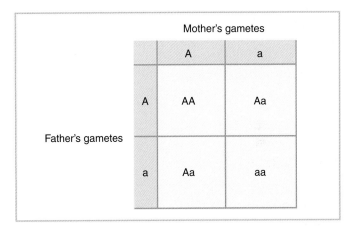

3. If $q = 0.025$, then $p = 0.975$. The number of affected individuals is expected to be

$q^2 = 0.025 \times 0.025 = 0.000625$, or 1 in 1600 individuals in the population are affected.

$2pq = 2(0.975)(0.25) = 0.049$, or about 1 in 20 individuals are carriers of the mutation.

As seen, affected individuals are less common than are carriers of the affected allele.

CASE STUDY 12

1. The proband has cystic fibrosis, an autosomal recessive disorder. Her parents are mostly likely carriers of the defective alleles inherited by the children. Two daughters died in infancy, suggesting that they also had CF. The sons are older and show no indication of the disorder.

2. Using the Punnett square, it is shown that the probability of gametes forming a heterozygote embryo is

Index

Note: Page numbers followed by f indicate figures; those followed by t indicate tables; and those followed by b indicate boxed material.